EVALUATING PUBLIC AND COMMUNITY HEALTH PROGRAMS

EVALUATING PUBLIC AND COMMUNITY HEALTH PROGRAMS

MURIEL J. HARRIS

JB JOSSEY-BASS™

A Wiley Brand

Published by John Wiley & Sons, Inc., Hoboken, New Jersey.
Published simultaneously in Canada.

This publication is designed to provide accurate and authoritative information in regard to the subject matter covered. It is sold with the understanding that the publisher is not engaged in rendering professional services. If legal, accounting, medical, psychological or any other expert assistance is required, the services of a competent professional should be sought.

For general information on our other products and services, please contact our Customer Care Department within the U.S. at 800-956-7739, outside the U.S. at 317-572-3986, or fax 317-572-4002.

Wiley publishes in a variety of print and electronic formats and by print-on-demand. Some material included with standard print versions of this book may not be included in e-books or in print-on-demand. If this book refers to media such as a CD or DVD that is not included in the version you purchased, you may download this material at http://booksupport.wiley.com. For more information about Wiley products, visit www.wiley.com.

Library of Congress Cataloging-in-Publication Data:

Names: Harris, Muriel J., 1955- author.
Title: Evaluating public and community health programs / Muriel J. Harris.
Description: 2nd edition. | Hoboken, New Jersey : Jossey-Bass & Pfeiffer
    Imprints, Wiley, [2017] | Includes bibliographical references and index.
Identifiers: LCCN 2016025319 (print) | LCCN 2016026276 (ebook) | ISBN
    9781119151050 (pbk.) | ISBN 9781119151074 (epdf) | ISBN 9781119151081 (epub)
Subjects: | MESH: Community Health Services–standards | Program
    Evaluation–methods | Data Collection–methods | Evaluation Studies as
    Topic | Community-Based Participatory Research
Classification: LCC RA440.4 (print) | LCC RA440.4 (ebook) | NLM WA 546.1 |
    DDC 362.1072–dc23
LC record available at https://lccn.loc.gov/2016025319

Cover Design: Wiley
Cover Photo: © Mats Anda/Getty Images, Inc.

Printed in the United States of America

PB Printing   SKY10026566_042621

This edition is dedicated to the memory of my father, Dr. Evelyn C. Cummings.

CONTENTS

PREFACE

You may not know what the term *evaluation* means, and, like me all those years ago and many of my students now, you are probably still a little wary of the term and wondering where this is all leading. No matter where you are in your understanding of program and policy evaluation, my hope is that whether you are a practitioner, a student, or both, you will find this book helpful on your journey and on your path to understanding. Just as I did many years ago, you probably evaluate what you do all the time without giving it a name. Evaluation is often an unconscious activity that is carried out before choosing among one or many options, both informally and formally. Informal evaluations range from selecting a restaurant for dinner to selecting a course of dishes off the menu. All the decisions you make along the way have implications for the success or failure of the outing. At the end of the evening, you go over the steps you took and decide whether the trip was worth it. If it wasn't, you may decide never to go to that restaurant again. So it is with program evaluation. We assess the resources and activities that went into a program, and then we determine whether the program or policy achieved what was intended, was worth it to those who experienced it and to those who funded it.

Evaluation activities occur in a range of work-related settings including community-based organizations, coalitions and partnerships, government-funded entities, the pharmaceutical industry, and the media. Program evaluations assess how an event or activity was conducted, how well it was conducted, and whether it achieved its goal. Evaluation determines the merit of a program or policy, and it forms the basis for evidence-based decision-making.

Evaluation is the cornerstone of program improvement and must be carefully planned and executed to be effective. It helps make the task of assessing the appropriateness of a public health intervention or the success of a program or policy explicit by using appropriate research methods. In evaluation, a plan is developed to assess the achievement of program objectives. The plan states the standards against which the intervention will be assessed, the scope of the evaluation, and appropriate tools and approaches for data collection and analysis.

There are many opportunities to conduct an evaluation during the life of an intervention, and the approaches to conducting the evaluation in each case will differ. The methods and tools for an evaluation that is conducted during the first few months of a program are different from those used when the program or participation in the program ends and the effectiveness of the program or policy is being assessed. In addition, during the life of the program, evaluation tools and approaches can be used to record program and policy participation and progress.

This book presents a model for evaluation and describes the approaches and methods for evaluating community health program and policy interventions. It is aimed at public health and community health students as well as practitioners who are new to program and policy evaluation. This book makes no assumptions of prior knowledge about evaluation. The approach to evaluation that is presented allows for the development of simple or complex evaluation plans while focusing on practical approaches. It encourages a critical thinking and reflective approach with the full involvement of multiple stakeholders throughout the evaluation process. This book provides learners with a systematic, step-by-step approach to program evaluation.

The book is organized into 13 chapters. It discusses the community assessment and the development of the public health initiative as the precursors to the four-step participatory model for evaluation with stakeholders at the center of each component. It frames program evaluation in the context of community-based participatory research. This edition also includes a chapter on process evaluation. Two case studies help the reader experience virtual evaluations, and mini-case studies and opportunities to "Think About It" allow the reader to reflect on the material and improve critical thinking skills. Valuable Takeaways provide simple reminders of important concepts covered in the chapter. An appendix provides some additional resources for evaluation.

ACKNOWLEDGMENTS

This edition is dedicated to the memory of my father, Dr. Evelyn C. Cummings. My sincere appreciation for all their support over the years also goes to my mother and all members of my family in the diaspora. To all the friends who have been a part of my amazing journey and have inspired me to explore the world and follow my passion, thank you. I have had the pleasure of working and teaching in Liberia, Sierra Leone, South Africa, the United Kingdom, the United States, and most recently, in Ghana as a Fulbright Scholar, from where I draw much of my inspiration. I would, however, be remiss if I did not also remember the person who gave me the opportunity to write this book. Sadly, he passed away just as we started working on this edition. Dad, Andy Pasternak, and all the departed, continue to rest in perfect peace.

EVALUATING PUBLIC AND COMMUNITY HEALTH PROGRAMS

CHAPTER

1

AN INTRODUCTION TO PUBLIC AND COMMUNITY HEALTH EVALUATION

LEARNING OBJECTIVES

- Identify the uses and approaches of evaluation.

- Describe preassessment evaluation.

- List the principles of participatory evaluation.

- Describe the links among community assessment, program implementation, and program evaluation.

- Explain the ethical and cultural issues in evaluation.

- Describe the value and role of stakeholders in evaluation.

Public health may be assessed by the impact it has on improving the quality of life of people and communities through the elimination or the reduction in the incidence, prevalence, and rates of disease and disability. An additional aspect of public health is to create social and physical environments that promote good health for all. The Healthy People 2020 goal describes health as being produced at multiple levels: households, neighborhoods and communities. In addition, it describes the importance of social and economic resources for health with a new focus on the social determinants of health. Its overarching goals are as follows:

1. Attain high quality, longer lives free of preventable disease, disability, injury, and premature death.

2. Achieve health equity, eliminate disparities, and improve the health of all groups.

3. Create social and physical environments that promote good health for all.

4. Promote quality of life, healthy development, and healthy behaviors across all life stages. (http://www.healthypeople.gov/2020/About-Healthy-People)

Public health, therefore, has an obligation to improve conditions and access to appropriate and adequate resources for healthy living for all people, and it includes education, nutrition, exercise, and social environments. Public health programs and policies may be instituted at the local, state, national, or international level.

The Committee for the Study of the Future of Public Health defines the mission of public health as "fulfilling society's interest in assuring conditions in which people can be healthy" (Institute of Medicine, 2001, p. 7). Public and community health programs and initiatives exist in order to "do good" and to address social problems or to improve social conditions (Rossi, Lipsey, & Freeman, 2004, p. 17). Public health interventions address social problems or conditions by taking into consideration the underlying factors and core causes of the problem. Within this context, program evaluation determines whether public health program and policy initiatives improve health and quality of life.

Evaluation is often referred to as applied research. Using the word *applied* in the definition lends it certain characteristics that allow it to differ from traditional research in significant ways.

- Evaluation is about a particular initiative. It is generally carried out for the purposes of assessing the initiative, and the results are not generalizable. However, with the scaling up of programs to reach increasingly large segments of the population, and with common outcome expectations and common measures, evaluations can increase their generalizability. Research traditionally aims to produce results that are generalizable to a whole population, place, or setting in a single experiment.

- Evaluations are designed to improve an initiative and to provide information for decision-making at the program or policy level; research aims to prove whether there is a cause-and-effect relationship between two entities in a controlled situation.

- Evaluation questions are generally related to understanding why and how well an intervention worked, as well as to determining whether it worked. Research is much more focused on the end point, on whether an intervention worked and much less on the process for achieving the end result.

- Evaluation questions are identified by the stakeholders in collaboration with the evaluators; research questions are usually dictated by the researcher's agenda.

Some approaches to evaluation, such as those that rely on determining whether goals and objectives are achieved, assess the effects of a program; the judicial approach asks for arguments for and against the program, and program accreditations seek ratings of programs based on a professional judgment of their quality and are usually preceded by a self-study. Consumer-oriented approaches are responsive to stakeholders and encourage their participation. This book focuses on the evaluation of public health programs primarily at the community and program level.

OVERVIEW OF EVALUATION

Rossi et al. (2004) describe evaluation as "the use of social research methods to systematically investigate the effectiveness of social intervention programs in ways that are adapted to their political and organizational environments and are designed to inform social action to inform social conditions" (p. 16). In addition, these authors caution that evaluation provides the best information possible under conditions that involve a political process of balancing interests and reaching decisions (p. 419).

Evaluation is the cornerstone for improving public health programs and is conducted for the purpose of making a judgment of a program's worth or value. Evaluation incorporates steps that specify and describe the activities and the process of evaluation; the initiative and why it is being evaluated; the measures needed to assess the inputs, outputs, and outcomes; and the methodology for collecting the information (data). In addition, an evaluation analyzes data and disseminates results in ways that ensure that the evaluation is useful.

This definition of evaluation as adopted by the social sciences and public health reflects a long tradition of evaluation that takes different approaches to evaluation and are applied across a wide field of study. Each has its own criteria, and the evaluator chooses the approach that best suits their field, their inclination, or the purpose for which the evaluation is being conducted.

The next section provides a brief overview of the most widely used approaches. These evaluation approaches include the consumer-based, decision-based, goal-free, participatory, expertise-oriented, and objectives-based.

Consumer-Based Approach

In the consumer-based evaluation approach, the needs of the consumer are the primary focus and the role of the evaluator is to develop or select criteria against which the initiative or product is judged for its worth. The focus of this evaluation is on the cost, durability, and performance of the initiative or product being evaluated.

Decision-Based Approach

This approach adopts a framework for conducting evaluation that includes the context, inputs, process, and product. It is also referred to as the context, input, process, and product (CIPP) approach. In including the context in the evaluation, this approach considers both the problem that is being addressed and the intervention that addresses it. In the context of public health, adopting this model requires understanding the public health problem being addressed and the program or policy intended to address it. The community or needs assessment forms the basis for developing the intervention. The input components of the evaluation assess the relationship between the resources available for the program and the activities identified to address the problem. Process evaluation, which is the third component of this model, asks the question, "Is the program being implemented as planned?" The last component, the product, assesses the extent to which goals and objectives have been met.

Goal-Free Approach

A goal-free approach to evaluation is just that. The evaluation does not start out with any predefined goals or objectives related to the initiative being evaluated. It is expected that the initiative will have many outcomes that are not necessarily related to the objectives that may have been crafted when the initiative was initially conceived and started. Therefore, not having defined objectives allows the evaluator to explore a wide range of options for evaluation.

Participatory Approach

The participatory approach to evaluation adopts an approach that values and integrates stakeholders into the process. Stakeholders in this process are the beneficiaries of the initiative's interventions. In this case, the evaluator serves as technical advisor allowing the stakeholders to take responsibility for most aspects of the evaluation process. The aim of this approach is to transfer skills in a co-learning setting and to empower stakeholders to become evaluators of their own initiatives.

Expertise-Oriented Approach

The expertise-oriented approach expects the evaluator to be a content expert who draws on his life experience to judge a program's worth. It may or not be accompanied by specified clearly defined and explicit criteria. This approach is often used in judging competitions and in public health and other fields in accreditation. However, in accreditation, such as the accreditation of schools of public health, although the institution provides the self-study narrative based on predefined criteria, the judgment of the program's merits and the decision to grant accreditation is made by the accrediting body.

Objectives-Based Approach

The objectives-based evaluation is the most commonly used in public health practice especially recently as responses to calls for proposals for funding now invariably require the applicant to include objectives. The objectives for an initiative are developed following the community assessment, and form the bases on which the initiative is developed focusing on risk or protective factors that would have an impact on the problem being addressed.

Additional objectives that may address concerns of the evaluator or the implementing team may be written as necessary to guide the evaluation and for the framework upon which the evaluation questions and the evaluation are designed.

LEVELS OF EVALUATION

Evaluation at the Project and Program Level

Evaluation may be conducted at the project or program level. Public health organizations and agencies may achieve the overall mission of the organization through a number of stand-alone projects that together make up a program. For example, a local service organization of an agency may have activities that address many of the determinants of health—for example, low literacy, access to health insurance, low levels of physical activity and poor nutrition. Addressing each of these determinants of health may occur in a department of health promotion, yet each may have an independent set of activities to achieve an overall goal to improve the health of minority, low-income populations within a jurisdiction. At the project level, process evaluation may be concerned with how the set of activities is being implemented and the extent to which each is being implemented according to a previously established plan. The link between literacy, lack of insurance, healthy nutrition, and physical activity is fairly well understood, so that, in combination, it is assumed that sets of activities at the project level will, over a specified time, address common objectives, such as reduce the percentage of individuals who are diagnosed with heart disease or increase the number of individuals with diabetes who achieve HbA1c levels of less than 7%. This evaluation takes place in the context of a carefully selected set of activities based on theoretically sound community assessment, which provides the framework for an intervention designed to achieve a stated set of goals and objectives.

Evaluation at the Organization Level

Evaluation may not only be concerned with the project and programs that are run out of the organization, but the organization may also have needs for its own development in order to provide needed services. Evaluating the organization may involve assessing the extent to which the organization is able to implement its strategic plan, the extent to which it is achieving its stated mission and reaching the populations it intends to serve. It may also assess its organizational capacity and relationships with others. Organizational development components that may be assessed include the capacity of its staff to address present and emerging health problems in the community and the extent to which projects and programs are institutionalized for long-term sustainability. Organizational culture, climate, and competency to deal effectively with the populations it serves may be the foci of evaluation. Policy development and implementation that occurs at the organizational level may also form the basis for evaluation.

Evaluation at the Community Level

Community-level engagement in projects and programs in the community and provision of services may form part of an evaluation, as well as might the social norms of the community. Using community organization theory as the basis for the evaluation, the extent to which communities have embraced new ideas, the extent of social networking and the level of social capital may be critical components of an evaluation. The empowerment continuum described by Rissel in 1994 assesses individual and community capacity to act in ways that bring about change and ultimately engage in collective political and social action.

Evaluation of Local, State, and National Level Policies

The evaluation of local, state, and national levels is generally carried out by organizations that have the capacity to coordinate, collect, and analyze large amounts of data from across jurisdictions. At the local or state health department, a research unit may have the responsibility to collect statewide data for the purpose of evaluating the impact of community-wide efforts. The Centers for Disease Control and Prevention (CDC)-supported Behavioral Risk Factor Surveillance System (BRFSS) survey serves the purpose of continual assessment of healthy-people goals by determining risk factors and disease-related outcomes. When state and national level policies are enacted, the BRFSS may serve to monitor changes at the population level in addition to other forms of data collection that may be required for evaluation. For example, when the State Children's Health Insurance Program (SCHIP) was enacted by Congress in 1997 and Title XXI of the Social Security Act was created, they aimed to design programs to expand health insurance for low-income children less than 19 years of age who were uninsured. The evaluation plan was designed with seven assessment components:

- Analysis of SCHIP enrollment patterns
- Analysis of trends and rates of uninsured children
- Synthesis of published and unpublished literature on retention, substitutions, and access to care
- Special studies on outreach and access to care
- Analysis of outreach and enrollment effectiveness
- Case study of program implementation
- Analysis of SCHIP performance measures (https://www.cms.gov)

As with all evaluation, state and national level evaluations focus on the effect on the larger population (impact) rather than at the more limited outcome level of risk factors. However, special studies as evidenced by the SCHIP evaluation may focus on program implementation and attempts at assessing changes in risk factors (for example, assessing enrollment effectiveness) rather than just assessing trends and rates of uninsured children alone or the four core health measures, well-child visits for children 15 months and ages 3–6, the use of appropriate medication for asthma, and visits to primary care providers.

PREASSESSMENT EVALUATIONS

One major assumption in evaluating an initiative is that it was well planned and fully implemented. This, however, is not always the case, and the evaluation team may find it must balance the expense associated with undertaking the evaluation with the likely result of the evaluation. If the evaluation is unlikely to provide information that is useful to the organization, it may be expedient to consider an alternative use of resources. An alternative use of the resources available for evaluation could be to answer a different question. The question becomes, "In undertaking this evaluation, will it provide useful information to the stakeholder for decision-making or program improvement?" This contrasts with the kinds of questions that precede a full evaluation of the initiative which are, "Is the initiative being implemented according to the plan?" and "Did the initiative have an effect on the beneficiaries?" If the evaluator is unable to provide the stakeholder with information that is useful for decision-making, program improvement, or replication, consultation may be necessary with regard to the type of evaluation that is required. The decision about the approach to the evaluation is made in consultation with the stakeholder. A decision to conduct a preassessment recognizes the need to assess the initiative's readiness to be evaluated rather than the initiative's implementation (process evaluation) or outcomes (outcome evaluation).

Components of a feasibility evaluation may include:

- Assessing the readiness of executives, staff, and stakeholders to support an evaluation and to use the results.

- Determining whether the stated goals and objectives are clear and reflect the intended direction of the organization.

- Assessing the logic of the program and its ability to achieve the stated goal and objectives given the initiative's activities and resources.

- Assessing whether data collected of the program's implementation activities are likely to be suitable for showing the effects of the program.

- Assessing whether processes exist or can be developed to provide sufficient information to assess the program's activities, outputs, and outcomes.

- Assessing access to program participants, program staff, and other stakeholders.

- Assessing the logistics and resources available to conduct an evaluation.

One of the detailed tasks in carrying out a preassessment is to work with the organization to understand the epidemiological and community data-based rationale; its interventions; the resources for the intervention; and the social, political, economic, and cultural context in which it operates. In assessing the interventions, the evaluator identifies the intervention components, understands the initiatives theory of change, and creates a logic model. The logic model shows the relationship between the activities implemented to achieve the objectives, and the resources devoted to them. The preassessment determines the existence (or nonexistence) of specific, measurable, realistic, achievable, and time-oriented short-term, intermediate, and long-term outcome objectives.

Whether preassessment is completed formally or informally, the result may be either that the evaluation is able to go ahead or that it has to be delayed until various conditions are met. Meeting the conditions for evaluation varies from one organization to the next. One organization may not have a document detailing its structure or processes with regard to its interventions, and it may require the evaluation team to work with them on developing the documents describing the community assessment findings, the goals and objectives, the theory undergirding the intervention, activities to address the problem and achieve the

FIGURE 1.1. *Components for Preassessment of Program's Readiness for Evaluation*

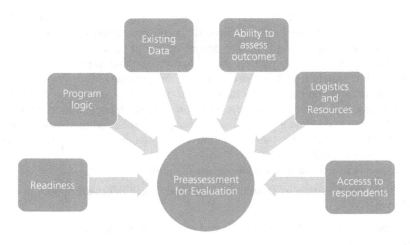

goals and objectives or tools for carrying out an evaluation. Another organization may only require data-management and evaluation tools that allow for appropriate and adequate data collection, whereas another may need help with ensuring that the plans for data analysis are developed. On the analysis of the existing documents, it may become clear that the initiative requires restructuring to ensure it uses a best-practice approach and has the capacity to get to outcomes. Such actions ensure that in the future the organization and the intervention have the components and tools essential for undertaking an appropriate and meaningful evaluation. Components for preassessment of a program's readiness for evaluation are depicted in above Figure 1.1.

THE PARTICIPATORY APPROACH TO EVALUATION

A participatory model for evaluation views evaluation as a team effort that involves people internal and external to the organization with varying levels of evaluation expertise in a power-sharing and co-learning relationship. Patton (2008, p. 175) identifies nine principles of participatory evaluation:

1. The process involves participants in learning skills.
2. Participants own the evaluation and are active in the process.
3. Participants focus the evaluation on what they consider important.
4. Participants work together as a group.
5. The whole evaluation process is understandable and meaningful to the participants.

6. Accountability to oneself and to others is valued and supported.

7. The perspectives and expertise of all persons are recognized and valued.

8. The evaluator facilitates the process and is a collaborator and a resource for the team.

9. The status of the evaluator relative to the team is minimized (to allow equitable participation).

A participatory model for evaluation embraces the stakeholders in the process and utilizes approaches to help the organization develop the capacity to evaluate its own programs and institute program improvement (Fetterman, Kaftarian, & Wandersman, 1996). The community-based participatory-research (CBPR) approach (Israel, Eng, Schulz, & Parker, 2005) proposes nine guiding principles that support effective research, which are easily incorporated into participatory program evaluation of public health initiatives. CBPR principles require that researchers

1. Acknowledge community as a unit of identity in which people have membership; it may be identified as a geographical area or a group of individuals.

2. Build on strengths and resources of the community and utilize them to address the needs of the community.

3. Facilitate a collaborative, equitable partnership in all phases of research, involving an empowering and power-sharing process that attends to social inequalities with open communication among all partners and an equitable share in the decision-making.

4. Foster co-learning and capacity building among all partners with a recognition that people bring a variety of skills, expertise, and experience to the process.

5. Integrate and achieve a balance between knowledge generation and intervention for the mutual benefit of all partners with the translation of research findings into action.

6. Focus on the local relevance of public health problems from an ecological perspective that addresses the multiple determinants of health including biological, social, economic, cultural, and physical factors.

7. Involve systems development using a cyclical and iterative process that includes all the stages of the research process from assessing and identifying the problem to action.

8. Disseminate results to all partners and involve them in the wide dissemination of results in ways that are respectful.

9. Involves a long-term process and commitment to sustainability in order to build trust and have the ability to address multiple determinants of health over an extended period. (Israel et al., 2005, pp. 7–9)

Important outcomes of CBPR approaches are building community infrastructure and community capacity, knowledge, and skills (O'Fallon & Dearry, 2002). The participatory model, through its engagement of stakeholders throughout the process, fosters the ideals of cooperation, collaboration, and partnerships, and ensures co-learning and empowerment.

THE PARTICIPATORY MODEL FOR EVALUATION

The Framework for Program Evaluation developed by Milstein, Wetterhall, & the Evaluation Group (2000) has six evaluation steps: Step 1, engage stakeholders; Step 2, describe the program; Step 3, focus the evaluation design; Step 4, collect credible evidence; Step 5, justify conclusions; and Step 6, ensure use and share lessons learned. The framework is associated with four standards: utility, feasibility, propriety, and accuracy (Figure 1.2). It has been adopted and used in the evaluation of public health programs since its development, and its subsequent publication as a monograph by the Centers for Disease Control and Prevention. The participatory model for evaluation that is introduced and expounded in this book builds on this approach to evaluation. Like the framework for program evaluation, the participatory model for evaluation uses an objectives-based approach to evaluation and draws on concepts from the other approaches outlined earlier.

The participatory model for evaluation incorporates community-based participatory research principles (Israel et al., 2005) and supports a collaborative, equitable partnership in all phases of the evaluation process. It fosters co-learning and capacity building while acknowledging and utilizing existing experience and expertise. It incorporates all the elements of the evaluation process but does so in a flexible and simplified way. It recognizes the often iterative and integrative nature of evaluation in designing the evaluation; collecting, analyzing, and interpreting the data; and reporting the findings. It links the

FIGURE 1.2. *Framework for Program Evaluation in Public Health*

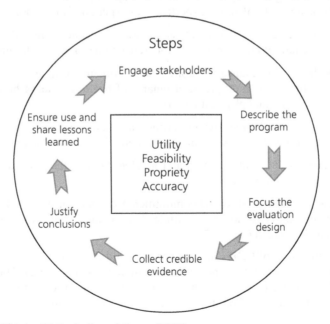

Source: From Milstein, Wetterhall, and Group (2000).

evaluation process to community assessment and program planning and implementation in a deliberative and iterative way. Stakeholders' active participation in the entire process provides flexibility in the evaluation and allows it to be customizable to the users' needs. Because conducting an evaluation depends on a thorough knowledge and understanding of a program's development and implementation, this book provides an overview of these critical precursors to evaluation, the community assessment, and development and implementation of programs. This model recognizes the dynamic nature of programs and the changing needs of the evaluation over time; hence, the cyclical nature of the process.

The participatory model for evaluation consists of four major steps:

1. Design the evaluation.

2. Collect the data.

3. Analyze and interpret the data.

4. Report the findings.

The participatory model for evaluation (Figure 1.3) used to evaluate public health community or policy initiatives and the focus of this book acknowledges the participatory nature of evaluation, recognizes that the community assessment and the public health initiative are precursors to an evaluation, and adopts an objectives-based approach to evaluation. In this model for evaluation, stakeholders who have a vested interest in the program's development, implementation, or results are part of the evaluation team and involved in each step of the evaluation process. In addition to acknowledging the inclusion of stakeholders as good practice in evaluation, the Public Health Leadership Society (2002) recognizes their inclusion as being ethical. Its third principle states that public health "policies, programs, and priorities should be developed and evaluated through processes that ensure an opportunity for input

FIGURE 1.3. *The Participatory Model for Evaluation*

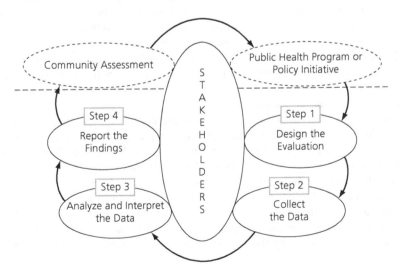

from community members" (p. 4). Stakeholders provide multiple perspectives and a deep understanding of the cultural context in which an initiative is developed and an evaluation is conducted.

THE PRECURSORS TO PROGRAM EVALUATION

When a community or individual identifies a public health problem among a population, steps are taken to understand the problem. These steps constitute community assessments, which define the problem using qualitative and quantitative measures. They assess the extent of the problem, who is most affected, and the individual and environmental factors that may be contributing to and exacerbating the problem. Community assessments determine the activities that will potentially lead to change in the factors that put the population at risk of disease and disability. Programs are planned and implemented based on the findings of the community assessment and the resources available. The Merriam-Webster dictionary describes community as "a unified body of individuals" who have common interests; history; or social, economic, and political interests. The unified body of individuals may occur in homes, workplaces, or houses of worship, and community assessments may be expanded to also include assessing organizational structures through which initiatives are developed and implemented.

The terms *initiative* and *intervention* are used in this book to refer to a program or policy that addresses a health or social concern identified by the community assessment. The health or social concern may be influenced by a variety of factors at the individual, interpersonal, community, organizational, or policy level. Details about conducting a community assessment and developing initiatives are discussed in Chapters 2 and 3. Examples of initiatives are a program for low-income families to increase their knowledge and skills with regard to accessing health care and an after-school program to improve physical fitness. Initiatives may also be based on the development of a public or organizational policy that also addresses a public health concern. Programs may modify the environment to improve access to conditions that support health, such as improving conditions for walking in a community or improving access to fresh produce. At the organizational level, factors that influence access to services may be subject to development and training and related initiatives. Initiatives can also develop or change public policy so that more people can have health insurance and improved access to health care. Another policy that you are no doubt familiar with is the seat-belt policy that was enacted to reduce the risk of injury and mortality associated with vehicular accidents.

An initiative or intervention may have multiple components such as activities, programs, or policies associated with it. One example is prevention of the onset of diabetes, which requires a multipronged intervention for those at risk. Individual components that constitute the initiative may include physical activity, diet control, outreach education, and policies that increase the availability of fresh produce and access to opportunities for physical activities. In addition, access to health care to ensure that screening is available and case management and care when needed is a critical component of assuring health. Evaluating a multipronged initiative requires assessing both process and outcomes for each component as well as assessing the overall effect of the initiative on preventing diabetes among the target population.

Evaluation activities may occur at multiple points on a continuum, from planning the initiative, through implementation, to assessing the effect on the populations served and meeting the goals outlined in the Healthy People objectives (U.S. Department of Health and Human Services, 2020). The Healthy People documents identify the most significant preventable threats to health and establish national goals to reduce these threats. Individuals, groups, and organizations are encouraged to integrate the Healthy People objectives into the development of initiatives. In addition, businesses can use the framework to build worksite health-promotion activities; schools and colleges can undertake programs and activities to improve the health of students and staff. Healthcare providers can encourage their patients to pursue healthy lifestyles; community-based organizations and civic and faith-based organizations can develop initiatives to address health issues in a community, especially among hard-to-reach populations, and to ensure that everybody has access to information and resources for healthy living. Determining the effectiveness of the implementation of programs and policies and the impact of such initiatives on the population that is reached is the task of program- or policy-evaluation activities. Although evaluation activities may use different approaches, their function is similar across disciplines. Formative evaluation is the appropriate approach during the program planning and development phase of an initiative; process monitoring and evaluation are useful during the implementation phase and when the aim of the evaluation is to understand what went into the program and how well it is being implemented.

Outcome evaluations are carried out after programs have been in place for a time and are considered stable; such an evaluation can assess the effect of a program or policy on individuals or a community. Outcome evaluation aims to understand whether a program was effective and achieved what it set out to accomplish. Impact evaluation is the last stage of the evaluation continuum. It is used when multiple programs and policy initiatives affect the quality of life of a large population over a long period. Multiple interventions on the population or subpopulation are assessed for changes in quality of life and for the incidence and prevalence of disease or disability within a jurisdiction. A jurisdiction is a legally defined unit overseen by political and administrative structures. Discussions of impact evaluation may be found in other texts. Figure 1.4 illustrates the context of evaluation; the specific kinds of evaluation are discussed in detail in the next section.

The Evaluation Team

The evaluation team is led by an experienced evaluator who may be internal or external to the organization. Historically, the evaluator has been an outsider who comes in to give an independent, "unbiased" review of the initiative. This approach to evaluation has limited evaluation to a few institutions and specifically when funding is available for evaluation. Evaluators may have titles that are more akin to researchers and who may be associated with a local university or community college. More recently, agencies and large nonprofit organizations have hired in-house evaluators or modified the roles of staff to provide evaluation and thereby strengthen the overall capacity of the organization. A significant advantage is that the agency may be able to provide a more sustained evaluation conducted at lower cost. Irrespective of the approach used, participatory models include stakeholders as part of the evaluation design and implementation in order to facilitate the use of the findings.

FIGURE 1.4. *Evaluation in Context*

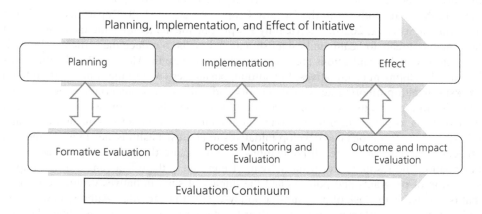

There are advantages and disadvantages to choosing an internal or an external evaluator. An internal evaluator who has the expertise to conduct an evaluation and who knows the program well may also have easy access to materials, logistics, resources, and data. However, internal evaluators are often too busy, may be less objective than those external to the organization, and may have limited expertise to conduct a full and complete evaluation. However, an internal evaluator is an important and valuable resource for an external evaluator who may be contracted with to conduct the evaluation.

An external evaluator is often viewed as being more credible, more objective, and able to offer additional insights for the development of the program and to serve as a facilitator than someone from inside the organization. An external evaluator may also be able to provide additional human and material resources and an expertise that may not be available within the organization. Additionally, external evaluators may not know the program, policies, and procedures of the organization, may not understand the program context, and may be perceived as adversarial and an imposition. This may be particularly true since in the process of conducting the evaluation, the evaluator will require access to staff and other stakeholders. The participatory approach to evaluation encourages and supports all stakeholders' engagement in the process from start to finish and the relationship between an internal evaluator and the external evaluator may be the difference between an evaluation considered to be useful and credible and one that is dismissed and left on the shelf to gather dust. It is important, therefore, to nurture this relationship should an internal evaluator be involved.

Whether an evaluator is internal or external, the person who has the primary responsibility for the evaluation should have these essential competencies:

- Know and maintain professional norms and values, including evaluation standards and principles.

- Use expertise in the technical aspects of evaluation such as design, measurement, data analysis, interpretation, and sharing results.

- Use situational analysis, understand and attend to contextual and political issues of an evaluation.

- Understand the nuts and bolts of evaluation, including contract negotiation, budgeting, and identifying and coordinating needed resources for a timely evaluation.

- Be reflective regarding one's practice and be aware of one's expertise as well as the need for professional growth.

- Have interpersonal competence in written communication and the cross-cultural skills needed to work with diverse groups of stakeholders. (Ghere, King, Stevahn, & Minnema, 2006; King, Stevahn, Ghere, & Minnema, 2001)

In addition, five ethical principles of program evaluation were adopted and ratified by the American Evaluation Association. These principles reflect the fundamental ethical principles of autonomy, nonmaleficence, beneficence, justice, and fidelity (Veach, 1997) and as such provide an ethical compass for action and decision-making throughout the evaluation process. These principles are the following:

1. *Systematic inquiry*: Evaluators conduct systematic, data-based inquiries. They adhere to the highest technical standards; explore the shortcomings and strengths of evaluation questions and approaches; communicate the approaches, methods, and limitations of the evaluation accurately; and allow others to be able to understand, interpret, and critique their work.

2. *Competence*: Evaluators provide competent performance to stakeholders. They ensure that the evaluation team possesses the knowledge, skills, and experience required; that it demonstrates cultural competence; practices within its limits; and continuously provides the highest level of performance.

3. *Integrity/honesty*: Evaluators display honesty and integrity in their own behavior and attempt to ensure the honesty of the entire evaluation process. They negotiate honestly, disclose any conflicts of interest and values and any sources of financial support. They disclose changes to the evaluation, resolve any concerns, accurately represent their findings, and attempt to prevent any misuse of those findings.

4. *Respect for people*: Evaluators respect the security, dignity, and worth of respondents, program participants, clients, and other stakeholders. They understand the context of the evaluation, abide by ethical standards, conduct the evaluation and communicate results in a way that respects the stakeholders' dignity and worth, fosters social equity, and takes into account all persons.

5. *Responsibilities for general and public welfare*: Evaluators articulate and take into account the diversity of general and public values that may be related to the evaluation. They include relevant perspectives, consider also the side effects, and allow stakeholders to present the results in appropriate forms that respect confidentiality, take into account the public interest, and consider the welfare of society as a whole. (American Evaluation Association, 2008, pp. 233–234)

(The full text of the American Evaluation Association Guiding Principles for Evaluators is available at http://www.eval.org)

The second principle, competence, refers to providing skilled evaluation. "Evaluators should possess (or ensure that the evaluation team possesses) the education, abilities, skills and experience appropriate to undertake the tasks proposed by the evaluation" (American Evaluation Association, 2008, p. 233). In addition, the evaluation team develops cross-cultural skills in order to understand the culture in which both the initiative and the evaluation are embedded (Ghere et al., 2006; King et al., 2001). Understanding the culture of the organization and its stakeholders will ensure that culturally competent evaluation is undertaken, which results in appropriately culturally competent interpretations of research findings.

Think About It!

As an internal evaluator in a small, not-for-profit organization that provides services to youth who have both physical and emotional disabilities, what are the essential professional norms and values, including evaluation standards and principles that you would adopt? To what extent does serving a population with disabilities present additional complexities for evaluation?

The Stakeholders

Stakeholders who are identified to be part of the evaluation team are individuals, groups, or organizations that have a significant interest in how well a program functions (Rossi et al., 2004). Involving stakeholders allows the initiative to be viewed in the appropriate administrative, epidemiological, political, and sociocultural perspectives.

Stakeholders provide funding for the program, management, or oversight or are participants in the program and benefit from program activities. In addition, some have an interest in the program but do not have any specific role in the organization and its initiatives. It is equally important to engage those community members who are not supportive of the initiative to understand their concerns and the competition that the organization faces. Involving multiple stakeholders in the process enhances the credibility of the evaluation, ensures that the appropriate voices are heard, and gives stakeholders ownership in the evaluation and its findings.

A stakeholder analysis will help identify the stakeholders who are associated with the program, their interest in the program, and their likely contribution to the evaluation tasks. The stakeholder analysis is conducted at the start and throughout the evaluation process to ensure that the right people are included at critical points, from developing the evaluation design to reporting the results. During the evaluation, the roles of the stakeholders change as they go in and out of the process and participate as is appropriate for their interest and expertise. Stakeholders in a public health or social services evaluation could include:

- The board of directors of the organization that has requested the evaluation to determine whether the organization is meeting the requirements for continued funding.

- The board of directors of a foundation that provides community grants and wants to be sure its grants are making a difference in achieving strategic goals.

- The executive director, who provides overall oversight and management for the program.

- The project manager, who provides the day-to-day management of staff implementing the program or the policy.

- Staff providing services to clients.

- Staff supervising logistical services.

- Persons receiving services who meet the criteria for the intended population sample.

- Persons who are affected in any way by the services or policies.

- Persons in the larger community who have an interest in the program's success.

Ideally stakeholders are involved in the evaluation from the start and throughout the process. In addition to their invaluable input into understanding program development and implementation, stakeholders have critical roles and responsibilities that include providing

- Access to databases, files, reports, logs, and publications.

- Administrative and logistical support for the conduct of the evaluation.

- Access to other stakeholders as necessary for recruitment and data collection.

- Support in implementing the evaluation plan.

- Insights into the results and interpretation of the data analysis.

- Support in disseminating the interim and final reports.

Keeping stakeholders engaged in the evaluation process involves developing meaningful relationships with them. Relationship development may be facilitated by understanding some of their issues, understanding the cultural and power issues that exist, and working to develop a trusting and ethical relationship.

CULTURAL CONSIDERATIONS IN EVALUATION

With the changing demographics of most countries, states, counties, cities, and neighborhoods, being sensitive to other cultures is important and may make the difference between an evaluation that produces useful findings and one that does not. It may be the difference between having a set of behaviors, attitudes, and practices that enables effective work and not being effective. Knowing there are differences among cultures and yet avoiding value judgments that undermine the integrity of a people is an underlying principle of cross-cultural engagement. Appreciating and embracing cultures different from our own facilitates an environment conducive to each person's growth and development.

Although there are many definitions of culture, it is generally thought to refer to a set of beliefs, traditions, and behavior that apply to a particular group of people. Cultural groups may be identified based on age, gender, religion, country of origin, race or ethnicity, sexual orientation, disability, family background, language, food preference, employment, or neighborhood community. These characteristics influence societal traditions, thought patterns, processes, and traditions. Sector (1995, p. 68) defines culture as "the sum of beliefs, practices, habits, likes, dislikes, norms, customs, rituals, and so forth that we learned from our families during the years of socialization." Yet, Mark Edberg (2013) identifies human culture as one in which behavior, beliefs, and objects interact providing meaning that is unique to that group.

Societal customs and traditions are passed through multiple generations and may include the way members of the group dress, sing, and dance or how they perceive and respond to the world around them. Traditions are passed down by word of mouth during periods of storytelling or less deliberately when societies perform traditions year after year. Indigenous Americans, for example, have many traditions that define their culture as do Africans and Asians both in their native areas and in the Diaspora. However, since culture is dynamic and is influenced by other cultures and technologies that surround them, the boundaries between cultural groups may be fluid and require that evaluators consider the nuances that might exist when working within a particular culture.

Certain practices are unique to a cultural group, but often we find similar traditions across groups. It is fascinating to observe that Black populations that live in America, the Caribbean, and Canada have traditions and thought patterns similar to those of Blacks who still live in Africa even though they have been separated for many generations. As cultures have become integrated through immigration and intermarriage, we see changes in cultural practices. Societies continue to eliminate those practices that are harmful and retain those that speak to the core values of their people.

Because culture gives people unique perspectives and often unique ways of doing, developing the knowledge and skills to work cross-culturally is critical to effective practice. To be able to fully appreciate and consider another person's culture, it is important to learn about that culture. Learning requires humility of spirit, openness and honesty, patience, and a willingness to share what we know with others.

When we take the culture of the people around us into consideration, we demonstrate

- A respect for others

- A willingness to listen to the perspective of others and to respect their views

- A willingness to learn

Culture plays an important role in program evaluation. Cultural context guides the methods and approaches that are used throughout the process as well as the interpretation of the results and how the conclusions are drawn. As a result, culture influences the validity of the evaluation findings (Johnson, Kirkhart, Madison, Noley, & Solano-Flores, 2008). Aspects of the evaluation process that culture affects include

- How the evaluation questions are asked

- The selection of the data sources

- The methods and approaches used to collect the evaluation data

- The techniques used in the evaluation

- The methods and approaches used in communication of the results (Kirkhart, 2005)

As in the case of being able to operate effectively cross-culturally, the development of human relationships through culturally competent evaluation processes ensures that research conclusions or program development are more likely to be valid and beneficial to the intended population. Standards of cultural competence have often been used to define the expectations of those working with a diverse population. Cultural competence incorporates the hope that the workforce has the knowledge, attitudes, and skills necessary to understand the beliefs, behaviors, and practices of the population being served. It is also necessary that they have demographic characteristics similar to those of the receivers of the services or, in some cases, that they simply be able to provide language-translation services.

Cultural competence has been defined in multiple ways. Batancourt, Green, Carillo, and Ananeh-Firenpong (2003, p. 294) suggest that cultural competence "acknowledges and incorporates at all levels the importance of culture, assessment of cross-cultural relations, vigilance towards the dynamics that result from cultural differences, expansion of cultural knowledge, and adaptation of services to meet culturally unique needs." Perez and Luquis (2008) identify three characteristics that are conducive to reaching mutual goals: cultural desire (the desire to work in a multicultural society), cultural awareness, and cultural sensitivity. Cultural competence may be characterized as knowledge, attitudes, and values that, when applied systematically, lead to the empowerment of others irrespective of their culture.

The 14 culturally and linguistically appropriate services (CLAS) standards (U.S. DHSS, Office of Minority Health, 2001) are provided primarily to healthcare organizations to address the inequities in health status and access to care seen among minority populations and have a focus on providing culturally and linguistically appropriate services by staff trained appropriately for culturally competent service delivery.

In recognizing the significance of paying attention to culture and valuing the input and expertise of others, the American Evaluation Association's Guiding Principles for Evaluators (2008, item D.6) reads, "Understand, respect, and take into account differences among stakeholders such as culture, religion, disability, age and sexual orientation and ethnicity." To do so, one must be culturally competent. Cultural competence in evaluation means

- Being open, respectful, and appreciative of another's culture

- Acknowledging the value of other cultures and the contribution of others

- Recognizing culturally based understandings

- Incorporating cultural understanding into each step of the evaluation process

Cultural competence is a journey and does not have a discrete end point because we never really become competent in another person's culture; however, cultural humility and the ability to listen to people from other cultures and to evaluate ourselves are important characteristics of evaluators who are culturally competent (Tervalon & Murray-Garcia, 1998). Cultural humility also includes understanding the impact of one's professional culture, which helps shape the relationship between the evaluator and the stakeholders. An important result of a relationship where there is cultural humility is likely to be full and equitable participation for all stakeholders.

The American Evaluation Association standards include two guiding competencies for evaluators that focus on cultural understanding (2008, items B.2 and D.14):

1. Demonstrate a sufficient level of cultural competence to ensure recognition, accurate interpretation, and respect for diversity.

2. Become acquainted with and respect differences among participants, including their culture, religion, gender, disability, age, sexual orientation, and ethnicity.

One of the earliest phases in the development of cultural competence is acquiring cultural sensitivity. In evaluation, cultural sensitivity dictates that the evaluation team

- Shed light on why a particular program works from the perspective of the participants and the stakeholders.

- Design an appropriate evaluation process.

- Interpret data with sensitivity and understanding.

- Promote social justice and equity.

In the application of cultural understanding to evaluation, Kirkhart (2005) describes multicultural validity in evaluation research as the recognition and application of understanding of cultural context to increase the validity of the research process from the formation of the evaluation question to the communication of findings. Kirkhart (2005) identifies five approaches through which differences in culture influence the validity of an evaluation:

1. *Interpersonal* approaches assess the quality of the interactions between and among participants in the evaluation process.

2. *Consequential* approaches assess the social consequences of understandings and judgments and the actions taken based on them.

3. *Methodological* approaches assess the cultural appropriateness of measurement tools and the cultural congruence of evaluation designs.

4. *Theoretical* approaches assess the cultural congruence of theoretical perspectives underlying the program, the evaluation, and the assumptions of validity.

5. *Experiential* approaches assess congruence with the lived experience of participants in the program and in the evaluation process.

In integrating cultural perspectives into its work, the United Nations Population Fund identified 24 tips for culturally sensitive programming (United Nations Population Fund, n.d.). Drawing on that work, I list here 10 of the tips that mirror the principles guiding the implementation of the Participatory Model for Evaluation:

1. Invest time in knowing the culture in which you are operating.

2. Hear what the community has to say.

3. Demonstrate respect.

4. Be inclusive.

5. Honor commitments.

6. Find common ground.

7. Build community capacity.

8. Let people do what they do best.

9. Provide solid evidence.

10. Rely on the objectivity of science.

(A full list of the tips may be found at http://www.unfpa.org/culture/24/cover.htm)

The Participatory Model for Evaluation incorporates an empowerment philosophy that integrates a cultural perspective and leaves the community with knowledge, skills, and an increased capacity and ability to conduct its own evaluation by including a community-based participatory research philosophy.

Think About It!

When have you worked on a project, been involved with an organization, or participated in an activity in which some people have been left out or ignored? How do you think that person may have felt? In your future work as an evaluator, how will you make sure to consider others' perspectives in order to accurately reflect their viewpoints? How will you ensure that every viewpoint is reflected in an unbiased way without reference to your own vested interest?

SUMMARY

- Evaluation is conducted by a team that consists of evaluators and stakeholders who share responsibility for the evaluation from the start of the process to completing the report and presenting the results.

- The Participatory Model for Evaluation considers the community assessment and the public health program or policy initiative as precursors to evaluation.

- Participatory evaluation fosters the involvement of stakeholders in all aspects of the evaluation from describing the initiative's context to writing the final evaluation report.

- The guiding principles for performing evaluation are systematic inquiry, competence, integrity, respect for persons, and responsibility for the public welfare.

- Evaluation occurs at multiple levels—project and program level; organizational, community level, and state and national level.

- Culture refers to a set of beliefs, traditions, and behavior of a group of people that may be identified by personal characteristics, geographical area, or common interests.

- Cultural competency is a set of behaviors that professionals adopt in providing appropriate cross-culturally and linguistically appropriate services with a view to reducing health disparities.

FIGURE 1.5.   *Valuable Take-Aways*

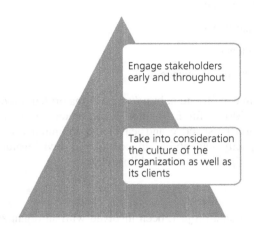

Engage stakeholders early and throughout

Take into consideration the culture of the organization as well as its clients

DISCUSSION QUESTIONS AND ACTIVITIES

1. Discuss the different forms of evaluation and their uses in evaluating public health programs.

2. Identify an article that uses a participatory approach to evaluation and another that adopts an alternative approach. Summarize the main points of each article and discuss differences between the approaches. What are other relevant perspectives you could consider as you review these differences?

3. Write a one-page paper discussing the main ideas of the relationship between culture and evaluation represented through a literature review. Write a short paragraph that explains the extent to which your paper's conclusions follow the evidence provided.

4. Identify a state or national evaluation report similar to the SCHIP evaluation and describe the evaluation approach that was used by the authors.

KEY TERMS

community-based participatory research
community health
cultural competence
ethical principles in evaluation
evaluation

initiative
participatory evaluation
participatory model for evaluation
preassessment evaluation
public health
stakeholders

CHAPTER

2

THE COMMUNITY ASSESSMENT

AN OVERVIEW

LEARNING OBJECTIVES

- Describe the relationship of community assessment to the implementation of public and community health programs and to program evaluation.

  - *Identify and describe approaches to conducting a community assessment.*

- Describe a literature review as a component of the community assessment.

- Explain the value and role of stakeholders in conducting a community assessment.

Public health concerns such as high or detectable rates of morbidity or mortality among a specified population may result in attempts to address the problem by proposing solutions and developing interventions. From the perspective of an evaluator, the intervention that is developed requires appraisal on two levels. First, it requires that the problem be specified: Who are affected? Why are they affected? How many members of the community are affected? Second, it requires an understanding of the assets and resources available for addressing the problem.

A community assessment determines the extent of the problem and proposes the most feasible, viable, and effective solution or combination of solutions to address the problem adequately and appropriately. A community assessment depicts the perceived and actual needs of a given population and their assets and resources for the development of a public health initiative. The community assessment precedes the evaluation process in the Participatory Model for Evaluation, as shown in Figure 2.1. This chapter provides an overview of the community assessment.

Community assessments are an important and integral part of program planning and are conducted with the community as the focus (Sharpe, Greany, Lee, & Royce, 2005). The community may be a geographical, faith, racial/ethnic, school, professional, or cultural community, to name a few. The community assessment is part of a cyclical and iterative process and precedes the selection, development, and implementation of the initiative (Figure 2.2). A community assessment may also be required following the evaluation of an existing program to identify additional community needs, assets, and priorities and to determine next steps for program development. The assessment may, in essence, herald the refinement of the initiative or the start of a new one.

FIGURE 2.1.   *The Community Assessment as a Component of the Participatory Model for Evaluation*

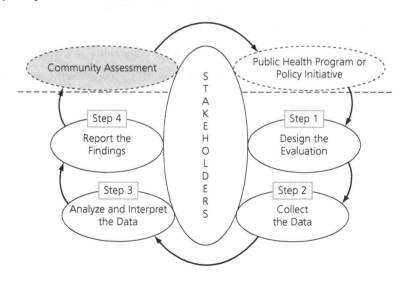

FIGURE 2.2.   *The Community Assessment, the Initiative, and the Evaluation*

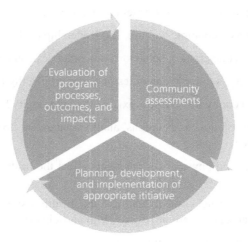

So, why conduct a community assessment? A community assessment is useful when your task is to

- Identify where the problem is most prevalent.

- Identify the people or groups of people who are most affected by the problem or involved with the problem.

- Identify the factors that produce the problem at the individual, physical, and/or social-environmental level.

- Assess individual and community needs and aspirations.

- Assess the community's readiness to address the problem.

- Assess the level of resources available within the community to address the problem.

- Obtain data that can be used to support the development of the initiative and provide the baseline against which any changes in the problem may be assessed.

A community assessment can also be described as a situation analysis that may produce an extensive appraisal of the affected community and organizations using a set of tools for assessing both the internal and external environments.

For the assessment process to be empowering and to benefit the community, Hancock and Minkler (2007) advocate that it be "of the community, by the community and for the community" (p. 138). An important aspect of this approach is that the community is involved in the process; the findings are provided to the community and can then be utilized by the community for decision-making.

Involving the community in a participatory process to identify and address their problems is likely to result in the development of sustainable, community-driven solutions to the problem. Hancock and Minkler (2007, p. 144) suggest incorporating questions that are important to the community in the assessment process. Such questions include

- What are the history, economic welfare, and leadership of the community?

- What individual characteristics, behaviors, and practices contribute to the problem?

- Do people have access to basic amenities that support healthy living?

- To what extent do equity and fairness exist in the community?

- What is the nature of civic associations, and to what extent do they support all facets of community life?

- How do the social and physical environments affect the health and well-being of the community?

- What is currently being done to address the health issues and concerns of the community? What services are provided? Who participates?

- What is the cultural life of the community?

- What is being done to minimize the impact of environmental hazards on the community?

- Who are the "movers and shakers" of the community, the people who get things done and whom others in the community rely on for information and resources?

So, what kind of information is collected?

The data used in a community assessment includes epidemiological data contained within reports and the literature review as well as primary data from interviewing a variety of stakeholders. This information includes

- The health problem, prevalence, and incidence of disease, and quality-of-life indicators.

- Risk and protective factors that influence the behavior of individuals.

- Sociocultural and political factors that reinforce or enable conditions that increase the public health problem and will affect any interventions.

- Assets and resources available within the community.

THEORETICAL CONSIDERATIONS

It is useful to conduct the community assessment using a theoretical framework because public health programs and policy initiatives are best developed using a strong theory. Examples of theoretical approaches for conducting a community assessment are available in the scientific literature. Community assessments may be based on one or a combination of individual, interpersonal, or communal theoretical models of health-behavior change. The conclusions that are drawn during the community assessment describe the relationships among the factors that cause the problem and the resources that are available. It is these conclusions that form the basis for the development of an appropriate intervention to address the problem.

Theories used in public health are related to the level of analysis to which they apply. For example, individual level theories apply to the theories that, when put in place, address the factors that affect changes in the individual. The most commonly used theories of individual behavior in public health are the transtheoretical model (Procashasca & DiClemente, 1983), social cognitive theory (Bandura, 1986), the health belief model (Hochbaum, 1958), the theory of planned behavior (Fishbain & Ajzen, 1975), and the social support theory (House, 1981). At the community and group level, community organization and community building are important concepts in the absence of a single unified model (Minkler, Wallerstein, & Wilson, 2008). The diffusion of innovation theory (Rogers, 2003) has at its central idea that an innovation (new idea) is first adopted by a small group or individuals within a social system and then it diffuses throughout the community. Table 2.1 provides an overview of the major concepts from these models; detailed descriptions can be found in Glanz, Rimer, and Viswanath (2008). Other theoretical frameworks have been used in public health, such as the Andersen model, which explains people's utilization of health services (Andersen, 1995). In building organizations and ensuring they provide needed services, the theory of organizational change (Goodman, Steckler, & Kegler, 2002) provides guidance. The theory is explained in four stages of change: awareness raising of high-level staff, adoption of the policy or program, and implementation of the policy or program, and institutionalization. In the last step, senior staff members ensure that the program or policy is sustainable through the establishment of systems to ensure quality control and continued investment.

When a theory or a theoretical framework is used for the community assessment, the same theory may be used in the development of the intervention that addresses the problem that was previously identified. The value in using a theoretical framework for program development is that it increases the likelihood of incorporating the factors (concepts and constructs) that are known to result in the change that the initiative is addressing. In addition, it is used in compiling the baseline data for future evaluations to determine if the evidence-based program that was instituted resulted in any changes to the problem.

Social marketing has been adopted from commercial marketing where it is used to analyze, plan, execute, and evaluate programs designed to influence the behavior of consumers. In public health, social marketing may be used as a part of the community assessment to understand the need for tailoring the intervention to the groups most at risk. The market analysis, which is the first of six constructs, is based on what are commonly referred to as the 4Ps: product, price, promotion, and placement, each helping to explain how behavioral change can be achieved by considering how the intervention is considered. Product represents the "what" of the intervention, whereas the real and perceived cost and benefits reflect the price; the "how" is represented by the promotion of the intervention and access to the product/intervention is described in its placement.

TABLE 2.1.   Commonly Used Theories and Models in Public Health

Theory	Major Concepts
Transtheoretical Model Based on individuals' changing behavior through stages of readiness	■ Precontemplation ■ Contemplation ■ Preparation ■ Action ■ Maintenance
Social Cognitive Theory Personal factors, environmental factors, and individual behavior operate in a dynamic, reciprocal way	■ Reciprocal determinism ■ Outcome expectations ■ Self-efficacy ■ Observational learning ■ Self-regulation ■ Rewards and punishments
Health Belief Model Based on individuals' perceptions of the problem and of the benefits, barriers, and factors influencing the decision to adopt a behavior	■ Perceived susceptibility ■ Perceived severity ■ Perceived benefits ■ Perceived barriers ■ Cues to action ■ Self-efficacy
Theory of Planned Behavior Based on individuals' intentions, attitudes, and perceptions of social norms and their ability to perform a behavior	■ Behavioral intention ■ Experiential attitude ■ Subjective norm ■ Perceived behavioral control
Social Support Based on individuals' perception and experience of support from those around them	■ Emotional support ■ Instrumental support ■ Informational support ■ Appraisal support
Community Organization Hypothesizes a community-driven process for addressing health and social problems	■ Empowerment ■ Critical consciousness ■ Community capacity ■ Social capital ■ Issue selection ■ Participation and relevance

TABLE 2.1.   (*Continued*)

Theory	Major Concepts
Diffusion of Innovation Theory (DOI)	■ Innovators ■ Early adopters ■ Early majority ■ Late majority ■ Laggards
Organizational Development	■ Network partnerships ■ Knowledge transfer ■ Problem solving ■ Infrastructure development including social and financial capital ■ Sustainability
Communication Behavior Change	■ The credibility, clarity, and relevance of the source ■ The content, delivery, length, and tone of the message ■ The medium of transmission ■ Audience segmentation and preferences
Social Marketing	■ Market analysis (4Ps) ■ Product ■ Price ■ Promotion ■ Placement

THE ECOLOGICAL MODEL

Historically, behavioral theories have been the primary drivers of initiatives to address public health problems. However, recognition of the social and environmental factors that influence health has led to use of an ecological-systems perspective, which incorporates in its analysis individual, social, and environmental factors. The assessment may incorporate concepts from theoretical frameworks at each of these levels. The ecological model allows the integration of multiple theories and models as needed. It dictates that it is not sufficient to look at individual factors in a community assessment because organizational, community, and public policy factors may play an important role in the problem itself or in addressing the problem.

The ecological model may be used to provide guidance for a comprehensive approach to the community assessment and program development across multiple domains of behavioral influence. At the individual level, behavior is influenced by biological, physiological, psychological, and emotional states. At the interpersonal level, structural factors and social and cultural norms of peers, family, and friends play a role. The organizational, community, and policy domains recognize the influence and impact of multiple environmental factors on behavior. Determinants at this level include economic, physical, and structural factors and systems that influence physical and emotional health outcomes. Where people live, work, and play significantly affects health outcomes. In addition, the social determinants of health (Commission on Social Determinants of Health, 2008) include conditions that lead to inequality and injustices that increase the risk for disease and disability and influence individual and collective health and well-being. Social cohesion, social inclusiveness, social capital, and trust are also factors in determining health outcomes (Marmot, 2004). Using the ecological model as the guiding framework allows these concepts to be included in a community assessment of factors that influence health. Incorporating core principles of the ecological model (Figure 2.3) in behavior-change models leads to behavior change through appropriate, behavior-specific interventions (Sallis, Owen, & Fisher, 2008).

Think About It!

Let us assume that you have just been hired by a local not-for-profit organization and you are anxious to develop a program for homeless men who are living under the bridge across town. However, you do not really understand the extent of the problem or the circumstances under which they have become homeless. In addition, you have little understanding of the conditions under which they live although you believe from reading the scientific literature that their health is affected by a number of factors. The factors that affect their health operate at the individual, interpersonal, community, organizational and policy levels. One example at the individual level is the level of smoking among this population,

FIGURE 2.3.   *The Ecological-Model Framework*

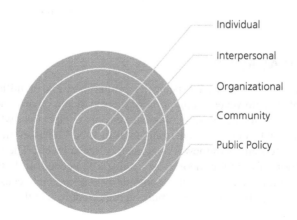

Individual

Interpersonal

Organizational

Community

Public Policy

which has profound impacts on their health but which we know is influenced by their peers, community norms, their access to services, and policies that might perpetuate the unhealthy behavior. You also do not know what organizations are in the area that would be supportive and willing to provide services to this population, relieving the burden on your organization, so together you can provide a continuum of care. Many of the men have recently become homeless as a result of the downturn in the economy, losing their jobs and their homes. You recognize that there are women and families that are also homeless but there are other organizations that already provide services for them. Your organization understands that the needs of men are sometimes different and an approach that recognizes the nuances and takes these factors into consideration is crucial.

Describe how you would go about getting the information you will need to move forward with your project. Where would you look for information? What information would you gather at the individual, interpersonal, community, organizational, and policy levels? What theoretical framework will you use to guide your thinking in developing a comprehensive intervention to provide secure, safe, and sustainable housing for men?

DATA COLLECTION

Data for a community assessment are collected from the population of interest to determine the incidence and prevalence rates of disease and the extent of the problem. Rates of disease and disability are described as the number of cases per 1,000 or per 100,000 of the population. In addition, risk and protective factors associated with the public health problem are identified and described. The risk factors are those personal and environmental factors or determinants that increase the likelihood of an individual's coming into contact with or being exposed to conditions that lead to disease or disability. Protective factors are mirror images of risk factors; when they are present, they provide protection against the risk of or the exposure to disease or disability. Most of our interventions and thinking in public health are about risk factors—for example, not eating healthy fruits and vegetables— yet we often fail to assess the behaviors that are protective of health such as drinking plenty of water, which is critically important when considering obesity as the negative health outcome.

Think About It!

What are some examples of risk and protective factors for a population that you serve either through your job or a project that you are involved with? Create a table to show the risk and protective factor for the same health outcome. Identify and focus on the most important aspects of the health condition you named. Table 2.2 shows one example when the health outcome may be heart disease.

TABLE 2.2.   **Risk Factor, Protective Factors, and Level of Influence**

Risk Factor	Protective Factor	Level of Influence
Smoking	Policies that limit access to cigarettes and other tobacco products	Individual & Policy

In addition to identifying risk and protective factors at the individual level, inter-personal community, organization and policy levels, a community assessment must identify human, material, and economic assets. These assets include formal and infor-mal community-based organizations, agencies, and networks that are available in the community (Kretzmann & McKnight, 1993) that will address the problem. The recent engagement in public-private partnerships allows this assessment to be expanded well beyond community-based organizations and public agencies to involve the business community, that is often willing to become engaged, but don't know how to. The assess-ment includes demographic, social, economic, cultural, structural, systems, and policy factors that affect the population of interest and the community. The assessment contains information about the state of the community, access to and delivery of services, cultural and social norms, policies and practices, as well as the economic situation at community, state, regional, and national levels.

Data on the economic situation of a community include not only the educational level of the population of interest but also the types and locations of jobs that the community offers to its residents (low paying versus high paying) and ones they have access to. With the expansion of Internet-based earning potential and opportunities to work from home, the job market has opened up well outside the community, making access to resources no longer dependent on what is available around the corner. Such characteristics of the community's structure and systems infrastructure are an important gauge of the community's ability and willingness to support public health efforts. Determining the resources in the community identifies important allies for addressing the problem and supporting sustainable, culturally appropriate initiatives that are congruent with the reality of the community and the lives of its residents. When the community is on-line, it may be even more challenging to provide public health interventions, but more and more practitioners and researchers are finding a way to do that and knowing their needs and assets is just as important.

The community assessment is conducted using both qualitative and quantitative approaches (Finifter, Jensen, Wilson, & Koenig, 2005). Data are collected to understand the community's expressed and observed needs for health and social services. Carrying out a community assessment requires that the researchers follow a process that involves multiple stakeholders and uses multiple data-collection sources and methods. The core components of an assessment determine what needs to be done to undertake the community assessment, gather and analyze the information, and make decisions about the kind of intervention and who will be involved based on the data (Figure 2.4).

A more expanded list of steps in conducting a community assessment include

1. Establish a team to undertake the community assessment.

2. Determine the availability of community, state, regional, and national data to assess the extent of the problem.

3. Determine which data are missing and need to be collected at the community level.

4. Decide on the data-collection approach.

5. Develop and/or secure data-collection instruments (surveys, interview guides, and so on).

FIGURE 2.4.   *Core Components of the Community Assessment Process*

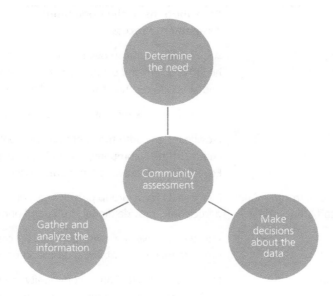

6. Develop the data-collection plan.

7. Secure human, material, and financial resources for implementing the data-collection plan.

8. Implement the data-collection plan (Gather the data)

9. Analyze and interpret the data.

10. Use the information to frame the intervention.

Step 1: Establish a Team

Conducting a community assessment based on a participatory model requires equitable involvement by the community. The first step in the community assessment process is to engage those who are most affected by the problem and professionals who provide community-based services. The team consists of people who live within the community or who have an interest in the assessment being conducted. They are known as stakeholders. Members of the team should include those who are familiar with the problem, research methods, data-collection approaches, and data analysis. It is important that the team also includes those who are most familiar with the problem and often those who are most affected. The team members' roles should be identified so each person is able to contribute to the process. Members of the community bring expertise and important perspectives with regard to the community, the population, and the risk factors associated with the problem being assessed. In the example in Table 2.3, the team comprises 12 people, half of whom are residents of the community and three of them are directly affected by the

TABLE 2.3.   The Community Assessment Team

Stakeholder	Contributions to the Community-Assessment Process
Project partners	Are key informants; provide insight into the public health problem and solutions; provide historical data and access to resources for data collection
Project consultants	Provide feedback regarding methods and tools
Community residents (parents of children and community members)	Provide insights into the public health problem and the culture of the community; review the instruments; are key informants; survey participants; collect data
Members of the faith community, local school staff, and students	Function as focus-group participants and survey participants; provide digital stories and photographs
Funders	Provide incentives for participants; cover costs of program management and data collection
Project manager and staff	Provide overall direction of community assessment; provide guidance in framing the questions; develop methodology

problem being addressed. It is important that the community members have a strong voice on the team to help guide the team as well as provide cultural translations for the team. It is often easy for some team members to be overlooked since they do not always have the same level of training as the others on the team. It is important that adequate training is provided so they can have a meaningful level of participation in aspects of the community assessment they feel most comfortable participating in.

The team decides on the tasks and specifies the aim of the community assessment: Should it be a broad assessment to determine the major problems or issues within the community or a narrow assessment of a specific problem? For example, if the problem is high rates of alcohol-related motor vehicle accidents, then the team may opt to spend its time and resources focusing on the groups that are most affected; how, when, and where the accidents occur; who might be facilitating the problem; and the best approaches for addressing the problem from the perspective of the community. The community assessment may be limited to youth between the ages of 15 and 21 rather than adults since they are categorized as drinking under the federal legal drinking age. Police-generated data might provide the first clues for focusing on this group.

In another application of this approach, conducting an organizational assessment would require teams at all levels of the organization to be involved in the assessment to provide appropriate and useful insights. The focus might still be on underage drinking, since this service-oriented organization hires individuals of all ages but especially college students who are often easy to find and available to work, in this college town where other higher-paying jobs are scarce.

Think About It!

Additional questions that the team members might ask themselves during the formation of the planning team and the beginning of the process are, "What are we taking for granted that forms the basis of our thinking?" "What assumptions are we making that limit our ability to think broadly about who needs to be involved in the team?" "What data need to be collected and what are the best approaches to understanding the problem?"

Step 2: Determine the Availability of Data

Once the aims of the community assessment have been established, the next step is to determine what information already exists. Data that are regularly collected by not-for-profit organizations and by state and local agencies should first be reviewed to determine what information is already available about the community and the public health problem of concern. These secondary data may be in multiple forms. They may be in data bases that have to be analyzed or in reports that have been compiled. The quality and the quantity of the data may be mixed and may be limited to small areas or one population group. On the other hand, the reports may not have disaggregated data of smaller population units. The team must assess how useful the existing data are and whether they serve the purposes of the group. If the intent of the group is to understand the factors leading to a problem in the whole community, but a previous assessment was conducted only in the local junior college of 500 students, it is important to collect additional data on other members of the community. Alternatively, given the example of underage drinking, data on the community may be available at the state level but not give any specifics for youth. Collecting primary data from youth would then be important to support the development of the intervention. Secondary data from local or state organizations and agencies may be available to answer some but not all of the questions, and the team may need to collect additional primary data.

Using human subjects in a community assessment requires that the team has its proposal reviewed by the Institutional Review Board of the organization. Usually, these boards are found in research universities, local hospitals, and medical councils. Sometimes they are called ethics boards.

Step 3: Determine Which Data Are Missing and Need to Be Collected

After a full review of the existing data, a determination is made by the team of the additional data needs of the project. Through group consultations, a list is compiled of the information that is available and of the questions that still need to be answered. Questions may include

■ What are the problems or issues in the community, in a specific area, or with a particular group?

■ How does the problem or issue affect different members of the community? Consider differences by ethnicity, sexual orientation, socioeconomic status, gender, age, and so on.

■ How prevalent is the problem among members of different groups—by age, gender, race, profession, educational level, socioeconomic status, and so on?

■ What are the factors that increase or decrease the occurrence of the problem for each of the groups?

■ What are the individual, interpersonal, community, organizational, or policy factors that influence the problem? Consider whether these factors vary by group.

■ What resources—human, material, and financial—are available within the community as well as outside the community that can be brought to bear on the problem?

■ Who are the people and what are the systems and structures available and ready to address the problem?

■ How does addressing the problem consider issues of social justice? Social justice expects that everyone irrespective of race, social status, religion, and so forth deserves the right to equal economic, political, and social opportunities to be successful. So, will addressing the problem ensure that those most affected are the targets of the proposed interventions?

Think About It!

It is important to collect only the information that is needed and answers the overarching research question. It is both a waste of resources and a waste of participants' time if data are collected that will not be used for program development and for which there is no clearly defined purpose. However, it is also important to ensure that all the information that is needed is collected and you don't have to go back to the community a second time. Consider the following questions: "What am I taking for granted?" and "What are the consequences that follow from not considering everybody's perspective in deciding what data should be collected?"

Step 4: Decide on the Data-Collection Approach

The data-collection approach that is used to conduct the needs assessment takes the needs of the project into consideration. The data that are collected may be quantitative or qualitative or a combination. The most suitable data are those that provide the evidence for answering the research questions. For example, if the question to be answered is, "What are the factors that influence youth drinking?" then the data-collection approach can include focus groups or individual interviews with youth and their parents as well as other key informants like community leaders and law enforcement. In addition a survey could give valuable information on the extent of the problem. In addition to the research question, the factors that determine the most appropriate approach for answering the question(s) and hence the most appropriate data to collect include the size and scope of the project, the study subject, the kind of information that is required, and the resources available for the project (Figure 2.5).

The Size and Scope of the Project The size and scope of the project influence the data-collection approach because the larger and more heterogeneous the population sample or the more factors being assessed, the more likely that a quantitative data method will be selected. Qualitative approaches may be used to complement quantitative approaches in large studies; in small studies, qualitative approaches may be used alone. Using the ecological-model framework, which includes an assessment of multiple factors that affect an individual's ability to be successful at a particular behavior increases the size and scope of the study in innumerable ways. Increases in both the size of the sample and the scope of the project have implications for the measurement approaches that may be appropriate for

FIGURE 2.5.   *Major Factors Influencing Data Collection in the Community Assessment Process*

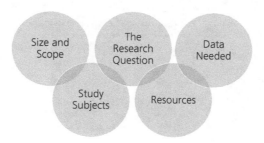

assessing each dimension. Such increases also result in significant cost. A mixed methods approach may be helpful to consider.

The Study Subject   The kind of subjects in the study also influences the approach used. In understanding the high rates of obesity in a community, for example, it is important to obtain information from individuals, as well as to do an environmental scan of the neighborhoods. In this case, the study subjects include both people and locations. Collecting data from individuals involves using surveys, individual interviews, and focus groups, among other methods. The environmental scan can take on multiple forms—for example, assessing the number and quality of community parks and opportunities for physical activity in the neighborhood or observing the type, quantity, and quality of food that people choose to eat or have available to them.

The Kind of Information Required   The kind of data that are collected is determined by the type of information that is needed. Studies of knowledge may be easily assessed using surveys, whereas understanding attitudes toward a behavior may be more easily assessed using focus groups or individual interviews. Behavior, however, may be less reliably assessed using self-reported surveys; observing the behavior provides more objective evidence, although for most behaviors it might be difficult if not impossible to make suitable and appropriate observations. Examples include assessing the use of drugs or condoms. A mixed methods approach assessing the extent to which healthy foods in grocery stores and farmers' markets are available and accessible within a community lends itself to using a combination of qualitative and quantitative measures. The kind of information required may suggest the use of photography and digital storytelling. Proxy measures for some data may be most appropriate, such as using blood tests to assess drug use.

The Resources Available   The financial, material, and human resources that are available for a project influence the amount of data that can be collected. The data-collection approach must also provide for the inclusion and the training of members of the community. Community members can be trained to develop the data-collection instruments and to collect and analyze the data. In general, it is critical to use the most appropriate and cost-efficient approach to collect the most useful data. It does little good to collect data using a survey and using up limited resources if using a survey will not help you answer the research question. Figure 2.6 summarizes the factors that are critical for determining the data collection associated with a community assessment.

FIGURE 2.6. *Major Components of a Community Assessment*

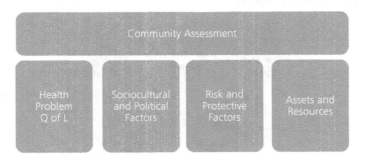

Think About It!

The data collection approach is dependent on a number of factors that include the research question; the knowledge and skills of the research team; the most appropriate approach for answering the research question; and the level of resources, the size and scope of the project, and the sample itself. At this stage of the process, two questions you can ask to ensure that data collected is the most valid data possible is, "To what extent am I considering the research question within the necessary contexts and relationships?" "To what extent will the methods used provide the evidence required to answer the research question?"

Step 5: Develop and/or Secure Data-Collection Instruments

The questions that need to be answered as part of the community assessment will determine the data-collection instruments that are most appropriate. In using a theory-based approach for the community assessment, existing or previously developed surveys allow the team to collect quantitative data and to draw conclusions about the problem using numbers (frequencies, means, Chi-square). Other instruments allow qualitative data to be collected on perceptions, depths of feelings, experiences, attitudes, beliefs, and behaviors using qualitative approaches. These instruments can also provide information on the quality of a product or an operation, exposure to an initiative or condition, and adherence to a task or behavior.

The mix of instruments selected will determine who should provide the data. Because data must be credible, it is important to ensure that the appropriate persons and sites are selected. Participants who experience a problem are likely to be the most credible for describing the problem, but in the assessment of assets to address the problem other people may provide different yet useful perspectives. Data obtained from multiple sources and collected using reliable tools increase the validity and the credibility of the research. Some of these tools are the following:

■ Focus-group discussions are useful for obtaining information quickly and for understanding broad perspectives. Focus groups are homogenous groups of six to eight individuals who convene to answer open-ended, predetermined questions.

■ Individual key-informant interviews are used to gather information from individuals who either are affected by the problem or can provide an independent perspective. Individual interviews are often carried out with opinion leaders who need to be included in the community assessment because of their unique perspectives but whose status in the community makes it preferable that they not be included in focus groups. Individual interviews are often quicker than focus groups because interviews can be scheduled more easily with one person than with six or more together.

■ Photovoice is a qualitative data-collection technique in which the data are collected by members of the community using cameras. The photographs are discussed to highlight issues that the photographer identifies as relevant for describing the problem.

■ Digital storytelling, which utilizes audio or video recordings, is developing into a popular approach in community-needs assessments. It allows the participants to document the problem and their experiences in their own words; they can provide strong testimonials that support the development of initiatives.

■ Social network analysis, which maps and measures relationships among people, groups, organizations, and so forth, allows the researcher to understand patterns of behavior and, in the case of disease transmission, can identify those at risk.

■ Asset maps can be used to identify and document physical or human resources within the community that may influence the problem and/or provide venues for the intervention—for example, churches, schools, health facilities, social services, and a variety of businesses. Assets are mapped to show the quantity, distribution, and accessibility of the resources to populations of interest. A mapping of stores in low-income neighborhoods could show the number and location of food outlets compared with shops that sell alcohol. In conducting a study of the accessibility of fresh fruits and vegetables in a community that has high rates of childhood obesity, an asset map might include the availability of produce in

 ■ Corner stores and convenience stores

 ■ Farmers' markets

 ■ Grocery stores

 ■ School vending machines

In addition, the skills, talents, and expertise of community leaders—heads of agencies, organizations, businesses, churches, schools—may be tallied to determine the level of resources available within the community for addressing the problem and developing the initiative.

Information on the instruments that can be used may be obtained by reviewing the literature and contacting others who have conducted similar studies. Local universities, health departments, and community-based organizations may have experience in using tools that might be helpful. Surveys and other data-collection tools may also be developed for specific initiatives, although the process is time-consuming, and developing a good instrument requires a certain amount of expertise. Quantitative and qualitative data-collection methods are described in detail in Chapters 8 and 9.

Step 6: Develop the Data-Collection Plan

A data-collection plan describes the steps that are required to ensure that the data are collected; Table 2.4 is an example of such a plan. It includes the following components:

■ Data to be collected

■ Methods for collecting the data

■ Source of the data

■ Persons responsible

Developing a data-collection plan may also be an activity that outlines the time frame for the data collection.

Step 7: Secure Resources for the Data-Collection Plan

Once the team has decided on the design for the community assessment and has developed the plan, the resources for implementing the plan must be secured through grants, donations, or existing budgeted activities. Required resources include:

■ Personnel (staff and volunteers) for conducting the study

■ Salaries and stipends for staff and volunteers

■ Incentives (participants if required)

■ Transportation (staff, volunteers and/or participants)

■ Data-collection instruments (purchase, duplication, and collation)

TABLE 2.4.   Example of a Data-Collection Plan

Data to Be Collected	Methods for Collecting the Data	Source of the Data	Person(s) Responsible
Knowledge about HIV/AIDS transmission	Existing survey developed by federally funded project	Adults 18 to 25 years of age	Youth-development project director
Attitudes toward condoms	Focus-group discussion; interview guide developed locally	Adults 18 to 25 years of age	Graduate assistant; project manager
Availability of condoms	Survey; observation; photography	Store owners, pharmacy managers	Project manager; leader of community-assessment team

- Interview space

- Equipment, supplies, and materials

  In addition Institutional Board/Ethics Board clearance must also be secured.

Step 8: Implement the Data-Collection Plan

At the implementation stage, it is assumed that all the resources are available, the materials have been developed, the study participants have been notified or recruited as required by the method, and the instruments are available and ready to use.

Let us look at an example from the data-collection plan in Table 2.4. The person responsible for ensuring that data on the availability of condoms are collected is the leader of the community-assessment team. The leader may identify other members of the team to participate in the data collection or recruit and train others. The plan identifies the data-collection methods as surveys, observation, and photography. The survey includes items regarding the level and turnover of condom stocks in stores and pharmacies throughout the year. Observation forms and the protocol for collecting the data are developed. The protocol contains instructions for making the observation and forms for documenting the results. The criteria for completing the forms are clearly defined for each category. In addition, it contains instructions for obtaining photographs that will be helpful in making judgments about the availability and accessibility of condoms in the stores and pharmacies. Before any data are collected, the store owners and pharmacy managers are contacted to inform them of the study and the team's intention to complete a survey in order to document the availability of condoms in their stores. They are asked to provide signed consent.

Step 9: Analyze and Interpret the Data

Interpretation and analysis of data collected for a community assessment are determined by the type of data collected. Quantitative data can be analyzed manually if the sample size is small or by using computer-assisted mechanisms such as Microsoft Excel, SPSS®, or STATA®. Determining frequencies, means, and standard deviations for the data and describing the sample is the first step. Depending on the level of data collected—ordinal, nominal, scale, or ratio data—the sample size and questions asked, other types of analysis may be undertaken, including univariate, bivariate, and multivariate analysis as well as comparing data from pre and post measures. If the community assessment is completed at the beginning and at the end of an intervention, a t-test may be appropriate. Graphs, charts, and maps provide a visual representation of the results.

Qualitative data is also coded and can be analyzed using manual or computer-assisted approaches. Evaluating qualitative data requires content analysis to determine themes. The themes form the basis for the analysis and the report to provide answers to the research questions.

The interpretation of the findings is based on the information that the community assessment set out to get and the likely use of the data. If the focus of the intervention is behavior change in the population sample, then the report may include the following:

- Persons affected by the problem

- Frequency of the behavior

- Context of the behavior

- Environmental conditions under which the behavior is carried out

- Approaches to addressing the behavior and internal and external resources that might support the intervention

If, however, the approach is policy oriented, then the focus of the report is the information required to frame the policy and the populations or setting that the policy would need to target. It may also provide information on the context and any possible barriers to policy development and implementation.

A community assessment of the physical environment could include a photovoice approach to data collection and understanding multiple perspectives and the needs for specific population groups such as the elderly and children.

Policy leading to social change requires a process that includes community and policymaker education, advocacy, and community mobilization and action. Understanding the requirements of the initiative for each component is critical to undertaking a meaningful policy-change process. The analysis and interpretation of the data collected during the process is based on the needs of the project. For example data may be collected to assess community mobilization and action. Data collected might include who are mobilized, numbers, locations, and the number and type of actions that were taken as a baseline for future mobilization. Data to analyze may range from the level of participation at events to actions taken as a result of e-mail alerts. It may also include analyzing data collected from policymakers with regard to the outcome of their actions. This data may be in multiple forms, which include quantitative and qualitative formats, and must be analyzed in ways appropriate for the method used.

Step 10: Use the Information to Frame the Intervention

The usual final step in the community assessment is to use the information obtained from the research to frame the new or revised initiative. The data provide information regarding the people affected, where they live and work, the factors that predispose them to the problem, as well as those that enable or reinforce the problem. The data also include information about the human, material, and financial resources for addressing the problem. Figure 2.7 summarizes the steps outlined above and highlights the community assessment's cyclical nature.

DATA SOURCES

When community assessments are conducted, primary or secondary data may be used to assess the problem and to determine who is most affected. Primary data are collected for the purposes of the particular study, and secondary data are existing data collected for a previously defined purpose. Primary data for a community needs assessment are gathered using qualitative or quantitative approaches. It is especially important to use primary

FIGURE 2.7. *Summarizing Steps 1–10*

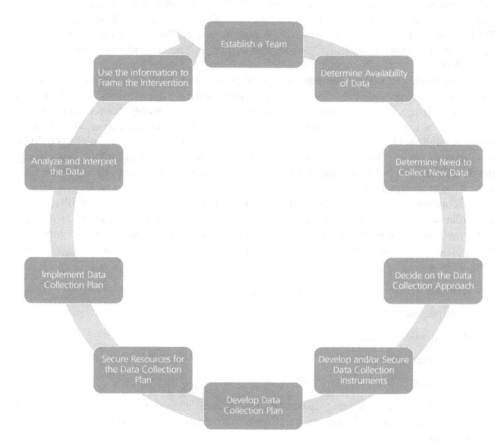

data when information about culturally diverse populations is limited and specific information is required to ensure the development of culturally appropriate interventions. Existing qualitative or quantitative data collected for other purposes may be available. Using secondary data is less time consuming and less expensive than collecting and analyzing primary data.

Primary-data collection utilizes a variety of methods, including self-administered surveys, case studies, observation, focus-group discussions, and individual interviews (Sharpe et al., 2005) and document reviews including the analysis of news items. Data may also be collected using face-to-face, telephone, or web-assisted technologies. Concept mapping (Trochim, 1989) may be used to assess how a topic is viewed in the context of a community assessment, which may be undertaken in person or using on-line mapping tools. Less formal assessments than these may take place when driving or walking through the community conducting an initial visual assessment, in community meetings, and when using participatory-research approaches, such as photo narratives (Bender & Harbour, 2001; Sharpe et al., 2005), photovoice (Wang, Burris, & Ping, 1996) or Visual Voices (Yonas et al., 2009) and theater, music, dance, puppet shows, and storytelling (Sharpe et al., 2005).

Large health-related assessments and existing local and state data bases in combination with census data provide valuable information for estimating the extent of a public health problem. In using secondary data, it is important to check its validity, source, sample size, and nature of the sample. If the population that was included in the data is not similar to yours, it might not be appropriate to rely on since its reliability (Cronbach's alpha) could be considerably lower. Other considerations in the use of secondary data include how closely the data match the public health problem being assessed and the extent to which the data reflect the local situation.

Secondary data may be obtained from death certificates; disease, disability, crime surveillance; hospital and health records; and surveys. Useful indicators are vital statistics: births and deaths, age-specific death rates, and disease-specific morbidity and mortality rates. Secondary data that may be available at state, county, and in some cases zip-code level include:

- HIV/AIDS infection rates and AIDS diagnoses

- Teen pregnancy rates

- Birth and death rates

- Obesity rates

- Crime rates

- Data related to the leading causes of death among a given population such as heart disease, unintentional injuries, cerebrovascular diseases, lower respiratory diseases, and cancer

In addition, health and wellness data may be available with indicators such as socioeconomic, environmental, and behavioral factors that influence disease risk, access to health care, access to resources for healthy living, and utilization of health and social services. Factors may include:

- Educational levels

- Household income levels

- Environmental levels of contamination of air and water

- Service utilization

Quality-of-life indicators such as educational attainment, employment, income, housing, safety, and human rights provide information about the public health problem and opportunities to consider holistic approaches. Census data (www.census.gov) provide demographic information for the United States down to the county level, and other community-level data may complement census data. Complementary census data and household surveys may provide useful information in other countries.

Applications of Geographic Information Systems mapping technologies provide a unique profile of the community by combining information from primary and secondary sources with census data (Fazlay, Lofton, Doddato, & Mangum, 2003; Harris & López-Defede, 2004). In addition, specific points of interest can be mapped using these systems to produce an asset map of the local community at zip-code or, in some cases, street level. For example, local resources such as resources for healthy living or economic activity may be mapped to understand levels of access for selected populations.

Multiple models have been described for conducting a comprehensive community assessment, and data may be collected using a variety of tools. One example of a community assessment that is commonly used by local public health agencies is the Mobilizing for Action through Planning and Partnerships (MAPP) process (National Association of County and City Health Officials, n.d.). The tool was developed by the National Association of County and City Health Officials (NACCHO) in collaboration with the Centers for Disease Control and Prevention. The cyclical MAPP process is organized into six phases and contains four major components of the health assessment:

1. *Community themes and strengths* provide insights into issues such as perceived quality of life and the identification of assets and resources to address problems using a qualitative research approach.

2. *Local public health system assessment* assesses the structures and systems within the community that provide services and their capacities.

3. *Community health status assessment* provides quantitative data on a wide range of health indicators.

4. *Forces of change assessment* identifies forces and actions external to the health system that affect the health of the community.

(More information about this community assessment can be obtained from the NACCHO website, http://www.naccho.org/topics/infrastructure/mapp/mappbasics.cfm)

Think About It!

As an evaluator who has some experience in conducting community assessments, you are asked to conduct a community assessment by your organization using the MAPP approach described earlier. How will you go about it? What are the organizing ideas, theories, or principles that are likely to influence your thinking? How will you ensure that all stakeholders have a voice? How will you ensure that the information you produce is correct and without distortion?

CONDUCTING AN ORGANIZATIONAL ASSESSMENT

Preamble

In adopting the Ecological Model for addressing public and community health programs organizational factors may have a considerable effect on the behavior of individuals. It is, therefore, important to ensure that organizations provide access to services for individuals who need them. This may require that organizations look inward and determine how their operations and systems present barriers to utilization. This mini case study provides an opportunity to adopt the community assessment process and framework in getting to outcomes to improve the performance of organizations.

A midsize organization in the Midwest provides public health services to a community of approximately 100,000 people. It has a staff compliment of about 100 personnel. The executive director has been at the organization for one year and has observed that the productivity of the staff is lower than ideal and satisfaction surveys conducted by various projects and programs within the organization often reflect less than satisfactory performance among the staff. She would like to change that but must first conduct an assessment to determine where the problems lie and then develop interventions to appropriately address them. The executive director understood that the staff was busy and could not devote a lot of time to it, but she also understood that it was critical to get good information. Her goal was to understand the situation from a cross-section of the staff and consumers, but from one big enough to be representative. Her first task was to identify a team who would be responsible for organizing the assessment. They would be responsible to determine the size and scope of the study, the study population, the data needed, and what resources were available to undertake the study.

The executive director appointed one of the senior staff to oversee the process. She identified a team of four who she knew had a range of skills required for undertaking the study. She wanted to be sure that the team included individuals with strong research and data analysis skills. She thought a mixed methods design study would be the best approach and would yield the most amount of information given the resources that she had. She also needed a connector: somebody who would recruit study participants and be responsible to ensure that the integrity of the research was maintained as well as participate in other aspects of the research. Given the short time frame, everybody in the team had to be engaged in all aspects of the study. Once the team was engaged, they decided to meet weekly and have frequent e-mail exchanges using a shared group list. The next task for the team was to determine the aim of the assessment: they went back to the notes that the executive director had prepared and reviewed their charge. It was to understand the factors that influenced the low consumer satisfaction ratings that the projects and programs had received over the previous year. A mixed methods study would include both quantitative and qualitative data collection and would be the best approach for understanding consumer satisfaction.

Step 2 of the process was to determine the availability of data to assess the problem. Given the task at hand, the group discussed the existing information at length, reviewing all the consumer satisfaction reports they had received, and organizing the findings by project and program to see if they could determine any trends or specific groups that could be the focus of their study. They were always asking themselves the question, "What assumptions are we making that limit our ability to think broadly about this study." Through group consultations, a list was compiled of the information that was available and of the questions that still needed to be answered. In step 3 the team determined that not all their questions were answered and they needed to collect data specific to their needs. After extensive deliberation the team decided on the following research questions:

- How does consumer satisfaction play out across the organization?
- How prevalent is consumer dissatisfaction among members of different groups by age, gender, race, profession, educational level, and socioeconomic status?
- What factors influence consumer satisfaction for each of the groups?
- What organization and organizational policy factors influence consumer satisfaction?
- What resources—human, material, financial, and structural—are available within the community and the organization that may be available to improve consumer satisfaction following the findings of the study?

Although a mixed methods approach seemed like a good idea for answering the research questions, in step 4 the team reviewed all the methods and decided that the most appropriate methods would be to

- Conduct focus groups with staff to determine their perspectives and perceptions related to the services they provide.
- Conduct individual interviews with a cross section of consumers from across all the service areas being careful to select representatives from across all the demographic groups they serve.
- Conduct key informant interviews with selected members of the community and senior management of the organization to identify resources that are needed and available if training and other human resource development was required.

For step 5, the team was able to identify a few previously used validated surveys on line and reviewed them carefully to see if they had any of the items they needed for their study. They found one that worked perfectly for the consumer group but had to develop tools for the focus groups. They were able to identify questions from a variety of data collection tools that helped them design instruments specifically for

(Continued)

(Continued)

the individual and key informant interviews. As they identified questions, they also considered which theory to use so that they would have baseline data for the intervention. An earlier literature review identified the use of constructs from a couple of different theories. They wanted to consider theories related to organizational development as well as theories that related to individual behavior. At the organizational level, they included constructs from the organizational change theory (Goodman et al, 2002) and the social support theory (House, 1981). Using the social support theory, they were interested in understanding how support for each other within the organization would reduce tensions and improve relations with clients. They were sure that the study would reveal insights for an intervention later in the process.

Now they were ready to design the data collection plan that described who, what, when, and how the data would be collected (step 6) and identify resources to undertake it (step 7). They needed to secure financial resources to provide incentives, transportation, and refreshments for the focus groups, which consisted of six groups of six to eight persons each. They also needed to identify space where they could conduct privately the focus groups and the 25 individual and key informant interviews. Some of the interviews would be held in the respondent's office or a quiet space that was mutually agreed upon. Data gathering in step 8 is always the most exciting and fun part of a community assessment, but it needs to be done carefully ensuring that the data is both valid and reliable. The analysis of the data (step 9) is dependent on the type of data. The data analysis and interpretation are related to each of the research questions.

In this study, the qualitative data was coded and analyzed using a free open-source data-analysis software available on the Internet. The quantitative data was entered and analyzed in Microsoft Excel©. A detailed report was compiled that was reviewed by a few key stakeholders before being made public. At long last the team got to step 10 and, working in consultation with the executive director, members of the board of directors and key organization staff designed an intervention to improve consumer satisfaction. Their study found that staff were dissatisfied with their working conditions, which made them unhappy and affected their work and their relationships with the consumers. They drilled down deeper in the analysis of their data and discovered that staff were primarily unhappy for the following two reasons: (1) staff felt unappreciated and alone primarily due to a lack of inclusion, participation, and communication in the organization, and (2) staff frequently missed work due to stress and a feeling of isolation. It took many meetings prioritizing the issue that would be dealt with first. The team in consultation with the management agreed that they would first tackle the issues that left staff losing many days from work that were without doubt affecting their quality of life. An extensive review of the scientific literature helped them develop a theory-based intervention.

REVIEWING THE SCIENTIFIC LITERATURE

In addition to collecting primary data and compiling secondary data, a community assessment incorporates an extensive search of the scientific literature before the start of the study and sometimes following the study. This might be especially likely if the community assessment identified factors that affected the study population that they had not previously anticipated. The review identifies known behavioral, epidemiological, social, cultural, and environmental conditions associated with the public health problem at the local, state, and national levels. In addition, it identifies current conditions and historical trends. Local and web-based library resources and a systematic search of the published research provide an opportunity to compare problems in the local community with state and national trends and to understand the rationale for the initiative. The literature review is focused and specific and is used to answer the following questions:

- How does the community's assessment profile compare with the profiles of other communities of similar size and demographics across the state or nationally?

- What are the most appropriate, logical, and evidence-based ways to address the problem the community identified?

EXAMPLE

PART OF A LITERATURE REVIEW

"In addition to violence and death, youth violence affects communities by increasing the cost of health care, reducing productivity, decreasing property values, and disrupting social services (Mercy et. al, 2002). Exposure to violence, including exposure to violence from the media, in adolescents is a significant risk factor for youth violence. Denise Herd reported that exposure to violence by the media is associated with aggressive behavior in readers, viewers, and listeners (Herd, 2009)." (Culled from a class project by Maryam Ahmed, Kara Keeton, Emily Pacholski, Lisa Smith, & Brittany Sullivan, 2013)

Conducting a review of the literature is a systematic process that involves a number of steps, including identifying the topic and the search terms, researching the publications, and synthesizing the literature (Shi, 2008). Published peer reviewed literature is searched using traditional library or online resources such as Medline, PubMed, or ProQuest to find relevant books, professional-journal articles, and technical reports. Peer-reviewed research is also available through advanced scholar searches using the Internet search engine Google.

For example, if the research topics are heart disease among adults and the relationship between heart disease and physical activity, the search terms may include heart disease (incidence and prevalence), heart disease and adults, heart disease and physical activity,

FIGURE 2.8.   *Framework for Summarizing a Literature Review*

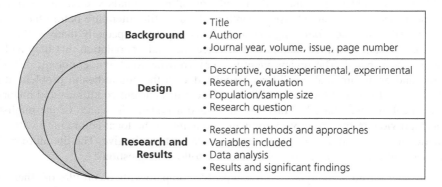

heart disease and exercise, heart disease and gender, heart disease and risk factors (age, obesity, nutrition, race). A more refined search using these categories but with women will provide a more focused review of the literature. In addition, the search may provide insights into theories that the program may adopt to provide an understanding of the public health problem at a local, state, or national level and into the relationship between the problem and the resources and activities needed to address it.

When the search is conducted and research articles are located, the researchers review references from the previous 5 to 10 years based on the topic and the articles' appropriateness and relevance for their work. Selected papers are reviewed closely and summarized by providing the following information: title, author, journal/book/report publication information, the study or intervention design (type of intervention or type of study, population or sample size, etc.). In addition, the summary contains the research question, the variables, the data-analysis approach and statistical methods, the results of the study, and significant findings. Issues of reliability and validity are also noted. Figure 2.8 provides a framework for summarizing a literature review.

When the search is complete and there are enough articles to provide a sufficiently detailed background to the problem and its potential solutions, the literature review is written. The literature review is a synthesis of all the papers reviewed with regard to a specific research question. The synthesis consists of "analyzing and interpreting [the article's] findings and summarizing those findings into unified statements about the topic being reviewed" (Shi, 2008, p. 117). The literature review may be organized under appropriate headings to capture the overall theme of a paragraph, and each paragraph must be linked to the previous paragraph by a suitable transition. The review of the scientific literature is a component of the community-assessment report and later will form part of the introduction and background section of the evaluation report.

THE REPORT

The public health related community assessment report is a summary of the results of the assessment and the review of the scientific literature. It is a discussion of priorities for addressing the public health problem in a considered and logical way. The results of the quantitative-data analysis are shown in narrative form as well as in charts, tables, and graphs to ensure easy understanding. Qualitative data are summarized, and samples of the data are presented as quotations to allow the reader to make independent interpretations. The easier the report is to follow, the more likely it is to be used. The report outlines the research approach, the results, and discussions of the results and their implications for an intervention. An outline of the components of an assessment report is provided here.

Literature Review Section

The literature review describes the public health problem(s) being investigated from the perspective of the existing literature:

- The rates of disease or disability (number of cases per 1,000 or 100,000 population) in the community compared with state and national rates

- Trends in the prevalence and incidence of disease and disability in the community compared with state and national trends

- The social, economic, and cultural environment that drive the problem/condition

- Risk and protective factors associated with the problem as seen in state and national data

- Peer, family, community, institutional, policy, structural, and systems influences associated with the problem

Methodology and Results Sections

The methodology used for the community assessment is described in the methodology section of the report and includes:

- The sample characteristics (primary data and secondary data)

- The data-collection approach (tools and methods)

- The data analysis

While the results section discusses the results of the community assessment. It organizes the results of the analysis in a systematic way. The results may be organized in order by answering each research question or by using the theoretical framework that was used to design the study. Alternatively the results may be organized to describe

- The extent of the public health problem(s) of the population and of population segments by age, gender, life stage, socioeconomic status, and ethnicity (if appropriate)

- Risk and protective factors associated with the public health problem

- Peer, family, and community influences associated with the problem

- Community, institutional, public-policy, structural, and systems factors that influence the problem

In addition, this section describes the human, material, and economic assets available in the community to address the problem:

- Individual knowledge, skills, and resources of community members, agency personnel, and others

- Interpersonal actions and norms

- Existing community resources and services

- Institutional resources (financial and material)

- Resources for developing public policy

From the analysis of the data, the results section also suggests supports for potential community-based, culturally appropriate ways to address the problem in the most comprehensive way. And, finally, it discusses limitations that may have resulted in bias in the study and in the conclusions—for example, small sample size, inappropriateness of the instrument, loss of study participants. Such issues may affect the researcher's confidence in the results.

STAKEHOLDERS' PARTICIPATION IN COMMUNITY ASSESSMENTS

There are multiple opportunities for stakeholders to participate in a community assessment. Consistent with the Participatory Model for Evaluation described in this book, identifying and engaging stakeholders occurs in the first step. Representatives of all stakeholder groups should be involved in the community-assessment process from the start so that they have a sense of ownership in both the process and the product. Including a mapping of community assets in the process allows stakeholders to identify and mobilize existing community resources to address community problems (Sharpe et al., 2005).

Stakeholders can have one or more roles in the process. They may initiate and conduct the community assessment, be a part of a research team, or serve as participants in the study. Stakeholder involvement may include designing the study, the data-collection methodology, and the instrument(s) as well as collecting or providing the data. Some stakeholders may not be directly connected with the program, but they can provide valuable perspectives. Savage and colleagues involved stakeholders as key informants in the analysis of emerging themes during their research (Savage et al., 2006). Some stakeholders are intimately connected to the problem, and they are able to bring the core values and unique culture of the population of interest into focus. They have insight into how they experience the problem, the risk and protective factors, as well as community, institutional, and policy structures that influence the public health problem.

An important stakeholder group that emerged in the early years of the HIV/AIDS epidemic was those who were infected and affected by HIV/AIDS. They became important advocates for their own needs and important partners in the fight against the spread of HIV and the provision of treatment for those infected. They are contributors to the process, providing guidance and resources in addition to being participants in research.

Stakeholder participation is critical for ensuring that the sample population is knowledgeable about the study and is willing to participate. In small and rural communities, previous knowledge of a research activity often facilitates data collection and ensures there is appropriately obtained informed consent. Information about impending community assessments can be provided in community meetings and in print and electronic media. It is important that the potential study respondents understand the value of participating in the study to ensure valid and reliable information to inform decision-making.

SUMMARY

■ Public health program and policy initiatives are developed in response to a public health concern when individuals, organizations, or agencies identify a problem to be addressed.

■ Conducting a thorough community assessment that includes both needs and assets ensures the identification and development of suitable approaches for addressing the problem.

■ The community assessment is part of a cyclical and iterative process; it precedes the initiative's implementation and/or follows the initiative's evaluation.

■ Using a participatory approach by including community members and those who are most closely associated with the problem ensures program development and implementation that are both culturally appropriate and sustainable.

■ Community assessments include factors that influence health at the individual, interpersonal, community, institutional, and public-policy levels.

■ Data for a community assessment may be primary or secondary data collected using qualitative or quantitative approaches.

■ Reviewing the scientific literature provides a broad perspective of the problem of who are affected and of why, how, and when they were affected. It also provides guidance for influencing the problem.

FIGURE 2.9.   *Valuable Take-Aways*

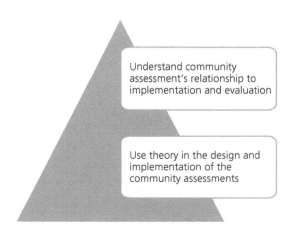

Understand community assessment's relationship to implementation and evaluation

Use theory in the design and implementation of the community assessments

DISCUSSION QUESTIONS AND ACTIVITIES

1. Community assessments collect data from members of communities to determine the extent to which, problems occur. Often the populations most at risk are not included in the assessment. Why might this be so and what steps would you take to address this issue?

2. Conduct a literature review focusing on the behavioral data related to a public health problem of your choice. In conducting a community assessment, what theoretical framework would you use to identify risk factors that influence the behavior? What conclusions would you draw regarding an appropriate intervention?

3. Community assessments include factors that influence health at the individual, inter-personal, community, institutional, and public policy levels. Discuss how addressing each of these levels of influence improves the likelihood of a comprehensive inter-vention to address the problem.

4. Do a tour of your neighborhood and identify any and all assets that might be available and accessible for addressing obesity. Use photography to support your study. What conclusions do you draw from your assessment?

KEY TERMS

community assessment
situation analysis
community organization
ecological model
diffusion of innovation theory
health belief model
literature review
MAPP
primary data

risk factors
secondary data
social cognitive theory
social support theory
theory of planned behavior
theory of gender and power
transtheoretical model
stakeholders
theory

CHAPTER

3

DEVELOPING INITIATIVES
AN OVERVIEW

LEARNING OBJECTIVES

- Identify and describe the elements in program planning and implementation.
- Explain how objectives are used in program planning.
- Describe a program's theory of change.
- Develop a logic model.
- Explain the role of stakeholders in program implementation.

Program development and implementation is the process through which people, conditions, and environments are changed to improve population health outcomes. Although priorities for intervening with programs or policy initiatives are identified during the community assessment, guidance for focusing the initiative and identifying targets for the intervention may be found in lists of national or international goals and objectives. Healthy People 2020 (U.S. Department of Health and Human Services, 2010) specifies four overarching health goals for the United States and identifies 10 leading health topics.

Overarching goals of the HP2020 objectives are

1. Attain high-quality, longer lives free of preventable disease, disability, injury, and premature death.

2. Achieve health equity, eliminate disparities, and improve the health of all groups.

3. Create social and physical environments that promote good health for all.

4. Promote quality of life, healthy development, and healthy behaviors across all life stages.

Healthy People 2020 identifies four cross-cutting measures that apply across the life span: (1) general health status, (2) disparities and inequity, (3) social determinants of health, and (4) health related quality of life and well-being.

In addition, 12 leading topic areas and 26 leading health indicators were identified to form the basis for measurement of progress across the health and public health sectors.

The 12 leading topic areas are

1. Access to healthcare services

2. Clinical preventive services

3. Environmental quality

4. Injury and violence

5. Mental health

6. Maternal, infant, and child

7. Nutrition, physical activity, and obesity

8. Oral health

9. Reproductive and sexual health

10. Social determinants

11. Substance abuse

12. Tobacco

(A complete report on the Healthy People 2020 goals, measures, and indicators may be found at http://www.healthypeople.gov/)

The Millennium Development Post-2015 agenda with a focus on sustainability builds on the previous eight Millennium Development Goals (MDGs), and has objectives ending poverty, promoting prosperity and well-being for all, and protecting the environment and addressing climate change (www.un.org). The 17 goals have specific targets to be achieved over the next 15 years.

Sustainable Development Goals for 2015–2030

1. End poverty in all forms everywhere.

2. End hunger, achieve food security and improved nutrition, and promote sustainable agriculture.

3. Ensure healthy lives and promote well-being for all at all ages.

4. Ensure inclusive and equitable quality education and promote lifelong opportunities for all.

5. Achieve gender equality and empower all women and girls.

6. Ensure availability and sustainable management of water and sanitation for all.

7. Ensure access to affordable, reliable, sustainable, and modern energy for all.

8. Promote sustained, inclusive and sustainable economic growth, full and productive employment, and decent work for all.

9. Build resilient infrastructure, promote inclusive and sustainable industrialization, and foster innovation.

10. Reduce inequality within and among countries.

11. Make cities and human settlements inclusive, safe, resilient, and sustainable.

12. Ensure sustainable consumption and production patterns.

13. Take urgent action to combat climate change and its impact.

14. Conserve and sustainably use oceans, seas, and marine resources for sustainable development.

15. Protect, restore, and promote sustainable use of terrestrial ecosystems, sustainably manage forests, combat desertification and halt and reverse land degradation, and halt biodiversity loss.

16. Promote peaceful and inclusive societies for sustainable development, provide access to justice for all and build effective, accountable, and inclusive institutions at all levels.

17. Strengthen the means of implementation and revitalize the global partnership for sustainable development.

Selection of the program and policy initiatives to be implemented is influenced by multiple factors that reflect the organization's overall mission. The organization's mission provides the direction for program planning and implementation. In a hypothetical example, high rates of poverty in a community led to the development of an initiative to address a number of health-related conditions that resulted when communities experienced high rates of poverty and individuals did not have access to opportunities for healthy living. The community assessment found that individuals who lived in this community had higher than expected rates of diabetes, but those most affected were Black and female. Most had not completed high school. In addition, it found that among those between the ages of 45 and 64 the number of new cases of diabetes was 6.9 per 1,000, and significantly higher than for 18 to 24-year-olds, whose rate was 2 per 1,000. Rates were even higher among those 65 and older. An additional finding was that women were more likely to be obese than men. The community decided to tackle the problem by developing a diabetes-prevention initiative.

Embedded within this information are a number of facts that would influence one or more organizations to develop program or policy initiatives to address the social determinants of health. The organizations most likely to take on the task of reducing the rates of diabetes in the population would likely have missions that encompass this population group and would have the capacity to effect change. This chapter discusses the development of public health interventions as a prelude to program evaluation.

Think About It!

The Healthy People 2020 and the Post Millennium Agenda have what appear to be different goals. What are the factors that might lead to a different kind of thinking for these two sets of goals? What similarities underlie both sets of goals? Given the scenario above, which goals would you chose to guide your intervention and why?

THE ORGANIZATION'S MISSION

The mission of an organization is reflected in its mission statement and mirrors the organization's charge, direction, and population focus. It is the foundation for the planning process and the development of goals, objectives, and activities to address the public health problem.

The mission statement announces the public health problem that the organization wishes to address in the broadest perspective. A strong mission statement for an organization contains the following components:

- The desired outcome of its programs or policy

- The population that will be the target of its work

- The geographical community it serves

An example of an organization's mission statement could be to "improve the quality of lives of African American women in Riverside County." Another organization's mission could be to "reduce the rates of chronic disease among women who live in the state." Both organizations could use their missions to address the high rates of diabetes among Black, low-income females. However, each organization might take a different approach to achieving the same goal. For example, one organization might chose to provide increased access to health care to improve treatment opportunities for those with diabetes; the other organization might focus on the prevention of the onset of diabetes through policy initiatives that improve opportunities for healthy nutrition and physical activity. Irrespective of the approach that is taken, the next steps in the process are planning and implementing the initiative.

PLANNING THE INITIATIVE

Build Community Support

The social, political, and cultural environment of the community provides a context for the organization's programs and policy initiatives. These factors determine the types of programs that the organization offers, its funding level, and community support for its initiatives. Community support influences initiative development and implementation in many ways.

When a community-based organization or a government agency identifies a problem and develops a program or policy, its ability to sustain the program is often influenced by social, political, and cultural factors in the community. In addition, the full implementation and maintenance of a policy initiative requires continuous monitoring and evaluation. Since policies operate in a much larger arena such as a jurisdiction, and unlike programs that serve relatively fewer individuals, this may prove more difficult, time consuming, and expensive. Policies that are intended to serve broader populations are influenced by political forces in ways that may affect the implementation of programs. Social and political factors influence people's attitudes toward population groups and causes.

When support for addressing the problem is high, programs are able to attract attention from many sectors, obtain adequate funding for program development, and to recruit participants. However, when support is low, the organization may have difficulty securing sufficient funding, and members of the community may not use its services or participate in its activities. Good examples of initiatives whose development is often limited because of low support (probably based on a combination of social and political factors) are providing community-based care for people with behavioral disabilities and providing shelter for the homeless. An additional program that also meets some resistance at community level is one that is intended to serve individuals who were previously incarcerated and aiming to build a new life.

Community support provides evidence for potential funders that the program is well accepted by the community. It ensures the credibility of the organization and demonstrates that community members believe that the initiative is making a difference. In addition, community support is critical for the development of coalitions to provide support to programs and policies. Conversely, a lack of support from key individuals, organizations, or sectors of the community works against the organization and negatively influences the public's perception of an issue and the organization's approaches to addressing it. It is, therefore, important to solicit the support of influential community members, other organizations that do similar or complementary work, people who are directly affected by the issue, and organizations and agencies that provide a voice for the community such as advocates and media outlets. Political leaders are also important stakeholders in the development of programs and the funding of initiatives. In addition to reliable community support, it is important to have strong institutional and administrative support.

Provide Institutional Capacity

Strong institutional and administrative capacity is important for developing and delivering quality programs. Administrative capacity influences the type of programs and the size and scope of program activities. Institutional capacity for program delivery includes having physical structures and staffing to ensure adequate and appropriate program implementation and oversight. Institutional and administrative capacity thus includes

- The physical structures that house the initiative components

- Managers, including board members, staff, outreach personnel, and volunteers

- Program operations and activities for each initiative

- Equipment and supplies suitable for program implementation

- Ability to address challenges posed by the initiative

Policy enactment and implementation also require strong administrative and community support of a different kind. Since jurisdiction-wide policies are intended to address a public health concern through laws, the administrative capacity required is first getting the law passed by the legislature or parliament and subsequently developing the guidance for its implementation. Additional administrative capacity is required for its enactment and adoption and often requires extensive media engagement. For example, in enacting a law for seatbelt use to prevent injury in vehicular accidents across the life span, once the law was enacted, it was the responsibility of staffers to write the rules for implementation. The media and other parties informed the public and law enforcement was expected to monitor its implementation. Each entity involved required both institutional and administrative support.

Use Community Assessment and Epidemiological Data

The community assessment and epidemiological data are used in determining the direction of the public health program or policy initiative. They provide a science-based rationale for the intervention and define the populations that, if targeted for the intervention, would benefit most. Furthermore, data that are used at the start of the program can form the baseline against which the proposed intervention outcomes can be assessed later.

Community assessment and epidemiological data contained within reports and the literature review provide information that is helpful for developing a detailed plan for the initiative (Figure 3.1). This information includes

- The health problem, prevalence and incidence of disease, and quality-of-life indicators

- Risk and protective factors that influence the behavior of individuals

- Sociocultural and political factors that reinforce or enable conditions that increase the public health problem and will affect any interventions

- Assets and resources available within the community

INCORPORATE THEORY

In Chapter 2, we reviewed the use of theory in community assessments and noted that when a theory or a theoretical framework is used for the community assessment, the same theory may be used in the development of the intervention that addresses the problem

FIGURE 3.1. *Outcomes of a Community Assessment Process*

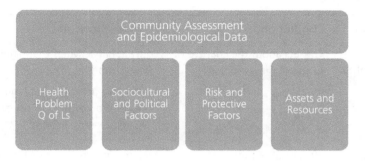

that was previously identified. Using a theoretical framework increases the likelihood of incorporating the factors (concepts and constructs) that are known to result in the change in environments and behavior that the initiative is addressing. It provides a structure upon which a health intervention can be designed and subsequently can be used to monitor changes. For example, if the health-belief model is selected for the community assessment, it assesses the perceived susceptibility, severity, benefits, barriers, cues to action, and self-efficacy and determines a baseline for each of these constructs within the population of interest. During the planning phase, each of these constructs is operationalized in order to develop an intervention that will result in the change of a behavior that reduces the risk of disease or disability. (See Table 3.1.)

When a more complex intervention is necessary, such as one based in the ecological model, it provides guidance for a comprehensive approach to program development across multiple domains of behavioral influence. At the individual level, behavior is influenced by biological, physiological, psychological, and emotional states. At the interpersonal level, structural factors and social and cultural norms of peers, family, and friends play a role. The organizational, community, and policy domains recognize the influence and impact of multiple environmental factors on behavior. Environmental determinants include economic, physical, and structural factors and systems that influence physical and emotional health. The ecologic model allows the program planner to incorporate theories at each level. For example, at the individual level, theories that are helpful for changing behavior are the transtheoretical model, the health-belief model and the theory of planned behavior. At the interpersonal level are the social cognitive and the social support theories, and at the organizational and community levels, the community organizing, organizational change, and diffusion of innovations may play a role in providing the supports and the motivations for behavior change (See Table 3.2).

When theory is used as the basis for the intervention, the goals and objectives follow the constructs of the theory and the community assessment data provide the base line for evaluation. For example, if the intervention were to improve health outcomes for low-income individuals with diabetes, the theories that might be helpful would be the health belief model and the social cognitive theory. The goals and objectives would be based on the need to assess the program's impact on the individuals with diabetes after a specified period.

TABLE 3.1.   Incorporating Theory in Program Planning using the Health Belief Model

Construct	Definition	Program Strategies
Perceived susceptibility	Beliefs about the chances of getting a condition.	Educational activities that highlight the populations at risk. Multimedia activities that highlight and increase perception of risk among vulnerable populations.
Perceived severity	Beliefs about the seriousness of a condition and its consequences.	Multimedia activities that highlight and increase understanding of the severity of the condition.
Perceived benefits	Beliefs about the effectiveness of adopting the recommended behavior to reduce risk or seriousness.	Educational activities that help explain what the potential benefits are from adopting the recommended behavior. Provide testimonials from those who have changed behavior and experienced the benefits.
Perceived barriers	Beliefs about the costs associated with taking action.	Educational activities to correct misinformation and provide incentives to reduce any barriers to adopting the new behavior.
Cues to action	Factors that influence the individual into taking action to adopt the new behavior.	Develop and use a reminder system to promote and encourage the new behavior.
Self-efficacy	Confidence in one's ability to perform the recommended behavior.	Provide skills building training for ensuring the individuals learn the skills for performing the new behavior. Provide opportunities for practice and mastery. Provide reinforcement of the new behavior.

TABLE 3.2. **Using Multiple Theories Within an Ecological Framework**

Ecological Level	Possible Theories	Program Strategies
Individual Level	Transtheoretical model, Health-belief model, Theory of planned behavior	▪ Educational activities to provide information to allow individuals to make an informed decision about the recommended behavior ▪ Educational materials to provide help to move individuals forward ▪ Role models ▪ Activities that reinforce new behaviors and prevent relapse ▪ Educational activities to correct misinformation and provide incentives to reduce any barriers to adopting the new behavior ▪ Activities to build self-efficacy for the desired behavior
Interpersonal	Social cognitive, Social networks, Social support	▪ Activities to ensure peer support ▪ Lay health advisors ▪ Building social support ▪ Modeling
Community	Community organizing, Social marketing, Diffusion of innovation	▪ Advocacy activities ▪ Building infrastructure for service provision ▪ Media initiatives ▪ Stakeholder engagement
Organization	Organizational development	▪ Leadership training ▪ Resource allocation ▪ Organization capacity building
Public Policy	Communication theory	▪ Media advocacy ▪ Policymakers training ▪ Materials development ▪ Policy analysis

The program's goals and objectives specify those benchmarks. Objectives that are more likely to reflect effective programs may include changes in the beneficiaries as a result of

- Educational programs with individuals, their peers, and families
- Community change activities aimed at changing community norms
- Organizational practices that increase access to services and utilization of opportunities for safe and healthy living
- Policies that support safe and healthy lifestyles and reduce risk associated with disease and disability

GOALS AND OBJECTIVES

Developing sound initiatives requires developing realistic goals and objectives. Unlike the mission statement, which is broad, *goals* provide clear direction, and *objectives* provide specific benchmarks for the initiative (see Figure 3.2). Objectives serve as the benchmarks for determining the level of implementation of the initiative and its outcomes. As mentioned earlier, the Healthy People 2020 (U.S. Department of Health and Human Services, 2010) and the Post-Millennium 2015 agendas and goals (United Nations, 2015) documents provide guidance for identifying specific targets of the intervention. Going back to our previous example of diabetes, we note that HP 2020 addresses achieving improved outcomes for diabetes through 16 specifically named objectives (D1-D16). Each can be used to identify evidence-based strategies, and together with the adopted theory they form the initiative to address the problem, which includes access to health services, formal health education, and preventive behaviors for those with prediabetes.

FIGURE 3.2.   *The Hierarchical Relationship of Goals and Objectives*

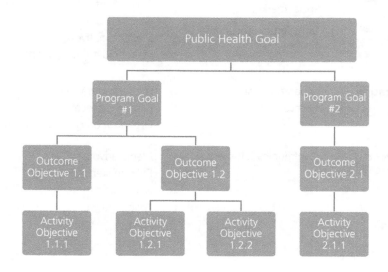

The Initiative (Public Health) Goal

The initiative's goal closely matches the mission of the organization and relates to the particular public health problem that is being addressed. The goal provides the initiative's direction and is a stated desire to meet an expressed and unmet population need. It is made up of three elements that

1. Describe who will be affected by the program or policy initiative.

2. Communicate the intentions of the program.

3. Specify broad changes that will occur as a result of the initiative.

If the mission of the organization is to "improve the health of women who live in the state," then the goal of the initiative may be to "reduce the rates of diabetes among and improve the quality of life for low-income African American women in Riverside County." In analyzing this goal we realize it contains all the components of a goal, as shown in Table 3.3.

Program Goal

The program goal reflects the initiative's goal but is written to be more specific. The program/health goal identifies

■ Who benefits from the program

■ The health benefits they will receive

■ When the benefits will be achieved

For example, if the program goal is to "reduce the proportion of low-income African American women who get diabetes by 2025 from 30% to 10%," the people who benefit are low-income African American women; they receive as a benefit a reduction in the incidence of diabetes among those who participate from 30% to 10%; and this benefit will be achieved by 2025.

TABLE 3.3.　Goal Analysis

Goal: Reduce the rates of diabetes among and improve the quality of life for low-income African American women in Riverside County.	
Describes who will be affected by the program or policy initiative	Low-income African American women in Riverside County
Communicates the intentions of the program	To develop prevention or policy initiatives that target the risk and protective factors that influence rates of diabetes
Specifies broad changes that will occur as a result of the initiative	Reduced rates of diabetes and improved quality of life

Initiative Objectives

The initiative's objectives are developed to support the program goal. There may be multiple objectives required to achieve one goal. The objectives outline the initiative's precise direction and define its planned purposes. Objectives provide

- Small steps (benchmarks) that, if completed, will achieve the goal; they define specifically the road to success

- Part of the blueprint for program replication

- Short-, medium-, or long-term benchmarks of the program's implementation

- Guidance for developing activities

- Guidance for program evaluation

Since the objectives are an important aspect of the evaluation because they are used to specify its focus, they must be consistent with the organization's mission and the initiative goal, and they must be realizable during the life and the funding of the program.

Well-developed objectives are defined as being specific, measurable, appropriate, realistic, and achievable in a specified time frame. A useful acronym for developing objectives and remembering their attributes is SMART. An example of the application of SMART attributes is provided in Table 3.4.

There are two kinds of initiative objectives: outcome objectives and activity objectives.

Outcome Objectives

Outcome objectives are written to guide the achievement of a program goal. They are important for assessing progress and the ultimate success of the initiative.

A *specific* outcome objective indicates what is going to change and by how much it is going to change. We can learn a number of things from the following hypothetical objective: "increase the proportion of low-income African American women who consume five portions of fruits and vegetables a day from 30% to 60% by 2020." First, we learn that the program developers intend to provide an intervention that will result in participants increasing their consumption of fruits and vegetables. Second, we learn that they expect that the proportion of women in their program who increase their consumption of fruits and vegetables will increase to 60%. Third, we learn that the baseline that the program is using, against which they will assess their progress, is a current proportion of 30%; in other words, nearly one in three low-income African American women eats fewer than five portions of fruits and vegetables a day without an intervention. In general, a specific objective contains the expected outcome against which the effectiveness of the intervention will be measured. In this case, the expected outcome is that women who participate in the intervention will consume five portions of fruits and vegetables a day by 2020. This provides an intermediate benchmark to reducing the proportion of women who get diabetes by 2025 (See Table 3.4).

The objectives set the stage for the level of intensity of the program. The intensity of the program determines the likelihood of its being able to accomplish the goals and objectives, so the higher the target the more intense the program needs to be. In the earlier example, if the program is of low intensity, the initiative may get the rate down to only 20% rather than 10%. To give another example, an education intervention that only provides information to change knowledge is likely to do that fairly easily, so expecting 90% of the participants to increase their knowledge of, let us say, methods of HIV/AIDS transmission is

TABLE 3.4. **Example of the Application of the SMART Attributes to an Objective**

Objective: Reduce the proportion of low-income African American women in the program who get diabetes from 30% to 10% by 2025.	
Specific: Does the objective clearly specify what will be accomplished?	Yes. The objective is a reduction in the proportion of low-income African American women in the program who get diabetes from 30% to 10%.
Measurable: Are the changes that are specified to occur measurable in appropriate and culturally sensitive ways?	Yes. Diabetes can be diagnosed using approaches that are culturally sensitive.
Appropriate: Do the changes that are to occur for the participant or in the environment make sense given what the intervention is trying to accomplish?	Yes. The changes that will occur for the women through the program will reduce their risk of progressing to diabetes.
Realistic: Are the changes achievable given the time frame, the population, the resources, and the experience of the organization?	Yes. Improved nutrition and regular exercise have been shown to improve health; the organization has the resources and experience to provide adequate programs.
Timed: Is the time frame for accomplishing the changes specified and realistic?	Yes. Setting the year 2025 as the end point is realistic given the changes that need to occur.

realistic even after a 3-hour session. This objective could read, "By the end of the training 90% of participants will explain all the methods of HIV/AIDS transmission." However, specifying a change in behavior with regard to preventing HIV infection would require a more intense intervention for a longer time and with a lower likelihood of success, so the target would be lower. Such an objective will be appropriately stated as, "By the end of the year, 60% of program participants will use condoms consistently." A policy-related objective requiring bikers to wear helmets would expect 100% of individuals to comply or face a fine or alternative punishment if caught.

Behavior change to improve health outcomes is influenced by multiple risk factors. These are the characteristics that we attempt to modify in order to achieve the behavior change. These factors occur in the individual and in the environment in which the individual lives, works, and plays.

Individual level: Intellectual ability, beliefs, values, skills, maturity, and health.

Interpersonal level: The relationships an individual has with family, peers, and significant others.

Organizational level: The resources, support, goods, and services provided by an organization or institution.

Community level: Societal norms, social networks, social capital, and access to goods and services.

Public-policy level: Laws and regulations that support or discourage healthy behaviors and access to goods and services.

Changes in risk factors may include increasing knowledge, changing peer norms, and improving physical structures to increase the likelihood of eating in a healthy way or of exercising. Changes in behavior may include increasing physical activity, eating healthier foods, obtaining health care, and enacting health policy.

To be *measurable,* outcome objectives should incorporate verbs that are action oriented and can be assessed using available measurement tools (Figure 3.3 provides examples of action-oriented verbs). Outcomes are measured using surveys, observation, interviews, photography, and so forth. Verbs such as *understand* and *appreciate* are difficult to measure using such tools and therefore should not be used.

Writing a specific, measurable outcome objective goes hand-in-hand with writing a *realistic* objective that has a *specified time frame,* the time it should take to accomplish the objective. An important aspect of writing objectives is recognizing that the time line is a temporal sequence of when changes can be made. The sequence represents a realistic expectation of when the individual or situation is likely to change. Setting a time line is dependent on the experience of the evaluator, the literature, or public health professionals who are familiar with the change model and the population or situation. For example, changing knowledge is fairly simple and can often be done in a single session, but changing behavior or enacting legislation may take many and varied activities and great effort to accomplish.

FIGURE 3.3.   *Verbs for Writing Objectives*

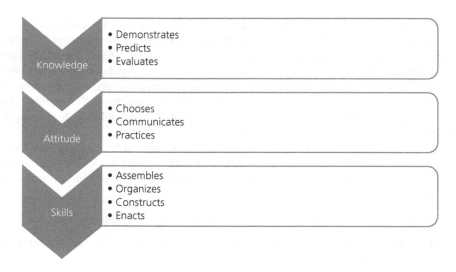

Objectives are short, medium, and long term. Consider a time frame of 10 years. Short-term objectives would fall within the first 1 to 2 years; intermediate objectives, between 3 and 5 years; and long-term objectives, between 6 and 10 years.

Objectives that focus on the individual level and on knowledge gain as the outcome are generally short term and have limited effect in reaching overall goals. Skill-building objectives are generally short to medium term, and behavior-change objectives are medium to long term. Behavioral objectives when achieved are much more likely to be a good indication for attaining the goal. Objectives at the interpersonal, organizational, or community level may also have different periods of time depending on the outcome expected. For example, changing community norms or improving access to resources may require short-, medium-, and long-term outcome objectives that provide benchmarks for change over an extended period. Policy outcome objectives are usually written for the longest time frames because they require a considerable amount of effort to achieve. Changing policy first requires increasing knowledge and understanding of the need for the policy at multiple levels such as the general population, policymakers, and the media. This first step leads to the development of coalitions and advocacy strategies. The actions of coalitions lead to procedures for the development or change of a policy. Only after these steps is the policy enacted. The time it takes to enact a policy will depend on the type of policy, the level at which it is enacted (local, state, or national), and the political climate. Table 3.5 demonstrates how to write time lines into objectives.

In adopting the ecological model for addressing a public health problem, an organization chooses to develop initiatives at multiple levels. The more levels that are included in the initiative, the more likely the health problem will be addressed from a holistic perspective and take into account not only individual factors but also, for example, peer influences

TABLE 3.5.   **Writing Time Lines into Objectives**

Type of Change Required	Time Frame for Change	Objective
Policy	Short term	By 2018, 90% of coalition members will know how to contact their legislators.
	Medium term	By 2019, 50% of coalition members will take at least one action per month in support of legislation for children to have 30 minutes of exercise during the school day.
	Long term	By 2021, state legislation will be enacted to ensure that children in all 50 counties get at least 30 minutes of exercise during the school day.
Individual	Short term	By 2018, 90% of women will know the importance of having a mammogram for the early detection of breast cancer.
	Long term	By 2021, 90% of women over the age of 40 will have a mammogram once a year.

on community norms and services, organizational structure and functioning, and local or national public policy.

Think About It!

Consider that you have been asked to develop a program for individuals with disabilities in a residential complex of males and females ranging from 18 years of age to 80 years of age. You have the task of designing an intervention that improves their quality of life. What quality of life indicator will you select? (Select one of the HP2020 leading health indicators). Write six important but SMART objectives at the individual, interpersonal, and organizational level (two at each level) ensuring that the easiest objectives to accomplish are short term and the most difficult or far-reaching to accomplish are long term. To what extent have you considered the complexity of working with this population? To what extent have you used the scientific literature to guide your thinking?

Activity Objectives

There are a small number of outcome objectives, but there are many activity objectives that are directed toward achieving each outcome objective. The activity objectives specify the activities for carrying out the initiative. Ultimately, it is the activities in the initiative that result in the outcomes specified. Together the objectives and the activities are the blueprint for replication of the initiative.

Activity objectives are the most frequently written objectives and the most familiar. They specify organizational and administrative tasks that need to be accomplished as a part of ensuring the implementation of the initiative. They guide the implementation of the initiative and become the process objectives in the evaluation. They are used to monitor and evaluate the initiative's level of implementation and progress.

Activity objectives should answer the following questions:

- What activity will be carried out to support the outcome objective?

- Who will conduct the activity?

- When will the activity be carried out?

- Where will the activity occur?

EXAMPLE

ACTIVITY OBJECTIVES

1. Fitness staff will conduct a three-day interactive educational and skill-building workshop starting on day 1 of the Regent Gym Cycling intervention in the gymnasium.

2. Thirty women 40 to 60 years old will participate in the 90-day Regent Gym Cycling intervention in the gymnasium.

3. Women 40 to 60 years old will identify a buddy to walk with for 45 minutes each day.

4. Volunteers from the Regent Gym will provide information and outreach activities in the community surrounding the Regent Gym for 60 days prior to the start of the Regent Gym Cycling intervention to raise awareness of the importance of exercise for cardiac health and increase participation.

5. Advocates for improvement in access to health care for refugee women will organize a training session for legislators.

THE INITIATIVE'S ACTIVITIES

The activities that are selected for the initiative should be the best approaches for achieving the objectives. For example, it is well recognized that to reduce obesity, both healthy eating and exercise are required; so initiatives and their activities are developed to address both. If obesity is associated with a health condition such as heart disease or obesity, increasing access to care may also be considered. Activities are based on a number of factors, including the demographic characteristics of the beneficiaries of the initiative; the risk and protective factors involved; the human, financial, and material resources available. The most appropriate approaches for achieving an outcome are adopted from conducting a review of the research literature and consulting with local, state, and national organizations

- Identifying theory-driven programs that address the same or similar issues

- Identifying or developing evidence-based best-practice models

- Consulting with experts doing similar work

The activities must be appropriate for achieving the objective. For example, if the objective is to improve the skills of young people to perform a certain task, then the activities that are identified must provide skill-building opportunities so that the youth learn and then practice the skill to proficiency. Likewise, if the outcome objective is to enact a policy, then the activities that are undertaken must clearly and logically lead to involvement and actions by policymakers. Activities to change policy may include:

- Education to change knowledge, beliefs, and attitudes

- Advocacy to increase understanding and relevance of the topic area

- Media communications to expand the reach of the message and to change public opinion and perceptions

- Message development to target the message for particular groups

- Training to develop a cadre of advocates, message champions, and new leaders

- Outreach to increase the volunteer core

- Meetings with policymakers to facilitate increased ownership of the issue

- Development of information sheets and briefs

- Building the capacity of the organization to handle the work (increasing staff, technology, infrastructure, staff development)

Overall, appropriate activities have the following characteristics:

- They are likely to lead to the change that is specified in the objective.

- They can be completed during the specified time frame.

- They are conducted by an organization that has sufficient resources and personnel.

- They are appropriate given the culture and expectations of the population for whom they are intended.

- They form part of an overall plan to achieve a program's goal.

Activities should preferably be based on established public health theory-based approaches that have been shown to have an effect on risk and protective factors. Any theories that have been used as part of the community assessment should be used to frame the activities. There is a greater likelihood of incorporating all the factors that are known to result in a given change if the activities are based on theoretical constructs than if they are not. See Glanz, Rimer, and Viswanath (2008) for a detailed explanation of the use of theory. Theories that have been used to design the community assessment are ideal for incorporating into the development and framing the activities. For example, in basing the community assessment on the social learning theory (Albert Bandura, 1986), the evaluator takes into consideration the reciprocal dynamic model that incorporates the individual, the environment, and the expected behavior. It recognizes the need to ensure that factors that affect each variable are addressed and activities are incorporated to support the expected changes. It emphasizes the importance of modeling the expected behavior (www.instructionaldesign.org) to facilitate learning through attention, memory, and motivation. In developing an intervention based on this theory, it is important to ensure that the model is similar to the expected behavior, which must have value to the individual. Therefore, intervention activities will be those that incorporate opportunities for the expected behavior to be observed multiple times with occasions for practicing it. Another example of a well-used theory is the transtheoretical model (Prochaska & DiClemente, 1983). Although progression through the stages of change can occur in a linear fashion, a nonlinear progression is common. Often, individuals recycle through the stages or regress to earlier stages from later ones.

In the stages-of-change model individuals progress over time from precontemplation (not ready) to action and then to maintenance of the new behavior. At each stage of this five step model, to change individuals requires different activities. For example, individuals in the *precontemplation* stage have no or little understanding of the consequences of their behavior and require activities to provide information necessary for change and the motivation to accept and use it. On the other hand in the next step (*contemplation*) when individuals are ready to change, they may do so within a 6-month window. These individuals are a little further along the continuum of change, but may still have reservations and may weigh the pros and cons of the new behavior when they may require more intensive support through such activities as counseling and modeling the new behavior. The third stage (*preparation*), individuals are likely to make changes within a month as they increase their self-efficacy through practicing and skill building for the new behavior. In the *action* stage, individuals are actively engaged in the behavior, followed by *maintenance* when individuals work hard to maintain the recommended behavior and prevent relapsing into the previous bad behavior. Finally, individuals get to the point where they are not likely to relapse and have fully adopted the new behavior.

One example is individuals such as those with diabetes. In the precontemplation and contemplation phases, individuals need guidance that is provided using educational materials about diabetes, its causes, and methods of preventing the further deterioration of health. Skills-building exercises, testimonials, and role modeling could increase their understanding of the disease and behaviors consistent with improving health. Activities may include regular visits to the doctor, eye specialist, and chiropodist, checking blood sugar levels, and, when necessary, consistently taking any prescribed medication. When maintenance is reached, all the activities recommended in the action phase are undertaken consistently.

DESIGNING THE INITIATIVE

The mission of the organization was to serve the people of the Hillside Community of 100,000, but it had a large refugee population from Eastern Europe and the Middle East who had been relocated to the United States after many years of conflict. They were primarily foreign-language speaking and had a deep sense of loss, since they had left their homes under very difficult conditions. The majority of the population served by the Hillside Community Center were women and children. Most of the children were between the ages of 5 and 18 and had also experienced episodes of depression. The executive director and her staff worked hard to make them comfortable, but the staff were unhappy and repeated consumer satisfaction surveys reflected that staff were not as patient or kind as they needed to be with their patients. It was time to plan an initiative that would address both these issues.

Building Community Support

The executive director knew that to have a well-received initiative she would have to build support for it. She already had the support of the community assessment team but she needed support of the board of directors and the leadership team of the organization in order to develop a set of activities that everybody would be supportive of. She wanted to build a strong, caring, and learning organization so they could continue to provide world-class service to their clients.

(*Continued*)

(Continued)

Providing Administrative Support

With the executive director and the board of directors fully on board, the assessment team quickly morphed into the planning team. An administrative assistant was appointed to join the group and the team was given a large room for planning purposes and had access to smaller conference rooms if they needed to plan activities for the intervention. They got to work, first reviewing the community assessment report.

Using Community Assessment Data

The assessment had revealed staff were under a considerable amount of pressure to serve this new immigrant population. In addition to the consumer satisfaction surveys, the assessment revealed that staff stress resulted in them being anxious and tired with recurrent headaches, stomach, and neck pains. There were two important reasons that an intervention was indicated. First, stress has serious consequences for an individual's well-being and quality of life, and secondly, the organization's clients were not satisfied with the service they were receiving. The risk factors identified in the study included a lack of emotional, instrumental, informational, and appraisal support within the organization and from management and sometimes from their peers. The organization and the community had resources that were needed in order to provide opportunities for staff to reduce their stress.

Goals and Objectives

The goal of the program was to, "Within a three year period, reduce from 40% to 20% the proportion of staff at the Hillside Community Center who report stress related disease or disability." The outcome objectives were:

1. By the end of the intervention period, 70% of staff will report lower levels of emotional stress

2. By the end of the intervention period, 90% of staff will report higher levels of instrumental support

3. Six months following the intervention, 90% of consumers will report high levels of satisfaction with the care they received at the clinic

The Initiative's Activities

The initiative's activities followed a theoretical model that had been used by Baqutayan (2011) to assess the effect of engaging students in 2-hour workshops weekly for 16 weeks. The topics of the workshops focused on the importance of social support in managing instrumental and emotional stress. The quasi-experimental design had shown that the intervention worked so it made sense to adopt it. The populations were different, but given other considerations such as time and resources, they decided that a workshop design was a good option. In addition to the workshops staff were encouraged to be more physically active. The committee and the staff worked hard to craft an intervention that was culturally appropriate for the staff they had at the clinic. They took into consideration the diversity of cultures as well as opportunities they would have for exercise and adapted the exercises as needed.

USE EXISTING EVIDENCE-BASED PROGRAMS

An alternative to developing initiatives from scratch is to identify and adopt already tested evidence-based programs that have proven to be effective (Figure 3.4). An evidence-based program is based on the most rigorous scientific evidence found through a well-designed intervention-research study that is supported by both qualitative and quantitative data. The evidence-based initiative selected for adoption should relate to the needs of the project and have similar goals and objectives.

FIGURE 3.4.   *Components of Evidence-Based Programs*

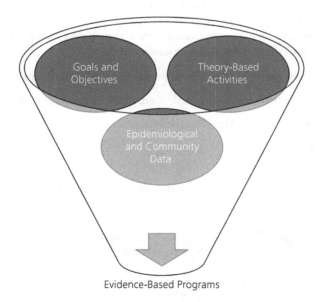

Evidence-Based Programs

Certain characteristics are associated with evidence-based initiatives:

- They specify the population that the intervention was tested with.

- They are based on research conducted using experimental or quasi-experimental designs with control groups.

- They identify the specific effects of the intervention on those who received the intervention compared with those who were in the control group.

- They provide sufficient information for replication.

Evidence-based interventions are now recommended in clinical and prevention programs in medicine, social work, and public health. For example, the Substance Abuse and Mental Health Services Association hosts the National Registry of Evidence-Based Programs and Practices, which contains a searchable data base of 137 substance-abuse and mental-health-related interventions (Substance Abuse and Mental Health Administration, 2008).

The Centers for Disease Control and Prevention developed the Tiers of Evidence conceptual framework (Centers for Disease Control and Prevention, 2007), which provides a system for classifying behavioral interventions based on the level of evidence for reducing the risk of HIV (Figure 3.5). The system has four distinct tiers: Tier I and Tier II interventions are those classified as evidence based. Tier III and Tier IV consist of behavioral-theory-based interventions. The system is based on the quality and rigor of the studies of an intervention and the strength of the findings. Tier I interventions are the most vigorously evaluated, whereas Tier IV includes programs with the least amount of empirical evidence. (Additional information about the Tiers of Evidence system can be found at http://www.cdc.gov/hiv/topics/research/prs/print/tiers-of-evidence.htm).

Sources of information regarding evidence-based and theory-based programs and principles that reduce the risk of a disease or disability include:

- Published articles and reports available on the Internet or in libraries

- Reports from or consultation with local, state, national, and international organizations

- Independent private and public research institutions

- Public health practitioners

FIGURE 3.5. *Classification System for Evidence-Based HIV/AIDS Interventions*

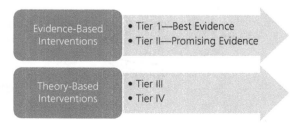

It is important to think critically about adopting evidence-based interventions because they may have been developed for a population different from your own. Questions to consider in determining whether an existing program can be adopted for your population:

■ What changes does the program target? Are these the same as those for the intervention being considered?

■ Does the intervention serve a population with the same or similar characteristics?

■ Are the appropriate resources available to implement the initiative?

■ Can the initiative be implemented as described by the developers of the intervention?

■ Are the intervention activities and delivery mechanisms culturally appropriate?

THE PROGRAM'S THEORY OF CHANGE

Irrespective of the approach used for developing the initiative, it is important to demonstrate a clear and logical relationship among the mission, goals, objectives, and activities in the program's theory of change, its operational theory. The theory of change is the theoretical foundation of the initiative. It explains what the organization is hoping to achieve with the initiative, the rationale for the program, and the program's goals, objectives, and activities. It describes how the resources and activities lead to attaining initiative objectives and goals. It is best developed by working with the stakeholders. Kirkhart (2005) cautions that it is important to consider the cultural context of the initiative and how it is represented in the theoretical perspectives.

THE LOGIC MODEL DEPICTING THE THEORY OF CHANGE

The logic model is a graphic or pictorial depiction of a program's theory of change (Frechtling, 2007). A logic model may be viewed as having multiple functions, which include being a flow chart that depicts program components and a planning tool for program evaluation.

The only requirement for a logic model is that it tell the story of the intervention in a condensed and understandable format. A detailed discussion of logic models is provided in Frechtling (2007).

A logic model is

■ A way to map a program during the planning or evaluation phase

■ A way to show the program developers' chain of reasoning and to provide a process for understanding the program's activities and how they link to the outcomes

■ A tool to facilitate stakeholder insight and reflection

■ A tool to inform monitoring and the development of benchmarks to focus the evaluation

■ A tool to help others understand the thinking of the program developers

An alternative use of the logic model may be in managing the project through a depiction of the activities and their implementation. Just to be clear, a logic model is not a theory; it only represents the theory that the program or policy depicts. It is also not an evaluation method or model. All it does in this context is provide sufficient understanding of the program components so that an evaluator is able to identify process and evaluation questions for evaluation.

Health-Related Intervention Logic Model

A logic model shows diagrammatically the initiative's basic components: resources, activities, outputs, and outcomes (Figure 3.6). To keep the purpose of the program in full view, the public health goal and the program goal are noted at the top of the logic model. In addition, the logic model identifies the points at which the process and outcome (short, intermediate, and long term) evaluation may occur.

A program logic model needs to include the following components:

Resources (sometimes called the inputs): The human, financial, and material resources that are used for the initiative. They include staff and other personnel who will be available to work on the program, grants and other monies allocated for the program, as well as office space, training materials, and other resources that are provided for the initiative.

FIGURE 3.6.   *Basic Framework for a Logic Model for a Health-Related Program*

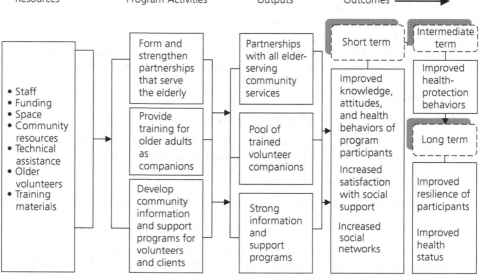

Public Health Goal: To improve the quality of life of senior citizens ages 55–75 in Regent Town
Program Goal: To improve the resilience of older adults and decrease health disparities for program participants by 2026

Program activities: The specific activities that participants take part in or are exposed to that will result in changes in the participants. Examples of activities are workshops, training, educational outreach programs, and other health enhancing activities that reduce risk factors associated with the problem being addressed. They may also include activities that influence the physical, social, or cultural environment and make behavior change more likely. Examples may include facilities and services.

Outputs: The initial products of the initiative, the results of the intervention. Examples of outputs are the number of people trained, the number of pieces of material distributed, the number of facilities built or made available to increase access, and the number of outreach activities.

Outcomes: Changes that occur in the participants in the program or those who are exposed to the policy. Outcomes may be developed as short term, intermediate term, and long term during the planning process. Examples of outcomes are an increase in knowledge, a change in attitudes, a change in behavior, increasing social support, increasing social networks, and improved access to resources.

Program goal: Based on the public health goal but focused on the population served by the initiative, it provides the specific direction for the program.

Public health goal: It expresses the expected improvement in the quality of life of the community's residents. The impact of the combined efforts of all the initiatives of all the organizations in the community that work to achieve a common goal.

Policy-Related Intervention Logic Model

A policy-related logic model also shows diagrammatically the initiative's basic components: resources, activities, outputs, and outcomes (Figure 3.7). To keep the purpose of the program in full view, the public health goal and the policy goal are noted at the top of the logic model. In addition, the logic model identifies resources; activities; outputs; short-, intermediate-, and long-term outcomes; and points at which evaluation may occur.

A policy-related logic model needs to include the following components:

Resources (**sometimes called the** *inputs*): The human, financial, and material resources that are used in developing the policy. They include staff and other personnel who will be available to work on the policy, grant, and other monies allocated for the policy development, as well as office space, training materials, and other resources that are provided for the initiative.

Program activities: The specific activities that need to be undertaken in order to design, enact, and implement a policy intervention. Examples of activities are training, coalition building, policy framing, advocacy, and media engagement.

Outputs: The initial products of the initiative, the results of the intervention. Examples of outputs are the number of people trained in advocacy skills, the number of pieces of material distributed or e-mails distributed, the number of media spots engaged, the number of legislative drafts written, and the number of legislators who support the policy.

FIGURE 3.7. *Basic Framework for a Logic Model for a Policy Related Initiative*

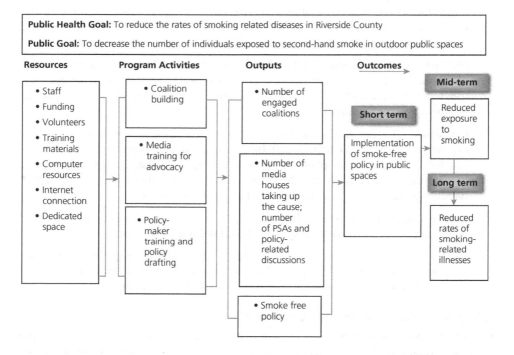

Outcomes: Changes that occur in those who are exposed to the policy. Outcomes may be developed as short term, intermediate term, and long term during the planning process and will result in the policy that is followed by implementation and monitoring. Examples include policies to increase physical activity for children in elementary school, policy to increase the number of homes that have lead abatement, policy to ban smoking in public parks. A policy at the organizational level could result in staff seeing the last client an hour earlier.

Program goal: Based on the public health goal but focused on the population served by the initiative. It provides the specific direction for the policy.

Public health goal: The impact of the policy on the public health goal. It expresses the improvement in the quality of life of the community's residents.

Criteria

A well-developed logic model may be used as a tool throughout the iterative process of program and policy development planning and is useful if it

■ Is detailed yet not overwhelming and contains crucial elements of the intervention

■ Clearly shows the relationships among the program inputs, outputs, and outcomes

- Is understood by the stakeholders

- Is complementary to other management materials

Note than an initiative may have more than one logic model and that the logic model will change as new components are added or changes are made to the existing intervention. The logic model is a dynamic tool.

CRITERIA FOR SUCCESSFUL INITIATIVES

In order to solve public health problems, initiatives (program or policy) for tackling them must be effective. Successful initiatives have the following criteria:

- They address one or more critical risk factors and the social determinants of health while recognizing and strengthening protective factors.

- They address the needs of the population specifically and are culturally sensitive and appropriate.

- They are sustained over a long period.

- They address problems that concern the community, which support funding solutions.

- They have well-trained, managed staff.

- They are well resourced.

Effective programs have the following characteristics:

- Activities are appropriate for accomplishing the objectives.

- Human, material, and financial resources are adequate.

- Activities reflect cultural sensitivity.

- Staff are trained and adequately prepared to deliver/support the initiative.

- A clearly articulated time line for developing and implementing the initiative is followed.

- Barriers to program implementation are recognized and solutions are identified.

- Effective strategies to promote the program are utilized.

- Monitoring and evaluation data-collection tools are developed and utilized to assess program implementation and effectiveness.

In addition, developing appropriate and effective initiatives to address public health problems requires input from a range of stakeholders. A critical stakeholder in the initiation of the program or policy initiative is the funder. The funder provides the resources for the program and oversight, often as a member of the board of directors. Other stakeholders include those who implement and those who will benefit from the initiative.

The development of culturally appropriate and sustainable programs that lead to empowerment (Rappaport, 1984) requires the establishment of effective partnerships with all stakeholders (Panet-Raymond, 1992). The partnerships are strengthened by the participation of stakeholders in multiple tasks, including:

- Reviewing the community assessment

- Developing the mission, goals, and objectives

- Identifying appropriate theories, theory-based initiatives, and evidence-based programs

- Identifying activities for program implementation

- Designing a program and developing the program's theory of change

- Identifying resources (human, financial, and material) for program implementation

- Initiating and overseeing program implementation

- Developing an evaluation plan, identifying an evaluator and ensuring a systematic evaluation of the intervention

STAKEHOLDERS' PARTICIPATION IN PLANNING AND DEVELOPING INITIATIVES

There are multiple opportunities for stakeholders to participate in planning and developing initiatives. Consistent with the participatory model for evaluation described in this book, identifying and engaging stakeholders occurs in the first step but continues throughout the process. Representatives of all stakeholder groups should be involved in the process from the start so that they have a sense of ownership in both the process and the product.

Stakeholders can have one or more roles in the process. They can be involved in the community assessment and continue their work to planning and developing the program. Alternatively, they can become involved at the point of identifying priorities upon which the program will be developed based on a previously conducted assessment. In developing the goals and objectives for the initiative, their participation will determine the extent to which the initiative is supported and/or adopted.

Stakeholder participation is critical for ensuring that the program or policy is sensitive to the needs and culture of the community it is intended to serve.

SUMMARY

- The mission statement reflects the organization's mission, direction, and population focus.

- The community is determined by a group of people and is not necessarily bounded by geographical limits.

- The initiative is developed based on the findings of the epidemiological profile; community assessment; the mission; and the social, political, and cultural contexts in which the program operates.

- Outcome objectives provide benchmarks for achievement of the program goal. Outcome objectives frame the initiative in multiple domains—individual, interpersonal, organizational, community, and public policy.

- Well-developed outcome and activity (process) objectives serve as tools in the evaluation.

- Initiatives include theory-based or evidence-based programs.

- Logic models depict the theory of change of an initiative in graphic or pictorial terms. The logic model informs the monitoring of the initiative and focuses the evaluation. Components of the logic model are resources, activities, outputs, and outcomes.

FIGURE 3.8. *Valuable Take-Aways*

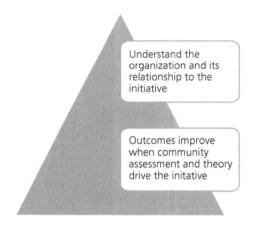

Understand the organization and its relationship to the initiative

Outcomes improve when community assessment and theory drive the initative

DISCUSSION QUESTIONS AND ACTIVITIES

1. Locate and read at least one article that describes an initiative that used a theoretical framework to design the intervention and one that did not use a theory. Draw the logic models for each. Review the conclusions for each initiative and discuss the authors' findings. What recommendations would you make to improve either or both initiatives? What are the consequences that follow from your line of thinking?

2. As an evaluator called in to help plan a new initiative, what advice would you give the planning committee? Give two examples each of SMART activity (process) and outcome objectives that you might consider for an intervention that addresses high-risk behaviors among high school students. Be sure the objectives relate to each other.

3. Develop a set of policy related objectives to tackle the environmental factors that trigger a common health problem of your choice using public policies. What activities would you plan? What resources would you draw on?

4.   Describe the challenges of developing a new initiative. How would you ensure that the project you develop is sustainable?

KEY TERMS

evidence-based initiatives
goals
logic models
mission
objectives

program activities
SMART objectives
stakeholders
theory
theory of change

4

PLANNING FOR EVALUATION

PURPOSE AND PROCESSES

LEARNING OBJECTIVES

- List the purposes of evaluation.
- Identify and describe the processes in managing an evaluation.
- Explain how evaluation standards and ethics underlie the evaluation process.
- Describe the role of stakeholders in evaluation planning.

The systematic collection of information about the activities and the outcomes of initiatives, which are an essential part of program evaluation, requires understanding the purposes and principles of evaluation as well as the appropriate management processes. This chapter describes how to plan an evaluation process.

When a group of program managers of public health initiatives were asked to define program evaluation, they provided these two definitions: (1) "Evaluation means finding out important pieces of information that will help provide quality of service based on the needs of the target population," and (2) "Evaluation means a process for learning how a program was actually implemented and what the impacts of a program are in the short and the long term."

Evaluation has these characteristics and more. Evaluation assesses the internal validity of an initiative and the extent to which an effect that is achieved is due to an intervention that was planned systematically. It is the cornerstone for improving public health initiatives because it provides information about the program through the conduct of culturally appropriate, carefully designed and executed research studies. The underlying assumption of public health interventions is that if an initiative is undertaken to address a problem through the conduct of a set of activities, the initiative will lead to a change in the participants or in the environment or in both. For example, if the community assessment finds that youth who have not had the benefit of a fulfilling education are more likely to use illicit drugs, then the root cause of the problem can be identified as poor educational attainment. A good education intervention, which is theoretically sound, will likely affect the proportion of youth who use illicit drugs. The purpose of the evaluation would be to document carefully the resources and activities of the intervention and determine changes that occur to the beneficiaries as well as to the social and physical environment over time. Evaluation activities will document changes in the short, intermediate and long term.

Evaluation is conducted for the purpose of making a judgment about a program's worth or value; it consists of a series of steps that must be matched with the needs of the project. The evaluation process is designed to answer a previously specified question by assessing the implementation of the program or policy and its outputs, outcomes, and impact. It provides feedback on the extent to which the initiative is achieving the organization's mission, goals, and objectives and makes recommendations for program improvements overall or for specific components of the program. In addition, evaluation studies attempt to determine whether the outcome was likely to have been caused by the initiative when the initiative's participants are compared with a control group.

THE TIMING OF THE EVALUATION

Two considerations influence when an evaluation is carried out: first, whether the program is ready to be evaluated, and second, the stage of program development and implementation.

Readiness for Evaluation

The readiness for evaluation is assessed early in the process. This may take the form of a simple assessment of a detailed program plan and a theory of change; or it may be a more formal pre-assessment including evaluation of the data and the data-collection tools. In the participatory model of evaluation, there is an excellent opportunity during the early discussions of the evaluation process and the contract to assess whether the program is ready for evaluation. The possibility of conducting the evaluation becomes clear once the program has been described and a theory of change and a logic model have been developed.

Stage of Development and Implementation

The timing of the evaluation is also determined by the stage of development and implementation of the initiative, which in turn determines the evaluation design and implementation. It influences which questions are most appropriate. A program in the early stages of development and within the first year or two of its implementation requires a different evaluation approach, focus, and time line than a program that has been fully operational for 10 years. In the first year of a program, it is important to determine that the resources and program components are being implemented with fidelity and according to plan and the tools for measuring outcomes are put in place and are functioning appropriately. Outcomes are not assessed until the full implementation of the program or at specified intervals during the initiative in order to determine trends in a longitudinal study or a single outcome in a cross-sectional study.

THE PURPOSE OF EVALUATION

The purpose of an evaluation is generally to provide information for decision-making or to provide information to improve evaluation practice.

- The evaluation may be undertaken in order to assess the extent to which the program is being implemented as planned or to determine whether the initiative is making or has made an impact on the beneficiaries.

- The evaluation may be undertaken in order to provide information for development of the initiative, to provide information for replication, or to determine its cost effectiveness compared with other programs.

- The evaluation may be undertaken in order to provide information about risk and protective factors or to assess alternative approaches for the prevention or treatment of health problems.

Although the primary purpose of an evaluation is to improve performance and to transform conditions, practice, structures, and systems, results from evaluations may serve other purposes:

- *Accountability* to the clients, community, funders, program management, and staff.

- *Social justice* to ensure vulnerable populations receive appropriate and effective services.

- *Program comparison* to determine best approaches.

- *Evaluation research* to test a hypothesis.

- *Program replication* at another site with another population.

In the earliest stages of the development of the initiative, the purpose of the evaluation is to understand how the program or policy is being implemented or to assess whether the initiative is likely to have the intended effect; such an assessment is known as a *formative evaluation*. Formative evaluation may be used in situations in which the dynamics, the participants, and the issues change frequently and program activities must adjust to the changing environment. It may also be used as a pilot test of a potentially larger program when the pilot consists of a subpopulation of the intended population or a shortened version of the full program. Formative evaluation provides early feedback and documentation to support a loop of assessment, planning, implementation, and evaluation. It answers the following questions:

- Do the program components work effectively separately and together?

- Is there suitable data for assessing process and outcomes?

- What are the factors that influence program implementation favorably and unfavorably?

- To what extent is the intervention likely to achieve the goals it has established?

- Is the logic of the intervention appropriate and consistent with scientific literature and sound theoretical models?

- Is the program culturally appropriate?

Formative evaluation may be used to pretest educational materials for an intervention and media messages prior to implementation of an educational campaign. In this case it may answer the following questions:

- Do the messages provide information that is useful for understanding the changes expected of the population for whom they are intended?

- Are the messages written in culturally appropriate ways?

- Are the images culturally appropriate and represent the diversity of the community?

- Do the messages provide information that is exact and specific to the necessary level of detail?

- Do the messages take into consideration the stage of development of the community and recognize when there is a need for simpler and possibly less esoteric messages?

In a recent formative evaluation study of messages surrounding a media campaign, focus group participants were asked to comment on a concept for reducing sweetened beverage (soft drink) consumption based on the number of calories it contained. The evaluation team reviewed the messages with residents of the targeted low-income minority neighborhoods to assess their cultural appropriateness and understanding. One of the comments about the original campaign related to the message about the number of calories in soda but it did not make any recognizable connections to why it was important. It was evident from the study that there was a need for clearer and more direct messages that highlighted the connections between the product and health consequences. The campaign was modified to reflect this (see Figure 4.1).

FIGURE 4.1. *Poster from the Revised Media Campaign*

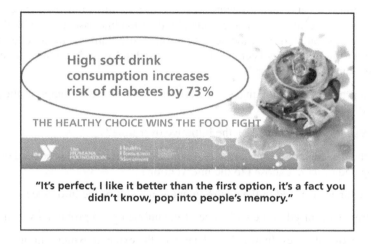

When the purpose of the evaluation is to determine whether the program or policy is being implemented appropriately or the extent to which the program is being implemented as planned, it is known as a *process evaluation*. However, process evaluation may not have been preceded by a formative evaluation; therefore, it may incorporate similar questions in addition to those more specific to formative evaluation. Formative evaluation focuses on reviewing documentation of implementation such as logs, meeting notes, registration documents, and any relevant databases when a program is stable and is intended to achieve specified objectives.

A process evaluation may review data-collection processes and outputs and the extent to which planned activity objectives are being achieved. It may also involve interviewing participants or project personnel to understand the process of implementation and its strengths and weaknesses. Improving the program of work in progress or an existing policy implementation is the purpose of process evaluation. Major questions during this phase include

■ Is the program/intervention being implemented according to the plan that was laid out before the program started?

■ Is the logic of the intervention appropriate and consistent with scientific literature and sound theoretical models?

■ What type, quantity, and quality of services are being provided?

■ What are staffing and training levels of those implementing the program?

■ How many meetings, trainings, and other activities are held and for whom?

■ Who is participating and how?

■ To what extent is the program considering the issue at hand in the context of the population being served?

If the purpose of the evaluation is to determine the effect of the program or policy, then it is known as an *outcome evaluation*. An outcome evaluation is performed at the end of the intervention or at a time predetermined by its outcome objectives. The appropriate time for an outcome evaluation is determined by the time line associated with the program objectives, by the completion of the activity, project, program, or, in the case of a policy initiative, after the policy has been in place for an extended period. Outcome evaluations answer questions such as these:

- Did the program or policy make a difference and produce a change in those affected directly by it?

- What results were produced by the initiative over time?

- What changes in knowledge, attitudes, beliefs, or behavior were produced in those who participated or were exposed to the intervention?

- What changes occurred in the environment as a result of the initiative?

- What trends occurred in the incidence of the public health problem over time?

If the purpose of the evaluation is to determine the extent to which initiatives have contributed to a population-level effect, it is known as an *impact evaluation*. The terms *outcome* and *impact* are often used interchangeably within different sectors of public health. In this book, *outcome* is used for short-, medium-, and long-term changes that occur during the first few years of program or policy implementation. *Impact* is used for long-term changes in quality of life that occur at the local, state, and national levels that are detected using surveillance methods, and that occur in the population at large from a plethora of activities that occur over time in multiple sectors. An impact evaluation answers this question: Did all the efforts of the combined initiatives influence rates of disease, disability, or mortality, or the quality of life of the population?

The purpose of an evaluation also may be *cost-benefit* or *cost-effectiveness analyses,* which allow evaluators to determine whether the cost associated with the program is worth the investment. These analyses answer the question: What were the benefits of the program relative to the expenditures?

THE CONTRACT FOR EVALUATION

Evaluations may be carried out by an internal evaluator when a contract is generally not required, but when an external evaluator is to be hired, the contract is negotiated by the initiator—the funding agency, the board of directors, the executive director, or other person designated by the agency or organization. Community-based and other low-resourced organizations will usually rely on in-house internal evaluators to conduct an evaluation, but when an organization can afford to hire an external evaluator or an evaluation team, local or national searches may be helpful although evaluators are often recommended through personal contacts. One situation in which the organization had the benefit of evaluation expertise and a person to conduct the evaluation was when a student of a university based research institute was assigned to evaluate a pregnancy-prevention organization's work; given the organization's meager budget, it was unable to afford an evaluator. The organization had the benefit of the expertise of the evaluator through her consultations with the student and most of the costs of travel and the evaluation were borne by the research institute.

The lead evaluator has primary responsibility for the evaluation and negotiates the terms of the contract based on previous experience, knowledge, skills, and orientation. Previous experience is, without a doubt, one of the most valuable assets. It ensures that the negotiator has almost certainly done this before and has the required knowledge and skills, and if the evaluator is very familiar with the needs of the different evaluations he or she is most likely to determine the needs of a contract. However, this does not exclude a novice from taking on a negotiation, it means the individual has to have a sound understanding of evaluation principles and practices and preferably be supported by a more experienced evaluator. This person may or may not be part of the team for the evaluation, but could serve as a consultant. The contract is a critical component of the process since it determines the scope of work and each partner's responsibilities in executing the evaluation. The role of the person who requests the evaluation is likely to be much smaller than the role of the evaluation team. Their primary responsibility is likely to be in ensuring that the evaluation team has access to stakeholders required for the research and logistics including access to data. The contract, which may be in the form of a letter or a formal legal document, contains the following:

- Name of the evaluator (as contractor) and the name of the contracting agent.

- Statement of the purpose and some explanation of the process of the evaluation and expected outcomes.

- Statements about access to management and staff, initiative beneficiaries, resources, and logistics for the time period during which the evaluation will be carried out.

- Specific expectations and timelines for reports and other documentation of the evaluation.

- Amount budgeted for the evaluation.

- Overall time line for the evaluation which may be a single one-off evaluation or an ongoing multiyear evaluation involving process and outcome evaluation.

- Dated signatures of all parties to the contract.

THE EVALUATION TEAM

Following the execution of the contract, the lead evaluator, working with the contracting agency or organization, identifies members of the evaluation team. The team should include stakeholders with the expertise to develop and implement the evaluation plan, although roles may shift during the evaluation process and training may be required for community members. Members of the team may also require specialized training.

The evaluation team must have evaluation expertise in multiple areas and the knowledge and skills required for completing the task. The size of the team is often determined by the budget. If necessary, ad hoc teams may be formed to carry out specific tasks related to the evaluation. A commitment to training stakeholders and to providing the necessary skills during the process is likely to lead people to participate (Travers et al., 2008). Such a commitment ensures equity across the team and buy-in from the start and is likely to lead to the organization using the findings (Patton, 2008). People on the evaluation team should include those with skills in

■ Working across disciplines

■ Cross-cultural communication

■ Critical thinking and evaluation

■ Research methodology

■ Data collection

■ Data management, analysis, and interpretation

■ Technical writing and reporting

As part of effective evaluation practice, the lead evaluator should ask who is not at the table, which voices will not be heard, and why. The team should make every effort to include those voices in the process.

The contributions of the stakeholders include providing an understanding of the program, providing input into the development of the evaluation plan, providing support to the implementation of the plan through data collection and analysis, and providing input into the interpretation of the results and writing the final report.

The evaluation-team leader has ultimate responsibility for ensuring the integrity of the evaluation process, that it is carried out with the highest ethical standards, and that it is completed within the time frame agreed on. The evaluator should "ensure that the evaluation team collectively possesses the evaluation abilities, skills, and experience appropriate to the evaluation" (American Evaluation Association, 2008, p. 233).

Once the team is assembled, the first step is to orient everyone to the team's approach to the evaluation. It is particularly important to orient the community members and newcomers to the art and science of evaluation. Encouraging evaluative thinking as part of the community's or the organization's culture increases the likelihood that data collection for evaluation purposes is incorporated systematically into initiatives (Patton, 2008). Orienting the team to the approach to evaluation may mean, for example, making sure all members of the team are familiar with and understand the principles of evaluation, the type of evaluation (preassessment, formative, process, outcome, or impact), the model for the evaluation, the participatory nature of the evaluation, and so forth.

The team must work through multiple steps in the process to complete the terms of the contract and provide the expected products within the specified time. It must define a plan of action with multiple components and steps that describe the activities that the team will undertake to complete the evaluation. Completing the evaluation requires the development of a well-functioning and effective team.

Think About It!

You have recently accepted a contract from a small but effective nonprofit organization that serves veteran groups. You have to build a team of evaluators to conduct an evaluation of an intervention to provide comprehensive public health services for veterans. What would be your primary considerations in building the evaluation team? What process will you use to assemble an effective team? How can you be sure that you have taken all the complexities of the program into consideration? Who is left out? How do you ensure cultural competency?

EVALUATION STANDARDS

The public health community adopted a set of evaluation standards (Milstein et al., 2000) put forward by the Joint Commission on Standards for Educational Evaluation (Joint Committee on Standards for Educational Evaluation, Sanders, & American Association of School Administrators, 1994; Patton, 2008) that inform the practice of public health today. The broad concepts of the standards of evaluation practice are utility, feasibility, propriety, and accuracy (see Figure 4.2).

> *Utility*: The utility standard requires that the information provided by the evaluation be useful to the stakeholders and those who will use the results. It addresses the amount and type of information that is collected, the interpretation of evaluation findings, as well as when and how the final report is produced. It encourages evaluation to be planned, conducted, and reported in ways that increase the likelihood of stakeholders' using the evaluation findings.

> *Feasibility*: The feasibility standard requires that the evaluation process be practical and nondisruptive, that it acknowledges the political nature of the evaluation, and that

FIGURE 4.2.   *Evaluation Standards*

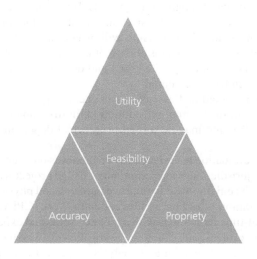

resources that are available for conducting the evaluation are used carefully to produce results. It specifies that evaluations should be efficient and produce information that justify their expense.

Propriety: The propriety standard requires that the evaluation be ethical and be conducted with regard for the rights of those involved and affected. It requires that the evaluation be complete and fair in its process and reporting. It also requires that the evaluation demonstrate respect for human dignity and avoid conflicts of interest; it cites the Tuskegee syphilis study as a reminder of the evaluators' responsibilities.

Accuracy: The accuracy standard requires that the evaluation uses accurate and systematic processes for conducting qualitative and quantitative research and that it produces technically accurate conclusions that are defensible and justifiable.

MANAGING THE EVALUATION PROCESS

An important consideration for evaluators is how an evaluation plan will be implemented and how the research will be managed. Evaluation projects are organized into five major phases. The first one is to recruit an evaluation team; the second is to review and confirm the terms of the contract and to make decisions regarding supervision and finances; the third is to develop an evaluation research plan; fourth is to develop a budget for the evaluation and lastly, implement the plan.

Recruiting and Developing the Evaluation Team

The first task of the lead evaluator is to recruit and assemble a team of people who will conduct the evaluation. The evaluation focus and the methods and funding determine team membership and the expertise required of team members. It is important to develop a multidisciplinary team for cross-discipline initiative evaluations that involve multiple domains. An evaluation that requires conducting a cost analysis may require different skills than one that requires the assessment of behavioral outcomes. The team must assess the needs of each evaluation carefully and throughout the process. If during the evaluation process new skills are needed, the evaluator must consider increasing the membership, either permanently or by using consultants. This decision will usually have funding implications that must be weighed carefully also. As teams change, it is also important to address issues that influence and change the dynamics of the group and decision making; ensuring equitable participation of team members is essential.

Once the team is recruited and assembled, the next step is to identify tasks for team members. Decisions regarding training and building skills to complete evaluation tasks must be made at this time. Training may be formal or informal depending on the needs of the project.

An example of an evaluation team I recently created was one that had a contract to conduct an evaluation of a jurisdiction-wide community-change project with a view to changing systems, policies, and the environment to improve nutrition and physical activity. The Evaluation Team for the Communities Putting Prevention to Work (CPPW) initiative consisted of 10 part-time and full-time individuals with a range of skills and experiences in evaluation or research. Most were professionals but a few were students who had specialized skills in biostatistics or qualitative data coding and analysis. A project manager and the principle investigator had 50% of their time dedicated to the project, whereas other members of the team had time commitments that ranged from 100% for 12 months to 10%, depending on their roles on the project. Part-time staff was hired for a limited period specifically to help with a large qualitative study. Staff of the local health department was an extension of the team and provided access to those implementing the program and policy initiatives and support for the evaluation. This fairly large team that met weekly was big enough to provide a range of skills and a good balance of qualitative and quantitative skills allowing it to take on both process and outcome evaluation. In addition, the team was involved in a formative evaluation of the media campaign that was launched to promote healthy eating and physical activity. It was impossible to do impact evaluation since it was only a two-year funded project and the evaluation was also compressed into that time frame.

Deciding on Contract Terms, Supervision, and Finances

The Contract The evaluation contract provides only a brief overview of the evaluation and its product, so the evaluation team needs to discuss and negotiate the details and the expectations with the clients and other stakeholders before the work begins. It is important to ensure that the contract expectations are clear on both sides, with some provision being made to amend the contract if necessary. The team has many responsibilities during these sessions:

- Discuss and decide on the overarching and specific evaluation research question(s). This discussion may cover previous evaluations of the program. An assessment of findings may provide insights and help identify questions that could be included in a new evaluation.

- Discuss data-collection options and access to research participants.

- Understand the climate for conducting the evaluation. Politically charged climates may make evaluation challenging. The team needs to understand the dynamics between the client and other local, state, and national stakeholders. These may include relationships with the board, funders, and the competition.

- Review the budget and determine the scope and scale of the evaluation. It is important to spend time developing a well-thought-out budget for the evaluation that will be adhered to closely. Evaluations are generally not well funded, and going back to the client for more money is usually not an option for the evaluation team, unless the scope of work changes significantly at the request of the client. If it is possible, the team should build in a review process to allow that flexibility and also should build in agreements with regard to moving expenditures within the budget—for example, from supplies to travel. If such changes need to be made, it is important to contact the funder. Generally, changes of 10% are acceptable and easily allowed.

- Identify roles and responsibilities for members of the evaluation team, staff, and key stakeholders. Discuss the principles of the participatory approach to conducting the evaluation and get buy-in from the team.

- Identify the logistics for the evaluation (support staff, office supplies, transportation, meeting space, data resources). Discuss how databases, reports, and publications will be made accessible to the evaluation team. This discussion may cover time frames and personnel. Staff is often busy and may find it difficult to accommodate the requests of evaluators, so allow plenty of time for requests to be honored.

- Discuss ownership of the evaluation data. Unlike data from traditional research projects, evaluation data often belong to the client. It is important to clarify data ownership early in the process to avoid any misunderstanding later. This discussion should also cover publication of the findings. Permission may need to be obtained to report at conferences and in other ways publish the findings.

- Discuss the expectations during the period of the evaluation for interim and final reports and check-ins, including formats and mechanisms for reporting.

Supervision Managing an evaluation project can be time consuming and requires different although complementary skills. It entails supervising staff and volunteers at each stage of the process as well as the day-to-day coordination of the team's efforts. It may include identifying and securing resources and ensuring that deadlines are met and that deliverables are developed. It may also require setting up meetings, following up on project commitments, and writing reports. In most evaluations, the management functions are carried out by the evaluator or a member of the team, but when the project is large, such as a large jurisdiction or statewide evaluation, it may be necessary to hire a project manager whose sole responsibility is coordination. When hiring a project manager, the skills of the individual are matched with the requirements of the specific evaluation. An individual with project management training or skills who might also be helpful in various aspects of the evaluation will be an asset to the team.

Finances During this period, the team must also consider how the finances will be handled. The team leader will usually have the final responsibility for ensuring funds are spent appropriately, but mechanisms should be designed to monitor and track spending. The level of monitoring and tracking will depend on the size, duration, and complexity of the project. The more complex the evaluation is, the more likely it is that an accountant needs to be involved.

Developing the Evaluation Research Plan

After the contract is signed by all parties, the evaluation team convenes and develops a detailed evaluation research plan. This plan will contain a number of components:

- Project evaluation research design

- Data collection and management

- Dissemination of findings

Project Design Undertaking the evaluation research project entails selecting the most appropriate design for answering the evaluation research question. The design is determined by the stage of the program to be evaluated, the evaluation question that is to be answered, the budget, the expertise of the team, and the time line. The primary determinant of the research design will be based on the purpose of the evaluation. A process evaluation, for example, will answer a different question from an outcome evaluation and will require different approaches. An outcome evaluation may require control or comparison groups in an experimental or quasi-experimental research design, whereas a process evaluation assesses the program's inputs and outputs. Information from a process evaluation, however, is important for making important decisions about replication, but the approach to data collection differs. The evaluation plan recognizes the difference in these evaluations and designs and reflects the needs and interests of the stakeholders.

The team develops a project action plan, which is essentially the implementation of the evaluation plan that encapsulates the project design. For the evaluation as a whole and for each major component, the action plan outlines the activities and the time frame for completing them. Activities in the action plan include those related to the research needed to answer the evaluation questions. As the project continues, the team may need different action plans that will fall within the scope of the project action plan. An action plan provides a graphic representation of the time line and required tasks and may also designate responsible persons. It differs from a logic model in that a logic model is a graphic representation of the initiative's theory of change; the logic model outlines the assumed links among the health problem, the activities used to resolve it, and the expected outcomes of the intervention. To be clear, the evaluation action plan outlines the specific project activities for conducing the evaluation with appropriate time lines. Examples of a basic action plan and of a plan for team recruitment and development are provided in Table 4.1 and Table 4.2. Consider also using project-management software, which facilitates the development and management of the plans.

Data Collection and Management   Based on the design selected and the type of questions to be answered, the most appropriate data-collection methods are identified. In an optimal evaluation

- The best data-collection methods are used.

- The data that are collected are both valid and reliable.

- The analysis of the data is appropriate and accurate.

Selecting the best approach to data collection and the best data requires that researchers be oriented toward the specifics of the project; hence, training must be built into the time

TABLE 4.1.   **A Basic Action Plan**

Major Project Activities	First Quarter	Second Quarter	Third Quarter	Fourth Quarter
1. Team recruitment and development	x			
2. Make contract, supervision, and financial decisions	x			
3. Project design	x	x		
4. Data collection and management			x	
5. Dissemination of findings				x

TABLE 4.2. An Action Plan for Team Recruitment and Development

Team Recruitment and Development	First Quarter			Responsible Person(s)
	Month 1	Month 2	Month 3	
Identify potential team members	x			Kwaku
Invite stakeholders to be on the team	x	x		Tina
Conduct orientation for team members			x	Jean and Sam

line and the budget. Divisions of the National Institutes of Health, the Centers for Disease Control and Prevention, and foundations now fund Community-Based Participatory Research intervention projects that require the involvement of multiple partners, many of whom have no experience with research. Members of the community who form part of the team and others who want to participate in the evaluation may need extensive training to develop their skills in research and data collection and in data analysis.

In addition, the data-collection approach selected must be credible and provide valid and reliable data. The evaluation team assesses the options and decides on the most appropriate methods. It develops or assembles appropriate data-collection instruments and decides on the needs for analysis, which may include personnel and logistics. Once the evaluation project is complete a final step is evaluating the evaluation itself to understand the strengths and weaknesses of the design, data collection, and the evaluation process overall. This evaluation assesses the validity of the conclusions and their relevance to stakeholders.

Dissemination of Findings As the evaluation team plans the evaluation, it must also discuss important aspects of sharing the results with stakeholders and their wider dissemination including:

■ The stakeholders' expectations of how the results will be used

■ The timing of evaluation reports that may be provided periodically during the evaluation process or at the end as a final report

■ The audience characteristics that will influence the presentation formats and style

■ The venues and formats of dissemination

Budgeting for the Evaluation

Using the budget approved in the contract process, the team develops a working budget that is based on the specifics of the evaluation plan. Table 4.3 is a sample budget. It includes costs for personnel, equipment and supplies, printing, and participants. The data-collection approach may have additional costs associated with it. A budget justification explains each budget line. For example, it specifies the number of staff, the level of staff, and the salary

TABLE 4.3.   **Sample Budget**

Budget Item	Yr 1 $	Yr 2 $	Yr 3	Yr 4	Yr 5
Staff Salaries and Benefits	119,925	125,921			
Project coordinator (1) 10% @ $60,000 + 23%					
Interviewers (2) 25% @ $50,000 + 23%					
Data analyst (1) 50% @ $50,000 + 23%					
Consultant Fees (if required)	2,000	2,100			
10 days @ $200 per day					
Travel (project team and study participants)	7,000	7,000			
Out of state $2,000					
In state $5,000					
Equipment and Supplies	3,800	1,000			
Computer $1,300					
Software $1,500					
General office supplies $1,000					
Communication	1,800	2,000			
Internet					
Telephone					
Participants	5,000	5,000			
Stipends $500					
Transcriptions 15 @ $300 per interview					
Printing	100	100			
Surveys 200 @ $.50 per copy					
Photocopying	100	100			
Subtotal	139,725	143,221			
Indirect costs (depending on funder) @ 25%	34,931	35,805			
TOTAL	$174,656	$179,026			

and benefits. In the table, the project coordinator earns $60,000 per year with fringe benefits calculated at 23% and works on the evaluation 10% of the time. The budget will reflect the cost of the project director with a possible increase in succeeding years. The cost of equipment and supplies in this example decreases in succeeding years because computer and software expenses are necessary in the first year only.

FACTORS THAT INFLUENCE THE EVALUATION PROCESS

A well-designed and implemented program or policy evaluation depends on a variety of factors that the evaluation team may have more or less control over. It is important that the evaluation team consider the possible limitations in order to provide the most cost-sensitive and useful evaluation.

Factors That Cannot Be Controlled

Once the contract negotiation is complete and the contract signed, there may still be factors that influence the evaluation but that the evaluators have limited or no control over. These include:

■ *The level of funding and of the resources allocated for the evaluation.* The higher the funding and the more resources available for the evaluation the more comprehensive the evaluation will be.

■ *Personnel support.* An adequate level of support is important to ensure access to resources, to the study population, to data, and to logistics that support the evaluation.

■ *The time line.* One that limits the type of data or the quantity and quality of data that can be collected will limit the evaluation.

■ *Access to the study population and to program data.* The degree of access may influence a number of parameters of the evaluation. It may affect the amount and the quality of the data that are collected; low amounts and poor quality of data introduce bias and affect the validity of the study.

■ A sociopolitical environment with little or no support for the evaluation makes the process difficult and results in difficulty in collecting the information, limited access to resources, and difficulty in sharing and utilizing evaluation findings. The sociopolitical environment is influenced by who requested the evaluation and who has a vested interest in the results.

Factors That Can Be Controlled

There are also factors that the evaluator has control over and must take into consideration during the planning process and beyond contract negotiation. These factors may include the level and type of expertise on the evaluation team and the management of the evaluation process.

Level and Type of Expertise on the Evaluation Team   The level and type of expertise on the evaluation team will influence the type of evaluation that is conducted and access to the study population. It is important to ensure that members of the team have knowledge and skills to contribute to some part of the process, while recognizing that not all members will contribute to all parts of the evaluation. For example, a stakeholder may be influential in the community but may know nothing about the evaluation process. Nevertheless, he or she may be able to contribute significantly to developing the research tools and to providing input to ensure the tools and approaches are sensitive to the study population. That member may also be instrumental in another stage of the process, recruiting members of the community to complete the surveys and participate in the focus groups or in photography and digital storytelling. Without that member's contributions, the evaluation may take longer than planned and may even not collect valid and reliable data.

The evaluation team also requires skills in evaluation, which will depend on the nature of the project to be evaluated. If, for example, the evaluation calls for a cost-benefit analysis in addition to the usual outcome evaluation, it is important that the team recruit a member who has skills in conducting such an analysis or that the team be willing to pay a consultant for that expertise.

Management of the Evaluation Process Apart from having the appropriate expertise on the evaluation team, the team must also be managed appropriately to complete the project and fulfill the requirements of the contract. For example, if the agreement is to provide a midyear interim report to coincide with a midyear review of the project by the board of directors, the evaluation team has the responsibility for meeting that deadline. To do so, the team has to complete all the tasks of data collection and data analysis and write a report that is appropriate given the status of the project. Resources and logistics have to be secured and made available for the evaluation project.

Recruiting the right people and providing the necessary training are crucial to the success of the endeavor. It is always necessary to ensure that each person on the team has a good understanding of the project and especially if team members are being hired to be a part of the data collection team but having not participated in the earlier work of the group.

Training of the Research Team Adequate and appropriate training is critical when planning for evaluation. Training can be accomplished in a variety of approaches. Webinars may save time and allow participants to view the material in their own time. Group training over one or two days provides opportunities to role-play, and print and video materials may also be provided for review.

Training comprises evaluation concepts, definitions, structure, and process for the study and topics include

- Background to the project

- Epidemiological profile of the health problem being investigated

- The purpose of this evaluation

- Sites of the evaluation

- Timeline and data collection schedule

- Description of the sample

- Sample size and characteristics

- Data collection methods and tools

- Number of data collection tools and descriptions of each
- Guidelines for interviewing
- Contacting respondents
- Introducing yourself to a respondent
- Confidentiality
- Building rapport with your respondent
- Ethical practices in evaluation research
- Best practices in data collection

Best practices for data collection are listed below:

- Learn about the community.

- Respect cultural norms. Before starting data collection introduce yourself, and explain the purpose of the study.

- The written consent of individuals is required. A parent or guardian must give consent before interviewing children. Children provide assent to be interviewed.

- When interviewing children, always have a member of the family or community or teacher that the child trusts present. Do not take a child to a secluded spot. See them as individuals with their own thoughts and concerns.

- Choose a space for the interview where your respondent is comfortable and one that offers privacy, whether it is an individual interview or a group interview.

- Make sure you are at the same level as your respondent(s). Sit so your respondent can see your face. If the respondent is sitting on the floor, sit on the floor. Conduct focus groups in circles.

- Respect confidentiality and use the name an individual gives to him/her self. It does not have to be their real name.

- Listening is the key to good interviewing. Do not interrupt to ask questions. Wait for the answer to the question. Be particularly sensitive when asking personal or probing questions.

- Use appropriate language. Listen to how they speak. Make sure they understand you. Don't use jargon.

- If the interview is not going well, take time to find out what the problem is.

- Make sure a translator is familiar with the needs of the project and reduce the risk of questions being misinterpreted in translation.

- Always ask permission both to photograph the individual as well as his/her home or property. Consider how your actions will be perceived by the individual or the community.

- Ensure that your photographs portray people, both adults and children, with dignity.

▪ Ask the interviewee if they have any questions or if there is anything they have said that they don't want published. Make sure that you share your findings with the participants in your study.

PLANNING FOR ETHICAL PROGRAM EVALUATION

In planning for an evaluation that is ethical, the researchers must consider first and foremost the risk and benefits associated with the research. It requires consideration of the risks to the respondents, the time and effort they will put into providing information for the study in order to answer the research questions for whatever type of evaluation is being conducted. Participants' risk in participating in evaluation studies may include their loss of privacy, stigmatization, and a breach in confidentiality could mean a loss of employment or benefits so it is critical that the evaluation team considers the real risk to respondents. If, for example, an evaluation is being conducted in an organization that has been faltering, but one in which there may be considerable blame on a few individuals, disclosing who provides this information may threaten an individual's ability to stay in the job. Every effort is made to maintain confidentiality.

In preparing a consent form for review and signature, the risks and benefits associated with the study are clearly stated; however, it may be impossible to know the emotional consequences for an individual to be interviewed particularly about sensitive topics such as previous child abuse or domestic violence, or exposure to war or other form of aggression. Therefore, in preparing for evaluation, careful consideration must be given to the likely effect on the respondents and steps taken to ensure their safety. This may be in the form of ensuring there is a psychologist to whom a research participant may be referred, or brochures that provide information about services that can be accessed. It is also important to maintain confidentiality of data collected from individuals who participate in an evaluation.

The term *confidentiality* refers to our guarantee that information that identifies a person by name, address, or any other identifier is not released to anybody outside the project team and is not used in any reports. Names and other identifiers do not appear on any surveys and materials that allow a link between the individual and a survey, focus group discussion, or individual interview data. It is also important to restrict the use of photography since it may be even more difficult to maintain confidentiality or anonymity. Also, do not reveal any information that is obtained during the course of an interview to an unauthorized person. Authorized persons are restricted to individuals working directly on the project and within the project team. To assure confidentiality you are asked to protect the interview form, consent form, and any other documentation related to the interview. Access to the survey and focus group data for the purposes of entering, analyzing, and reporting is restricted to the research team. In rare legal circumstances it may not be possible to guarantee confidentiality. Respondents must be advised of their likely vulnerability and given the option to not participate. Maintaining anonymity of the data and keeping any consent forms that have names and signatures delinked from the data that is collected also helps to protect confidentiality.

The Federal Health Insurance Portability and Accountability Act (HIPPA) of 1996 was designed to make it easier for people to maintain the privacy of their health care information. It requires that researchers get special permissions to collect HIPPA protected physical and mental health information. In addition, designated researchers should be trained in Human

Subjects Protections. Training is often obtainable on line through universities and research institutions.

The ethical principle of "respect for people" (AEA, American Evaluation Association, 2008, p. 233) requires that evaluators respect the security, dignity, and worth of all stakeholders with the expectation that evaluators limit the length of participation of individuals to the minimum, limit the use of emotionally charged questions that could cause undue embarrassment, and provide compensation for the time spent or for expenses incurred. For example, women who are invited to participate in a study may have to pay somebody to look after their young children or give up an income-generating activity. It is important that compensation is fair. Ethical responsibility also dictates planning for the physical safety of participants, especially for women and children before, during, and after participation in a research study. In addition, flexibility must be allowed in scheduling interviews allowing for individuals to continue their normal activities without undue interruption.

Protecting individuals' identity is important in writing reports and publishing findings. In qualitative research in which quotes are often used to illustrate a point or to provide an example, the use of quotes that allow an individual to be identified is unacceptable. So, for example, rather than identifying the individual as "Mary Jo, Riverside," one might say, "MJ, Riverside" or to be even less specific, "Female, Riverside." If the age of the individual is important to report, then, "MJ, 49 years, Riverside" or "Female, 49 years, Riverside" may suffice. If the place does not need to be named and the report will result in that community being stigmatized, then the community may also be left off, so "MJ, 49 years" may also be sufficient. Using the respondents's characteristics increases credibility of the research and helps the reader recognize the range of respondents.

INVOLVING STAKEHOLDERS

All those who have an interest in the program and the evaluation are the stakeholders and the audience for the evaluation. They are involved in both the process and the management of the evaluation. As mentioned earlier, extensive stakeholder involvement increases the level of oversight for the evaluation project, improves its credibility, and increases the likelihood that the evaluation results will be used. As in previous components of conducting the evaluation, stakeholders play a critical part in designing the evaluation. They are important contributors to

■ Framing and selecting the appropriate evaluation questions

■ Identifying the concepts that are critical to measure

■ Developing and executing the evaluation plan

In this participatory evaluation and empowerment model, all members of the evaluation team advance their knowledge and skills during critical thinking and decision-making processes that go on. It is important for the team to

■ Choose the most important and appropriate evaluation questions for making decisions and improving effectiveness

■ Balance the need to assess implementation and process with the need to assess effectiveness and outcomes

■ Select the most appropriate measures, approaches, and tools, taking into consideration the expertise of the group, time frames, and the budget

CREATING AND MAINTAINING EFFECTIVE PARTNERSHIPS

Effective partnership development is as critical for program evaluation as it is for the outside community and its institutions. Panet-Raymond (1992) suggests that partnerships are successful when they have

■ Established power and legitimacy (and strive for an equitable relationship)

■ Well-defined missions, a clear sense of purpose, and common goals

■ Respect for each other, and clear expectations of the partnership

■ Commitment to the partnership approach

■ Open-mindedness, patience, respect, and sensitivity

In addition, partners benefit from having written agreements clarifying objectives, responsibilities, methods, and approaches for the partnership and its work (Panet-Raymond, 1992).

Establishing and maintaining healthy partnerships during evaluations can be both difficult and time consuming, yet the partnership is critical for participatory evaluation and must be nurtured (Fitzpatrick, Sanders, & Worthen, 2004). Suggestions for nurturing the partnership include the following (see Figure 4.3):

■ Prepare evaluation sponsors and other stakeholders by framing evaluation in an understandable way.

■ Encourage and support stakeholder participation and teamwork.

■ Plan sufficient time for the evaluation process.

■ Encourage and support active participation of stakeholders.

■ Ensure adequate communication across the group.

FIGURE 4.3.   *Nurturing Strong Evaluation Partnerships*

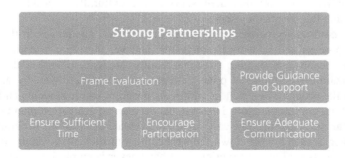

Stakeholder support and participation is enhanced through providing multiple opportunities for input during the evaluation process. Such input occurs when stakeholders have wide and varied experiences, knowledge, and skills, and when they have been provided with appropriate and timely training. Constructive critique and negotiation are also important strategies (Fitzpatrick et al., 2004).

In successful groups, members rely on and involve each other in planning and decision-making. Achieving a common goal also requires that the group members possess task-related and positive socioemotional behaviors (Belcher, 1994). Task-related behaviors include providing opinions, evaluations, suggestions, and information or asking for suggestions, direction, opinions, or analysis. Positive socioemotional behaviors are showing solidarity, helping, showing satisfaction, laughing, and joking. In contrast, negative socioemotional behaviors are disagreeing, withholding help, showing tension, showing antagonism, defending or asserting oneself while deflating another's status (Belcher, 1994) and will, over time, undermine team spirit and cooperation.

Effective communication is critical for maintaining effective group dynamics. Such communication includes listening carefully and attentively to what other people are saying. It may mean paraphrasing to ensure understanding of what is being said. It also includes being attentive to body language and how it affects the interaction. When we look at the person we are talking to, we indicate that we are listening. Looking away or walking away indicates that we are not listening and more importantly we are not interested in what is being said. The approaches that are selected for communication are important and must take into consideration culture, reading levels, and language preferences.

Developing cultural competence to work with groups and communities is a lifelong process that requires examining one's own biases. It requires avoiding the use of stereotypes and recognizing that within cultures there are also individuals who may embody some but not all aspects of the culture that is being defined. Often we consider Hispanic culture to be monolithic and ignore the fact that people of many different countries make up the Hispanic population. Culturally, there are some significant differences, although there are also many similarities. Likewise, we may assume that all Blacks are the same; however, Blacks may come from a variety of continents and countries, each with its own cultures, beliefs, and practices although there is clearly some commonality across groups. Cross-cultural communication and developing cultural competence require that we also understand that within each cultural group there are social networks that support and protect its people. As societies change and people of different cultures access services, good cross-cultural communication becomes even more important, and evaluators have the responsibility to ensure that their services are culturally appropriate for both the organization and the clients they serve.

Both the community partners and the evaluators face challenges in the community-engagement process and in working in teams, and yet there are opportunities to learn through it all. I teach an evaluation class that requires students to work with a community-based organization to conduct a preassessment evaluation followed by an appropriate evaluation of the program or a project within the program where students build their skills for cross-cultural communication. The students develop an evaluation plan in consultation with the organization and in some cases go on to evaluate a part of the program. At the end of the semester, students write down their reflections of their involvement in the project. One of the students said of the experience, "I have never been put into a situation like the community-evaluation project that required me to use critical thinking and problem-solving skills for a variety of situations—whether it was communication problems we were having or problems with developing our suggested tool for our organization to use."

The community partners may face challenges of their own. Another student in her reflections made the following observation: "I was expecting these organizations and coaches to be very welcoming and excited about our work for their project. But, instead, I realize that maybe some organizations are a little fearful of what these evaluations will expose about how the organization is functioning. I try to put myself in their shoes, and think how I would react if I learned I wasn't doing what I claimed or what I was supposed to be doing, and, all along, I thought I was doing a great job. That would be very difficult."

Dealing with these challenges is part of the process of developing an evaluation team, cross-cultural communication, and competency. Using the participatory process of evaluation allows the team to take the time to help stakeholders understand the process and the merits of conducting an evaluation. It also allows time for issues to be resolved. The challenges of engaging stakeholders in the evaluation process are offset by the gains that are achieved that make the team stronger and ensure a useful product.

Think About It!

Suppose your proposal to conduct an evaluation in another country is funded and you have to develop an evaluation team and conduct an evaluation in that country. What particular cultural differences would inform your thinking? How would your understanding of culture and working with stakeholders influence your thinking and your work? How for example would you react to being asked to name one of your country partners as a CoPi on your request for IRB approval to undertake the research? Describe your immediate and then your delayed considered response? What self-talk did you need to get to the delayed considered response, if different?

THE EVALUATION PLAN

The culmination of the planning for evaluation process is the development of the evaluation plan that will guide the evaluation. The evaluation plan is a formal document that describes in clear language what the plan is for the evaluation. It is usually presented in draft form as part of the negotiation of the contract for the evaluation. The evaluation plan opens with a description of the problem and the attempts to address it by the organization or agency. It describes the precursor to program planning, the community assessment with supporting epidemiological profiles. It describes the program and a logic model depicting the program as well as it is understood at the time of the contract. The proposal to undertake the evaluation provides an outline of the evaluation design, the action plans, and time lines, the data analysis plan, and the strategy for reporting the results of the study.

(Continued)

(Continued)

In a recent study, the author was asked to provide what was called an inception report, which was in effect an evaluation plan. The plan was based on the guidelines contained in the request for proposals (RFP) that was advertised in the local paper. A subsequent meeting with the funders of the study clarified the expectations of the research study. The table of contents for the inception report contained similar items to what would appear in an evaluation plan (see Figure 4.4). The appendix contained copies of all the tools that were intended to be used for the evaluation. This level of detail may not always be required in an evaluation plan but the evaluation team must be guided by the needs of the contractor. It is important to be clear about the requirements of the board, organization, or individual funding the study at the outset to avoid misunderstanding and risk not being able to fulfill the contract. In this agency commissioned evaluation study, providing the extensive amount of information to the funders early on meant that logistics could be discussed in very real terms. The discussion resulted in adjustments to the time line for the study from 21 days to three months and the negotiation for the provision of logistical resources beyond what had been originally proposed. The agency commissioning the study was much more familiar with the terrain for the evaluation as well as the needed logistics than the evaluation team. Although the time line changed and the data collection team expanded from 2 researchers to 6, the terms of reference and the budgeted amount for the evaluation remained the same.

FIGURE 4.4. *Table of Contents for an Inception Report*

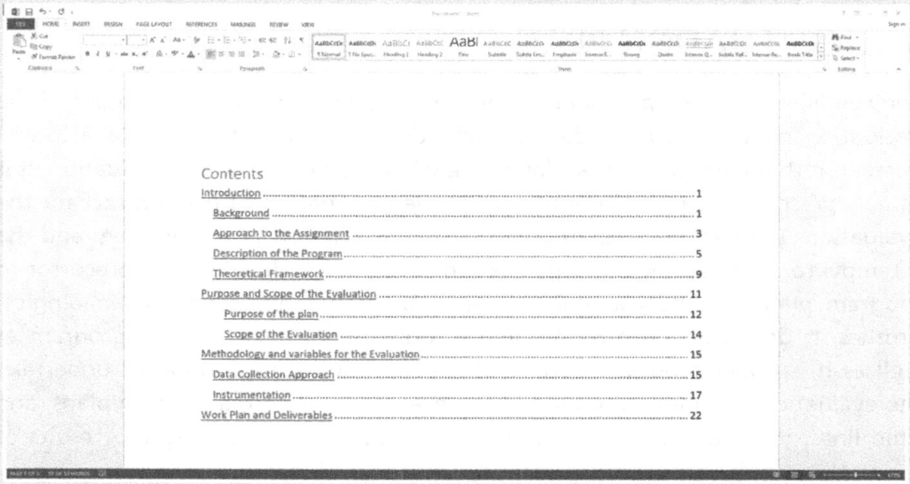

Contents

Introduction 1
Background 1
Approach to the Assignment 3
Description of the Program 5
Theoretical Framework 9
Purpose and Scope of the Evaluation 11
Purpose of the plan 12
Scope of the Evaluation 14
Methodology and variables for the Evaluation 15
Data Collection Approach 15
Instrumentation 17
Work Plan and Deliverables 22

SUMMARY

- Creating effective partnerships for evaluation requires effective cross-cultural communication; participation and teamwork; shared goals; and open-mindedness, patience, and sensitivity.

- Initiatives go through stages of development that determine the type of evaluation and the design of the evaluation. Process and outcome are types of evaluation that occur at different stages.

- The evaluation process includes specifying the initiative, the inputs, the outputs, and the outcomes that define the success of the intervention and specifying the methodology for collecting the information (data), for analyzing the data, and for disseminating the results so they are useful to the stakeholders.

- The type of evaluation is determined by the stage of development of the program. In the early stages of development and within the first year or two, a formative or process evaluation is required. After the program is fully implemented and stable, an outcome evaluation is generally undertaken. An outcome evaluation may be complemented by a process evaluation.

- Establishing and maintaining healthy partnerships can be both difficult and time consuming, yet partnerships are critical for participatory evaluation and must be nurtured.

- The evaluation standards put forward by the Joint Commission on Standards for Educational Evaluation are utility, feasibility, propriety, and accuracy.

- Ethical evaluations require that all respondents give informed consent for research, and that participant's privacy, confidentiality, and safety are protected at all times.

FIGURE 4.5. *Valuable Take-Aways*

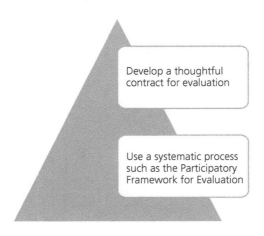

DISCUSSION QUESTIONS AND ACTIVITIES

1. Imagine you are the executive director of a large, not-for-profit organization that has multiple initiatives and has just received new funding for up to 5 years to address a single public health problem. You would like an evaluation plan developed for your organization. You do not have the expertise to carry out an evaluation yourself, but you know what needs to be done. What would be the advantages and disadvantages of hiring an external evaluator versus asking the person in your organization who is in charge of the data center to conduct the evaluation of the new initiatives?

2. Discuss the implications of using the standards of evaluation practice in developing an evaluation plan for a program offered by a community-based, youth-serving, minority organization with limited funding.

3. When planning for evaluation, what ethical challenges would you consider are important to address. Describe one ethical challenge and how as an evaluator you would address it.

KEY TERMS

accuracy
contract
cost-benefit or cost-effectiveness analysis
cross-cultural communication
evaluation plan
evaluation standards
feasibility
formative evaluation
hypothesis
impact evaluation

inputs
outcome evaluation
outcomes
outputs
process evaluation
propriety
inception report
utility

CHAPTER

DESIGNING THE EVALUATION

PART 1: DESCRIBING THE PROGRAM OR POLICY

LEARNING OBJECTIVES

- Explain why it is necessary to have a systematic process for describing a program.
- Describe the components involved in describing a program or policy.
- Explain the importance of a logic model in program and policy evaluation.

The participatory model for evaluation (Figure 5.1) described in this book identifies a four-step approach for ensuring a systematic evaluation:

Step 1: Design the evaluation.

Step 2: Collect the data.

Step 3: Analyze and interpret the data.

Step 4: Report the findings.

This chapter focuses on Step 1: Design the evaluation, which discusses in detail the background to the evaluation—the basis for the evaluation. Program or policy evaluation by definition requires that there is a program or policy initiative that has been implemented and there is a requirement to determine if it has been implemented appropriately and if it has an effect on the beneficiaries. It is the foundation for the evaluation. Too often we are tempted to begin an evaluation, or at least begin to frame the evaluation questions without first understanding the initiative to be evaluated. It saves a considerable amount of time if the first couple of questions that are asked are, "What is the program or policy that is to be evaluated?," "How did it come about?," "What does it intend to achieve?" The program or policy may be evaluated in a number of different settings where public health interventions take place, which include

- Community and faith-based programs that provide services across the public health and health promotion spectrum

- Hospital-based programs

FIGURE 5.1. *The Participatory Model for Evaluation: Design the Evaluation*

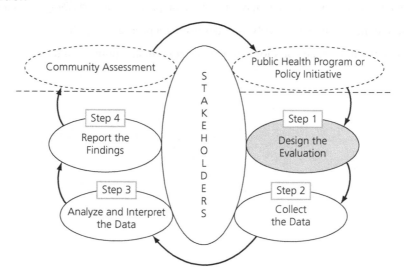

- Social justice and other rights-based programs

- Health education programs

- Organizations that provide services to address public health problems

- Healthy communities and those that strive to be healthy

The setting will often determine the focus of the evaluation because the questions asked of a community-based program may be somewhat different from questions asked of an organization. A program offered at a community-based organization, a hospital, or a school may serve only a small segment of the affected community, and the major questions asked are, "How are the persons served affected by the program?"

With health-related policy, however, these questions may reflect changes at the jurisdictional local, regional, national, or international levels. For example, health policies have included those to increase access to health insurance for children and low-income families, policies that have heavy penalties attached for drinking and driving, policies that require that children be restrained in cars, and policies to reduce speeds of traffic in built-up areas and on highways to reduce the risk of disability and death from road-traffic accidents. In recent years, that has been a focus on health in all policies, an initiative to ensure that all agencies consider the impact of policies on the health of individuals across multiple sectors. These policies have resulted in more green space in engineering designs and more sidewalks in road construction, as well as traffic-calming devices in neighborhoods. Each of these policies provides opportunities for evaluation. The process for conducting the evaluation, whether it is evaluating a program or a policy, is the same. Designing the evaluation begins with understanding and describing the initiative being evaluated. The chapter focuses on this first and important step of designing the evaluation—describing the program or policy.

It is important that the program or policy is well described and understood by each member of the evaluation team as well as stakeholders. This chapter explains how to describe the public health initiative. There are possibly two critical questions at this point: (1) Is there a project document that describes the initiative's planning, development, and implementation? and (2) What do stakeholders and especially those who are closely aligned with the program know about the development, planning, and initiation of the program? The role of stakeholders is critical here since many public health programs are developed with no guiding documents. They are often conceived and developed but with no formal record of any data that formed the basis for the development, clear goals and objectives, or understanding of the relationship among the community assessment, theoretical frameworks, goals, and objectives. However, the history associated with the program or policy's development often resides with the stakeholders, so the more they are involved at this stage in the process, the more information can be gathered. Programs change over time and that historical perspective, which might frame those changes in the context of political, social, and economic changes, is helpful in understanding the trajectory of the program, its strengths, and weaknesses.

In addition to discussing the program with stakeholders, all the available project documents are reviewed to ensure that the evaluation team gets insights into the initiative's planning, development, and implementation. The evaluators are especially keen to understand the details around the various processes.

Describing the initiative's resources and activities, its goals and objectives, its development, and its context allows stakeholders and the evaluation team to reach a common understanding so that appropriate research questions can be asked and answered (Figure 5.2). The importance of carefully describing a program to be evaluated is often not fully appreciated by new and seasoned evaluators alike. An initiative needs to be described for three reasons. First, describing the program provides evaluators with an understanding of the program's ability to produce the changes that are outlined in the goals and objectives (Centers for Disease Control and Prevention, 1999). Second, clear descriptions of programs are required for meeting the program evaluation standards of utility and accuracy (Joint Committee on Standards for Educational Evaluation et al., 1994). Third, describing the initiative supports the development of recommendations at the end of the process. The evaluators have an opportunity to develop both a working logic model, one that reflects the reality of the program and one that is based on the literature and best practices.

Policy development and implementation may look somewhat different from program development and implementation. As in the development of a program, the context in which the policy is developed is important, as is the process. However, the policy content is the primary driver of the changes to achieve stated goals and objectives, whereas in programs it is the activities that drive the changes. Another significant difference between programs and policies is the fact that programs are more likely to target small segments of the population, whereas policies are intended to apply across the whole population. The stakeholders involved in the process are individuals, groups, and organizations that have an interest in the policy being developed and implemented, most often based on a needs assessment using local and national data. In some cases, however, policy development may be initiated by a significant singular event that has strong advocates and, in the case of public policy, finds strong support within political corridors. The three major components (context, process, and stakeholders) in the development of health policy form a complex set of interrelationships.

THE CONTEXT OF THE INITIATIVE

During this stage of the evaluation process, the program or policy's context is described in several ways: The organization's mission; the social, political, and economic environment in which the program or policy is developed and implemented; the organizational structure and resources; the relationship of the project, program, or policy initiative to the organization;

FIGURE 5.2.   *Components for Reviewing the Program or Policy Initiative*

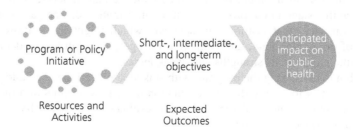

FIGURE 5.3. *Components for Understanding the Context of the Initiative*

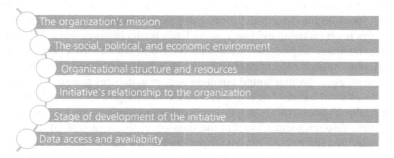

- The organization's mission
- The social, political, and economic environment
- Organizational structure and resources
- Initiative's relationship to the organization
- Stage of development of the initiative
- Data access and availability

the stage of development of the initiative; and the access and availability of data for the evaluation. See Figure 5.3.

An organization or agency that embarks on a public health program should have a mission defined by a mission statement. The mission statement is the first component in understanding the organization's motives and intentions for focusing on a specified population and provides a basis for understanding the context in which the initiative is developed and implemented.

The Mission Statement

The mission statement defines in clear terms what the organization sets out to do. One example is the mission statement of a service organization that intends to eliminate social and economic barriers to good health. According to its mission statement, it intends to accomplish this through policy change and evidence-based initiatives. Its approach to achieving this is through collaboration with communities and organizations.

EXAMPLE

MISSION STATEMENT

"To eliminate social and economic barriers to good health through policy change and evidence-based initiatives by collaboration among communities and organizations."

Although this mission statement is very clear, it does not tell us which population specifically it will serve. It leaves us believing it might be a national organization that will work with any and all communities wherever it is expedient for it to put down its roots. It also does not specify which social and economic barriers to good health it will focus on, leaving the door open for it to pursue a range of options and opportunities. A mission statement does not have to be specific. A mission statement only provides information about the values the organization has. In this case, the critical and expressed value is one that sees as significant a focus on the determinants of health, rather than the individual's behavior and one that prides itself on using evidence as the basis for its interventions. Another example of a mission statement may be this one from a ski resort, which reads, "Provide affordable, educational, and outdoor recreational activities in a safe, clean, and inviting environment for people of all ages through sound business and management practices." Mission statements can be as short as one line and a few words— "Empowering children and families to achieve lifelong successes"—to one that occupies many lines on a page. The common thread that runs through them all is that the mission of the organization does not change, even if the activities and patrons do. The experience of the author has been that many organizations do not have a clearly articulated mission and one role of the evaluation team may be to help them define a mission that reflects their values and their intent such that they have a basis on which to develop future programs.

Think About It!

If you were to develop an organization to serve a population of your choice, what would your mission statement be? Write down a mission statement that reflects your values and intent as a public health professional to make the world a better place.

THE SOCIAL, POLITICAL, AND ECONOMIC ENVIRONMENT

The second component to understanding the context is to understand the cultural, social, political, and economic environment in which it operates. The climate defines what the organization can and cannot do and the level of support it has for the initiatives it wants to offer. For example, in a low-income neighborhood with poor social and economic conditions, it may not be expedient to offer programs that may be politically unpopular since in a poor political climate and one that is less than supportive of this population funding for existing programs may be curtailed. The economic context and, therefore, current and past funding levels may shed light on the initiative's local and national support and its long-term sustainability. Other aspects of the organization's cultural, social, political, and economic climate include its demographic profile and the profile of beneficiaries, budget, assets, and the resources available to it and to the community at large for addressing the problem. In an effort to generate financial resources to ensure the sustainability of programs beyond the funded three- to five-year period of a grant, individuals are required to pay for their participation albeit it at discounted fees. However, in communities where disposable incomes are low, families must choose between participating in a program for which they may not value or understand the benefits in the short term and using those valuable resources for more practical and impending needs. The lack of economic resources in a community in which the program is likely to have a long-term impact on the individuals' health may very well be undermined and over time may no longer be available. As an evaluator, it is important to understand the constraints of the program, an understanding that will also guide framing and proposing recommendations at the end of the evaluation.

THE ORGANIZATIONAL STRUCTURE AND RESOURCES

The third component to understanding the context is to understand the organization's structure. Generally, a nonprofit organization has a board of directors that oversees its programming and provides recommendations for the organization's direction. Public agencies might have advisory bodies that provide recommendations. Other parts of an organization's structure are the staffing arrangements and the responsibilities of critical staff like the executive director and other directors and senior managers. In order to understand an organization's structure, the evaluation team can create an organizational chart (Figure 5.4 is an example) showing lines of authority. The figure presents the structure of a nonprofit organization overseen by a board of directors; the organization, with 35 staff members, has five funded initiatives. The executive director supervises four directors, one each for policy initiatives, finance, programs, and public relations. The office of the director of finance has an accounts manager, and the program coordinator reports directly to the director of programs. The program and volunteer staff are supervised by the program coordinator.

Understanding staffing arrangements includes understanding work responsibilities and the time and effort it takes to implement the activities of the initiative. In this first step of designing the evaluation, describing the staffing structure supports process evaluation, which assesses the resources available for the development of program and policy initiatives as well as to implement and oversee programs. The more staff members there are available with direct responsibility to the policy or program initiative, the more likely it is able to fulfill its mandate. Adequate staffing levels may also mean that an internal evaluator may be available who can join the evaluation team. In small organizations and agencies with only a few staff members, many tasks get left undone and resources for monitoring and

FIGURE 5.4.   *Organizational Chart*

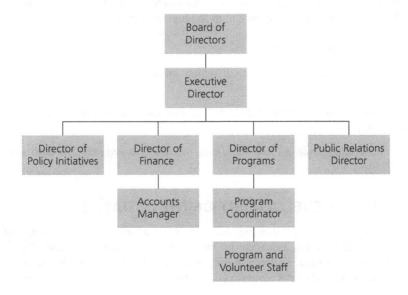

evaluation are the least likely to be supported. Describing the organizational structure and the allocation of staff is an important component of identifying human resources and the programs' ability to get to outcomes. It is important to assess the training and preparation of the program staff and their capacity to undertake the initiative.

In addition to the organizational structure and human resources for program planning, development, and implementation, financial stability and an established physical infrastructure are critical to well implemented and sustainable projects. The organization's ability to secure grants, as well as to oversee the administration of moneys allocated, increases the organization's credibility and provides a base from which additional project-related funding can be built. If the organization struggles to secure funding and staff from one year to the next, the likelihood of achieving its goals and objectives may also be threatened.

THE INITIATIVE AND ITS RELATIONSHIP TO THE ORGANIZATION

The fourth component to understanding the context is to understand the initiative's structure and its relationship to the organization. So, for example, if the initiative that is being evaluated is one of three programs, then it is important to understand how they relate to each other, specifically with regard to staff-time distributions, supervision, and funding. Although each program must relate to the overall mission of the organization, it may be that the initiatives bear little relationship to each other. For example, using the mission statement we reviewed earlier—"To eliminate social and economic barriers to good health through policy change and evidenced-based initiatives by collaboration among communities and organizations"—the initiatives that the organization elects to support may have very different outcomes and may require a large number of staff stretched across the organization, but a staff with little synergy and, therefore, a loss of opportunities for cost-sharing and maximizing benefits. The evaluation team should be careful to understand how the staff are distributed and how they contribute to individual projects and programs but specifically how they relate to each other.

The team of evaluators study

■   The characteristics of the initiative, which make it appropriate for addressing the problem.

■   The extent to which the intervention is compatible with other programs within the organization.

■   How the initiative reflects and builds on the assets, strengths, and attributes of the organization.

THE STAGE OF DEVELOPMENT OF THE INITIATIVE

The fifth component in understanding the context is understanding the stage of development of the initiative and assessing its role in program implementation. Public health programs mature over time, so knowing the maturity of the initiative helps the evaluator understand the likelihood of the program getting to outcomes. A more mature program may have already worked through the theory of change sufficiently for a more robust outcome evaluation to be conducted compared to a new program, which may not have been in place long enough to show any program effects or identify unintended consequences. Earlier stages of the program would benefit from process evaluation when outcome evaluation would be inappropriate. The stage of the initiative will often define the level of resources available as well as the level to which components of the program have been offered often enough so that a level of mastery can been achieved by staff implementing the program, thereby ensuring consistency across beneficiaries.

Policies that are enacted and implemented may also show changes over time as policy-makers tweak the program to ensure it achieves the intended changes in the population. It is often the case that public health professionals and advocates would rather wait until they can get a good bill, rather than risk implementing a bill that is unable to address the problem fully. For example, advocates in Kentucky are reluctant to push for a statewide smoking ban given that there is considerable resistance from various segments of the population and they fear having a bill with too many exclusions. The alternative approach to a statewide bill is to have bills developed county-by-county with the hope that, when sufficient counties have smoking bans, the statewide ban is more likely to be sustainable. Although this might affect the extent to which the state will achieve the health outcomes associated with lower smoking levels, an evaluator needs to understand and take into consideration the maturity of a smoking ban policy.

DATA ACCESS AND AVAILABILITY

The sixth component to understanding the context is to understand how data are collected and how they are utilized to draw conclusions within the organization. An organization that does not have access to data and does not have a management information system (MIS) is also unable to provide data for monitoring and evaluation. To evaluate a program or policy, it is important that data are available—data collected at the baseline and also data collected periodically since the initiative was started. Evaluators need to know the type of data, the quality and quantity of data, and the level of sophistication of the data-management systems. The level of sophistication may range from simple—a paper system with scratch pads for case histories—to sophisticated, in which all data are entered into a database by each member of staff allowing for integrated summaries of individual's participation and outcomes. The more advanced the system is, the more technically complex monitoring the organization can undertake.

THE PROGRAM INITIATIVE

Understanding and documenting the program or policy's justification, resources, activities, outputs, and outcomes is the most important component of this step. The program or policy logic model depicts the resources, activities, outputs, and outcomes in a graphic way and forms the basis for a shared understanding of the program components. It forms the foundation for the development of the evaluation process. The logic model clearly articulates the initiative's theory of change, which may be tested in the evaluation. The next two sections discuss these components for program and policy initiatives.

Justification for the Program

In justifying the initiative's development, the extent to which the public health problem affects sectors of the population and the factors that contribute to its existence at the individual, community, organizational, and policy level are assessed. During this phase of describing the program, the administrators and staff are asked about the motivations for the program. These justifications can sometimes be found in the organization's reports of community assessments or other documents. The results of the community assessments may be published in agency, local, state, or national reports, and may have been used for program or policy development. In some organizations, little is documented so convening staff, may be the best chance of finding out about the program. Where documents are available, an extensive literature review may turn up peer-reviewed publications and reports related to the community. On the other hand, there might be stakeholders in the community who were involved with any community assessments that were undertaken or who can provide names of individuals or organizations who might be able to provide some insight. The community assessment is a prerequisite for developing programs and policies. In Chapter 2, we learned that the community assessment determines the extent and magnitude of the problem among specific populations, the risk factors associated with the problem. It depicts the actual needs and resources of the community, and it provides a focus for developing the intervention. In addition to reviewing any documents provided by the program and stakeholders, the team reviews existing data and reports and conducts a review of epidemiological studies published in the scientific literature.

The literature review extends the program review to determine the incidence, prevalence, morbidity, disability, and mortality rates associated with the problem in the nation, in the state, similar communities as well as the community of interest. Such a review provides an opportunity to compare the program being evaluated with others that are similar and are based on similar population profiles. The literature review also provides information on the behavioral, social, cultural, and environmental risk factors and conditions associated with the public health problem. It describes in narrative form the nature of the problem, those who are affected by it, and why, how, and when they were affected, and it provides guidance for assessing the risk and protective factors associated with the problem at the individual, interpersonal, and environmental levels and also the social determinants of health that influence the problem. It provides the justification for the program or policy. The review of the scientific literature in this step of describing the program forms part of the introduction in the evaluation report described in Chapter 11.

The literature review answers the following questions:

- How is the problem described in the literature?

- What are behavioral and environmental risk factors associated with the problem?

- What are the characteristics of the population as defined by age, gender, ethnicity, socioeconomic conditions, and culture associated with the problem?

- How has the problem been addressed in other jurisdictions?

The Program

The most important constituent of the evaluation is the initiative itself since the focus of the evaluation is usually the initiative and the extent to which the initiative causes changes in the beneficiaries in order to address a public health problem that has been identified. It is important to understand the initiative and how it intends to get to outcomes.

The Program's Logic Model

Describing the program or policy for evaluation means that the theory of the change is clearly understood. The theory of change is the logic behind the *program* that essentially describes the assumptions that are made about how the inputs and program activities will result in expected outcomes. See Chapter 3 for a more detailed explanation of the theory of change. The logic model is the pictorial depiction of the theory of change, which is created during this stage of the process if one has not already been developed by the program developers.

The logic model for the *program*

- Is a tool to facilitate stakeholder insight and reflection about the program

- Maps a program during the planning or evaluation phase

- Documents program resources, activities, and external factors that might affect implementation

- Shows the program developers' chain of reasoning and provides a process for understanding the program's activities and how they link to the outcomes

- Is a tool to inform monitoring and the development of benchmarks to focus the evaluation

- Provides opportunities to discuss the program's strengths and weaknesses

Drawing or reviewing an explicit logic model as part of the process of describing the program is a precursor to deciding on the evaluation questions since it illustrates the relationships between program elements and expected changes (Figure 5.5). Describing the program provides the foundation for the process and outcome evaluation questions, but describing the program or policy especially provides direction for process evaluation as it discusses the resources available, the level of implementation, and the associated outputs. It is important to recognize and allow for the stage of development of the program during this process. It may also be necessary during the course of the evaluation to modify the logic model based on a changing program. This is most likely if the evaluator is involved in the program through its implementation. If the evaluation team is called in right at the end, the likelihood of changes is small.

In addition to the logic model described by the documents and stakeholders the evaluators may draw a logic model that reflects an ideal chain of reasoning for achieving the program's outcomes based on the literature. The logic model must also depict external factors such as social, economic, political, physical, or other factors that might affect the

FIGURE 5.5.   *Tips for Drawing a Logic Model*

- Start with the program in its simplest form.
- Limit the number of words in the diagram.
- Show only the most critical relationships among the resources, activities, outputs, and outcomes.
- Include external factors that influence implementation or the achievement of outcomes.
- Show a date for when the logic model was developed.

program's implementation (Figure 5.6). Another aspect of describing the program is understanding what steps are taken by the program to mitigate any of the potential barriers to the program's getting to outcomes. The logic model can be developed in sets so that each set of drawings represents a chain of reasoning. This is especially important if the program is made up of a collection of projects that may not contribute to the same outcomes.

Questions may be asked in the course of the evaluation to provide an overall understanding of the context of the program and its fit within the organization, the larger community, and public health. Questions may include

- How does the initiative reflect and build on the assets, strengths, and attributes of the community?

- To what extent does the intervention complement or build on existing programs within the larger community?

- To what extent is the initiative developmentally and culturally appropriate for the intended population?

- To what extent does this initiative form part of a synergistic whole and contribute to the community's overall public health goal?

In developing a program implementation plan and the subsequent logic model, program developers will generally start with identifying the need for the program and the outcome objectives, and, working backward, identify activities to achieve the objectives and then identify resources. In designing the evaluation, however, the process goes the other way. The evaluation reviews the logic model first and then the resources devoted to the program, followed by the program activities and outputs, before the assessment is made of the

FIGURE 5.6. *Basic Framework for Completing a Logic Model*

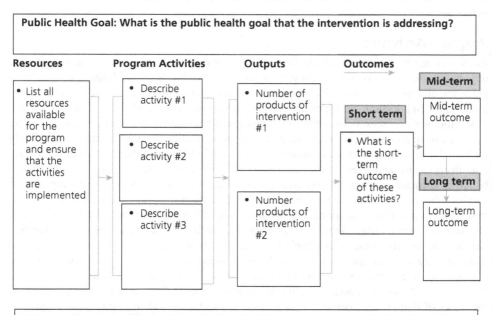

Public Health Goal: What is the public health goal that the intervention is addressing?

Resources — **Program Activities** — **Outputs** — **Outcomes**

Resources:
- List all resources available for the program and ensure that the activities are implemented

Program Activities:
- Describe activity #1
- Describe activity #2
- Describe activity #3

Outputs:
- Number of products of intervention #1
- Number products of intervention #2

Short term
- What is the short-term outcome of these activities?

Mid-term
Mid-term outcome

Long term
Long-term outcome

What are the external factors identified by the literature or the stakeholders that affect program implementation?

outcomes and their effects on the beneficiaries of the program. This logic also assumes a process evaluation has been conducted before the outcome evaluation is carried out.

The Program's Resources

The program's resources depicted by the logic model are those resources that are specific to the implementation of the program and getting to outcomes. They are part of the chain of logic that the model describes. The resources may include but are not limited to funding allocated to the program development and implementation, training materials, space, staff, volunteers for implementing the program, and logistics for ensuring the program is implemented as planned, and so forth. The evaluation is designed to assess the program inputs in quality and quantity. The quantity of the resources influences the extent to which program activities are instituted and implemented. For example, if a program's implementation relies on the provision of transportation for low income individuals with disability, but no provision is made for transportation either in the form of a fully functioning service, a participant collection mechanism, or the provision of fuel or vouchers for using independent transportation, then participation in a center's activities may be impossible, resulting in their not being able to benefit from the services and, therefore, the organization is unable to achieve the stated outcomes. The lack of adequately trained staff will also undermine the program. The assessment of the resources in the design of the evaluation may also lead to assessing the relative cost of one intervention compared to another intervention with similar outcomes.

Program Activities

Activities are the primary vehicle for programs and policies to achieve their goals and objectives. Activities may fall into one or more of the five levels of influence to achieve behavior changes that result in improved health of the individual and reach population level goals. In addition, activities are selected based on theoretical underpinning that provide guidance for how behavioral outcomes can be achieved. For example, in reducing the rates of diabetes in a population, based on best-practice models, activities will likely include the following strategies: improving self-care behaviors at the individual level; support from family and peers at the interpersonal level; organizations that provide comprehensive, culturally appropriate, adequate, accessible services; and community wrap-around services that promote and provide access to healthy nutrition and exercise through developing and supporting appropriately supportive social norms from the cradle to the grave. Organizational and public policies must support and reinforce access to services and opportunities for healthy living. The King's Fund and Nuffield Trust in 2011 defined integrated diabetes care as, "an approach that seeks to improve the quality of care for individual patients, service users, and careers by ensuring that services are well coordinated around their needs." A complex array of activities is also more likely to ensure the prevention of the onset of diabetes as well as the reduction in morbidity and mortality associated with diabetes. The Healthy People 2020 plan emphasizes the need to consider the social determinants of health such as poverty, education, and other social structures as risk factors that must be addressed in order to achieve improvements in health across all populations in addition to the more traditional clinically focused approaches. Ensuring satisfactory behavior change is based on a thorough understanding of the needs of the population and identifying the most important and most changeable factors that control the behavior that is being addressed. These most important and most changeable factors are selected for the intervention that is based on a myriad of strategies that together result in the behavior change over time. The extent to which intervention strategies are tailored to ensure they are culturally, age, and linguistically appropriate must be described since the tailoring of the program increases the likelihood that the strategies will be acceptable, provide appropriate information, and reach the population for whom they are intended. An additional element to report in describing the program for evaluation is dosage. Dosage is essentially the amount of the intervention that the individual receives. It often reflects the level of implementation of the program. Another aspect of the level of implementation, however, is the reach of the program, the extent to which it provided services to the intended population.

Describing the program requires that all aspects of program implementation are clarified including why program activities are believed to lead to expected changes. In describing the activities, the evaluator clarifies who is responsible for implementing various aspects of the program, implementation strategies, and associated outputs. Outputs reflect the immediate products of implementation. For example, outputs may include the number of workshops conducted, playgrounds built, farmer's markets established, units constructed and so on.

Program's Goals and Objectives

The logic model depicts the goal for the program in the box at the top of the model, and the objectives are shown in the outcomes column. (See Figure 5.6.) If there are no clearly defined objectives for the initiative, the evaluators work with stakeholders to clarify expected outcomes for the program and to formulate objectives that can be used for evaluation. The baseline for the objectives may be obtained from the community assessment, the description of similar initiatives in the literature or in reported research. This search may also yield targets for the intervention. Healthy People 2020 (U.S. Department of Health and Human Services, 2010) provides national targets, and the goals defined in the 2030 Agenda for Sustainable Development provide international targets. Without objectives, evaluators are in the dark regarding the targets for evaluation. If necessary, the evaluation team must develop them in consultation with stakeholders.

THE POLICY INITIATIVES

Policy initiatives are subject to the same level of scrutiny and the establishment of the logic of the intervention as programs. It is important to recognize that evaluating policies requires as much attention to detail. It may require a modified list of questions because of the nature of policy initiatives and their goals to reach whole jurisdictions, as well as the more political environment in which they occur. In developing and implementing policies, there are also multiple components with the context being one of them. For the purposes of this book, in describing the policy initiative, it is worth noting here that there are different types of policies often described as little p and big P policies. Little p policies are those policies that are developed and implemented within organizations and big P policies are those that generally refer to jurisdiction-wide policies that affect large populations and involve changing local, state, or national laws. As such, within the five levels of influence of the ecological model p policies occupy a different position than P policies and, therefore, take on different considerations for evaluation. Little p policies are found within the organizational level, whereas P policies are found within the public policy level (Figure 5.7). As a reminder, the ecological model consists of five interacting levels of influence on behavior. These are the individual, interpersonal, organizational, community, and public policy. The public policy domain refers to public health polices such as seat belt use, smoking in public places, and driving and texting. These policies, which are made by county, state, or national lawmakers are expected to provide protections across large populations unlike school board or organizational policies that generally only have an impact on a relatively small group of people.

Political systems and the extent to which lawmakers are open or closed to the need for the policy as well as the likelihood of community engagement in the issues related to the policy will influence the ease with which policy is developed. Implementation of policies is legally mandated ensuring that they reach all those to whom they apply in the organizational or community spheres. A policy initiative includes a varied group of stakeholders with often differing political interests and affiliations, with the media and community-based organizations playing a significant role in training and advocacy.

Although there may be many years of policy development that contain distinct pathways to policy implementation that include research and analysis, training, bill writing, and

FIGURE 5.7.   *The Ecological-Model Framework Showing P and p*

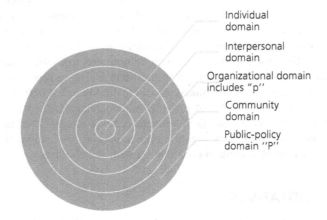

Individual domain

Interpersonal domain

Organizational domain includes "p"

Community domain

Public-policy domain "P"

enactment, this chapter will focus on the evaluation of the policy implementation, providing a parallel description to the process for evaluating programs.

Justification for the Initiative

Passing and subsequently implementing a public health policy follows many years of concerted efforts by a range of stakeholders, but the foundation of the work is the justification of the need for the policy based on a public health problem definition. For example, for many years it has been clearly documented through a series of research projects that tobacco is the most common culprit in the high rates of lung cancer. Lung cancer has been shown to occur both from the direct use of tobacco and in the passive acquisition and inhalation of fumes from others' smoking. Second-hand smoking is now also listed as an important risk factor. Many local efforts that have included projects and programs to help individuals stop smoking have not affected the rates of lung cancer, and it seemed that the best approach would be to have a policy that would limit access to tobacco products and exposure to the harmful effects of smoking. Social, cultural, economic, and political factors have thwarted efforts to enact universal policies to end the growing, production, and distribution of tobacco and its products. Many states have instituted policies, sometimes only in local jurisdictions, to limit exposure, but they have not enacted a statewide ban. In public places across the nation, smoking is severely restricted, and in airports, for example, individuals who want to smoke are relegated to one designated room. Smoking is no longer allowed on any aircraft, and there are advocates who would like to ban smoking in public parks; efforts have been made to achieve this. A recent proposal is to ban smoking in cars to prevent smoke exposure to children. Banning smoking in private homes and individuals' cars may prove harder to do given the expectation of individual rights. The need for a comprehensive policy that has the effect of curtailing smoking and exposure to second hand smoke is justified by the high rates of morbidity and mortality associated with lung and other cancers. Public health advocates are at the forefront of work to have policies that ban smoking.

Policies may also be developed and implemented at the organizational level when a policy might ensure that there is uniform practice. For example, the school board could institute a policy whereby all schools in a district get healthy meals of a specified evidence-based level. This policy may result in other policies—for example, those that specify what foods shall be purchased and even the quality of the food. In one school district, policies surrounded the purchase of local fruits and vegetables. School boards may also institute a policy that all students get no less than 30 minutes of physical activity while they are at school.

Policy Logic Model

The theory of change is the logic behind the implementation of a policy that describes the assumptions that are made about how the inputs, one of which is the policy itself, result in the expected outcomes. In a policy logic model, the policy may also be an output when many of the activities were related to the development and enactment of the policy; the related outcomes coming later. As in the case of a program, the logic model

- Is a tool to facilitate stakeholder insight and reflection

- Maps a policy's implementation and evaluation phase

- Documents resources, activities, and external factors that might affect implementation

- Shows the developers' chain of reasoning and provides a process for understanding the policy implementation activities and how they link to the outcomes

- Is a tool to inform monitoring and the development of benchmarks to focus the evaluation

- Provides opportunities to discuss the policy's strengths and weaknesses

Drawing or reviewing an explicit logic model as part of the process of describing the policy is a precursor to deciding on the evaluation questions since it illustrates the relationships between implementation elements and expected changes. It is important to recognize and understand the stage of development of the policy during this process since enacting a policy does not always mean it is a "good" policy that will result in the public health outcomes that were anticipated. Policy also has the risk of having unintended consequences for some population groups even as it addresses a public health need. Planning an evaluation of policy must consider the unintended as well as the intended outcomes. In addition to the logic model described by the documents and stakeholders, the evaluators may draw a logic model that reflects an ideal chain of reasoning for achieving the policy's outcomes based on the literature or the experience of others. The logic model must also depict external factors such as social, economic, political, or other factors that might affect implementation. Let us work thorough the example of instituting 30 minutes of physical activity across all schools in a school district. In this example, we assume that the policy has already been passed by the school board and it constitutes an input. Implementation across all the 100 schools may differ, but the policy requires that 100,000 students are physically active for at least 30 minutes a day as a primary outcome. See Figure 5.8.

FIGURE 5.8. *Policy Logic Model*

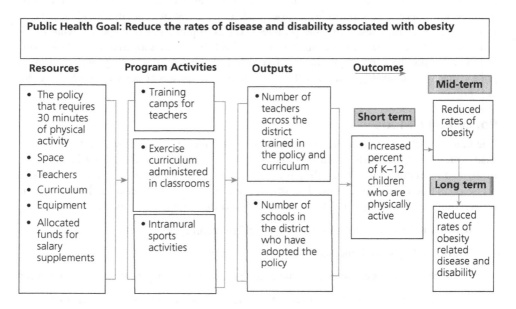

Public Health Goal: Reduce the rates of disease and disability associated with obesity

Resources
- The policy that requires 30 minutes of physical activity
- Space
- Teachers
- Curriculum
- Equipment
- Allocated funds for salary supplements

Program Activities
- Training camps for teachers
- Exercise curriculum administered in classrooms
- Intramural sports activities

Outputs
- Number of teachers across the district trained in the policy and curriculum
- Number of schools in the district who have adopted the policy

Outcomes

Short term
- Increased percent of K–12 children who are physically active

Mid-term
Reduced rates of obesity

Long term
Reduced rates of obesity related disease and disability

External Factors: Resistance to physical activity in schools from law makers; lack of equipment for physical activity; insufficient trained staff; few options for physical activity in school; poor funding of schools

Resources for Policy Implementation

As in the case of implementing programs, implementing policies also relies on the provision of resources. Policies may be enacted and implemented at a number of different levels, across jurisdictions, and within smaller communities of practice. The enactment of policies and their implementation require such resources as personnel for writing the rules where applicable. Once the rules have been written and each aspect of the policy has been explained to ensure appropriate and uniform implementation, it is ready to be implemented. Since policies are applied across large jurisdictions, an important resource is the institutions that are responsible for implementation. For example, the implementation of a partial smoking ban ordinance in bars and restaurants within the jurisdiction required them to create smoke-free areas at possibly some cost to the establishment. However, over time, realizing the importance of also limiting second-hand smoke exposure, the partial ban was converted to a full smoking ban. The evaluation team must consider all the resources that were expended throughout the jurisdiction. As implementation is effected at multiple establishments, inputs are distributed and may vary across sites, but the most important is letting people who are affected by the policy know about it through the use of print, audio, and visual avenues. Costs may be associated with the production of billboards, media messages, interviews and broadcasts, brochures, and books. Expenses associated with the implementation of the policy may also be required at the individual level as in the case of helmets and child restraints laws. Laws required the purchase of helmets for all motorcycle riders and their passengers as well as car seats for children through age 12 years. Going back to our example about physical activity policy in schools, there were considerable resources allocated for the implementation of the policy across the school district to ensure that 100,000 children in grades K–12 get 30 minutes of physical activity. Implementing the policy to achieve the intended changes associated with the policy required space, trained teachers, curriculum to train the teachers, curriculum that are required at the classroom level, equipment, and sufficient funds to provide salary supplements. Given the need to have a range of opportunities for physical activity, access to walking trails, basketball courts, soccer fields, and other individual and team sports must be considered. Unlike programs, because policies affect very large numbers of the population they also require larger amounts of resources.

Activities The theoretical underpinnings of policy initiatives are much less well defined than in programs since policies are a more dictatorial approach to changing behavior to achieve similar public health goals. For example, a policy to reduce carbon emissions relies less on evidence-based strategies as used in programs and instead through a mandate requires manufacturers to meet stated criteria within a specified time period. The implementation of the policy is expected irrespective of the management's attitudes toward the policy or indeed awareness of the public health issue that required the policy. A program approach, which is often the starting point for behavioral outcomes, may have taken into consideration the need to provide extensive amounts of information and supports within a well-designed set of interventions informed by theory. In reviewing the activities, however, for the achievement of policy-related outcomes, care must be taken to identify the activities that lead to the observed changes that complemented the implementation of the policy.

In order to get to outcomes, the school-based policy must be implemented through designated activities that may include training the teachers on the new policy, in-classroom, and out of classroom activities. It would be important to describe the activities across the whole school, classroom by classroom, as well as any out of school activities. Describing the policy implementation across the district will provide indications of its reach and hence its ability to achieve the public health goals. As in evaluating programs, it is the evaluation team that would determine the effectiveness of the implementation of the policy and the extent to which it followed the designated plan.

Activities surrounding reducing the extent to which individuals in the population smoke tobacco products include smoking cessation programs, but policies such as increasing taxes on cigarettes, banning smoking in public places, and reducing access to cigarettes for minors have had a more widespread impact. Increasing educational programs and media messages in and out of school and for the general public has had the effect of increasing information about the dangers of smoking as well as of second hand smoking. Designing an evaluation to assess outcomes related to just one of the policies provides a range of challenges including that of isolating the effects of a single policy. Evaluating the public policy must take into account the myriad of activities that may contribute to achieving the intended goals as policies are more likely to be assessed over periods of 5–10 years. Designing an evaluation for organizational level policy (p) is much less challenging. However, assessing the implementation of the policy may not differ significantly from assessing the implementation of a program given the determination of whether the policy was implemented as planned.

Goals and Objectives The logic model depicts the relationships between the expected public health benefits and the activities for achieving it. The goals and objectives provide the pathways and blue print for the design of the activities. Short-, medium-, and long-term objectives are reviewed in this step to understand the stakeholders' intents. In our example (see Figure 5.7), the three objectives are (1) increase the percentage of students K–12 who are physically active, (2) reduce rates of obesity, and ultimately (3) reduce rates of obesity-related death and disability, the assumption being that increasing physical activity in school will have a lifelong impact on individuals. In reality, in order to increase the percentage of students K–12 who are physically active at each grade of the school may require different approaches to implementation of the policy, whereas the short-, medium-, and long-term outcomes remain the same. It would also mean many years of tracking, although if all the children go to the same district and they all become adults and live in the town, we might be closer to being able to determine the effect of the policy. It would still be challenging, however, to assign any changes in obesity to this one policy. The logic model shows one expected change in the population in the short term with regard to physical activity, yet the logic of the intervention assumes that there are precursors, such as increased knowledge about the value of physical activity and providing environmental opportunities to be physically active both in and out of the classroom. The individual-level activities and environmental level supports provide the necessary climate, which results in a change in attitude before the subsequent change in behavior. Restricting the logic model to only critical pathways keeps it simple and easy to explain to stakeholders. However, in designing of the evaluation, the more proximal objectives may need to be considered.

Criteria for Describing the Initiative A well-developed description of the program or policy is required as a first step to designing the evaluation to allow for the identification of questions for evaluation. The authors Paul and Elder (2012) recommend intellectual standards against which a description of a program or policy can be assessed. These standards require that the document is clear, accurate, precise, and relevant, provides depth of understanding, is logical, provides information that is significant, is fair [objective], and avoids any bias. In addition, the evaluator assesses the quality of the logic model to ensure that it has the information that is required.

The level of detail should be sufficient to create an understanding of the elements of the relationship as well as identify contextual factors that might affect the implementation of activities or the achievement of stated outcomes. When contextual factors are identified (cultural, social, economic, or political), as well as individual factors—such as socioeconomic status, educational level, or ability—wherever possible the program/policy must take steps to minimize their impact on the outcomes through mitigation where possible. Where mitigation does not occur as part of the planning or implementation of the initiative, the effect on the outputs and outcomes must be noted. In describing the program, these mitigating factors and their solutions must be identified. In the future assessment of the program, they may provide helpful insights. Insights might be especially useful in designing the blue print for the intervention following the evaluation.

Think About It!

Consider an organization that you have been involved with. What problem can you think of that has been addressed by putting a policy into place that all staff and/or beneficiaries of that organization must adhere to? In understanding the policy aspect of this section, answer the following questions:

- What was the problem that the policy was intended to affect?

- What were the characteristics of the policy initiative that make it appropriate for addressing the problem?

- What was the training and preparation of the program staff to implement the policy?

SUMMARY

- Describing the initiative provides an understanding of the social, cultural, economic, political, and structural context of the organization. It supports the development of recommendations at the end of the process. Knowing a program's strengths and weaknesses allows the team to develop a feasible and useful evaluation.

- A thorough understanding of the program or policy is achieved only from the multiple perspectives of the program's administrators, funders, staff, and advocates, as well as its current and past participants.

- A logic model provides a tool for stakeholders so that they can have a shared understanding of the initiative, can clarify benchmarks, and can identify strengths and weaknesses.

- Successful program and policy initiatives are comprehensive, meet the needs of the population at risk, are well resourced, and based on theory-based strategies.

FIGURE 5.9.   *Valuable Take-Aways*

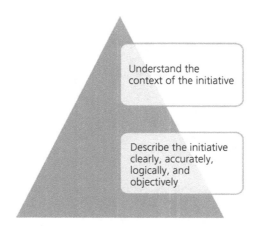

Understand the context of the initiative

Describe the initiative clearly, accurately, logically, and objectively

DISCUSSION QUESTIONS AND ACTIVITIES

1. Describe a public health initiative's organizational, sociocultural, political, and economic contexts. What questions might stakeholders have that would guide an evaluation?

2. Contact a local community-based organization that focuses on policy or the environment. Draw a logic model that provides a graphic representation of the theory of change for one of the organization's initiatives and describe what you learn about the initiative from doing so.

3. Review a description of a program or policy in the peer-reviewed literature and answer the following questions:

    a. Is the description sufficiently clear so you can determine the resources devoted to the program or policy?

    b. Are the goals and objectives clearly stated?

    c. Are the activities to achieve the objectives well defined and sufficient to achieve the stated objective?

    d. What information would you require to meet the criteria put forward by Paul and Elder (2012)?

 KEY TERMS

activities	intellectual standards
logic models	objectives
goals	theory of change

CHAPTER

6

DESIGNING THE EVALUATION

PART 2A: PROCESS EVALUATION

LEARNING OBJECTIVES

- Describe process evaluation and its purposes.
- Describe how to choose process evaluation questions.
- Apply indicators and methods to answer evaluation questions.

One of the earliest definitions of process evaluation was provided by Windsor, Baranowski, Clark, and Cutter (1984, p. 3):

> *Process produces documentation on what is going on in a program and confirms the existence and availability of physical and structural elements of the program.... Process evaluation involves documentation and descriptions of specific program activities—how much of what, for whom, when, and by whom. It includes monitoring the frequency of participation by the target population and is used to confirm the frequency and extent of implementation of selected programs or program elements.*

Chapter 5 discussed the importance of describing the program as the first component of Step 1 of the participatory model of evaluation. The next component in exploring Step 1 is designing the research study (see Figure 6.1). It is the part of the process that identifies what needs to be studied about the program or policy but specifically what questions need to be answered. The next two chapters expand on what it means to design the evaluation. This chapter will focus on how inputs, structures, and processes are assessed in process evaluation, whereas Chapter 7 explores outcome evaluations.

Many have described process evaluation as looking into the "Black Box" and in their discussion of evaluation challenges in the real world, Bamberger, Rugh and Mabry (2012) identify differences in program implementation that may be influenced by local

FIGURE 6.1. *The Participatory Model for Evaluation: Design the Evaluation*

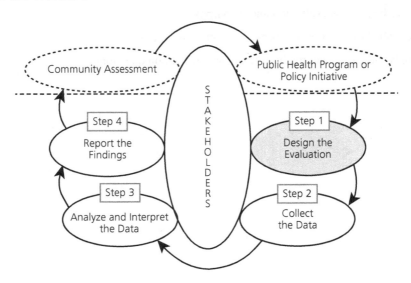

cultural, economic, administrative, and political factors and must be accounted for during the evaluation. In comparison, outcome evaluation assesses the effectiveness of the fully implemented and stabilized initiative on the beneficiaries and measures the extent to which the initiative made a difference to those who were exposed to it. If indeed the primary reason for conducting a process evaluation is to assess if the intervention is operating as expected and for purposes of program development or replicating the intervention, then it is reasonable to assume that a process evaluation must only be conducted when the intervention is fully developed and stable. Formative evaluation occurs to ensure that all the structures and processes are in place for full program implementation.

The basis for designing the evaluation questions is the logic model described in previous chapters. The logic model provides information about the program or policy inputs (resources) and activities and outputs that allow the formulation of questions for a process evaluation.

PURPOSES OF PROCESS EVALUATION

The primary purposes of process evaluation are to assess the extent to which the intervention is implemented with fidelity to the plan and to develop a sufficient understanding of how the intervention works to be able to develop it further or create a blueprint for replication (see Figure 6.2). In addition, process evaluation has been described as

- Documenting and describing program inputs and activities.

- Identifying program implementation, strengths, and weaknesses.

- Disentangling different components of a complex initiative.

- Assessing beneficiaries and their level of participation.

FIGURE 6.2.   *Primary Purposes of Process Evaluation*

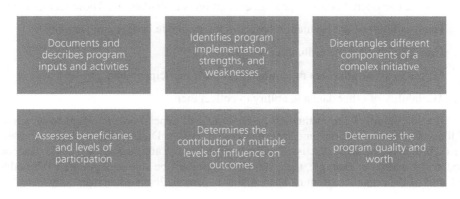

■   Determining the contribution of multiple levels of influence on outcomes.

■   Determining the program quality and worth.

There are other aspects of the evaluation that may have little to do with the implementation of activities or the provision of resources, but which is concerned about social justice. In this case, the evaluation team would assess whether the initiative is being delivered in a fair, equitable, and respectful manner. A set of evaluation questions might include,

■   To what extent are members of the intended population involved in program planning and development?

■   To what extent are members of the intended population participating in the initiative?

■   To what extent are populations who could benefit from the initiative being left out?

The assumptions that underlie the program are also assessed during process evaluation. Assumptions are those elements or conditions associated with a program's implementation that are thought to be available. When they don't occur, the result may be ineffective program or policy delivery and the initiative will not attain its stated outcomes. For example, public health staff at the local health department will educate policymakers in the hopes that they support legislation to ensure equitable access to opportunities for physical activity across the city. A number of assumptions are made. The first is that the staff will have the time and the resources required to do this work in addition to their other project responsibilities and that the policymakers are willing and able to be engaged in the process. In assessing staff responsibilities, it is clear that they do not have time for additional training. Since it is vital that staff are trained and have the time to implement the intervention, it means that the policymakers' education strategy will either not be delivered or will be delivered poorly. Not implementing the program with fidelity violates a critical component for getting to outcomes. Process evaluation that assesses assumptions as well as program implementation saves time and resources in conducting an outcome evaluation. It assesses if the intervention was implemented as planned, and when it was not implemented as planned it provides the reason. It also determines if the plan was flawed to begin with.

In spite of the value associated with conducting a process evaluation, there are factors that must be considered before a process evaluation is embarked on. These factors include

■   The feasibility of the evaluation based on the available budget and personnel

■   Time available for the evaluation process

■   Access to and availability of administrative and participant data

■   Availability of other data and ability to collect them

The likelihood of the evaluation proceeding will depend on the extent to which any of these factors is a serious and insurmountable barrier. During the contract negotiation period these issues can be discussed and where necessary, adjustments are made to accommodate the team. For example, the evaluation team must be able to negotiate a fair budget, and staff of the organization must be available to provide input when necessary.

KEY ISSUES IN PROCESS EVALUATION

There are eight key issues that are explored in answering the overarching question, "Was the program or policy implemented as planned?" The issues are

1. The level of resources allocated and expended (resources, inputs, and outputs)

2. The extent to which intervention activities were accomplished as planned (fidelity)

3. The quality of the intervention components

4. The level of implementation of the activities

5. The effectiveness of administration of the intervention

6. The intensity, reach, and dosage of the intervention

7. The level of participation of the intended audience

8. The effect of assumptions and external factors on implementation

Process evaluation documents whether the initiative is meeting participants' needs, it identifies any barriers to program implementation, it looks at participation satisfaction, and helps to disentangle complex interventions. It provides information that is used to improve intervention activities and operations. In process evaluation, the focus is on understanding the implementation of the initiative at any stage of the program. It asks the question, "Is the program or policy implemented as planned?" A process evaluation focuses on the hows and whys of a program or policy implementation and gets at the questions, "What is being done?" and "What works?" A well-conducted process evaluation precedes an outcome evaluation and is a useful addition to the evaluation should no program or policy effect be detected. Determining the level and scope of the initiative's implementation will provide information with regard to why the program is or is not effective and provide the context for an outcome evaluation. In a study by Jacobson and Wetta (2014) assessing breastfeeding interventions in Kansas, the researchers examined progress toward achieving the goals and objectives and problems that were encountered during program implementation, and they evaluated the measures that were used to assess the impact of the program. This approach expands the use of program evaluation beyond whether the program is implemented as planned, yet it contributes to the knowledge necessary to determine if the program is likely to achieve its stated outcomes.

Outcomes provide the rationale for identifying and implementing activities. For example, if the objective of the intervention is to increase access to fresh fruits and vegetables, then activities that would be required include contacting farmers and organizing farmer's markets. After a specified period, say 6 months after the program was implemented, a process evaluation would assess the progress that has been made toward achieving the objective of the intervention to increase access to fruits and vegetables. The findings of the process evaluation would provide the basis for determining if the intended outcome is met. See Figure 6.3.

FIGURE 6.3.   *Relationship Between Outcome and Activity Objectives and Outputs*

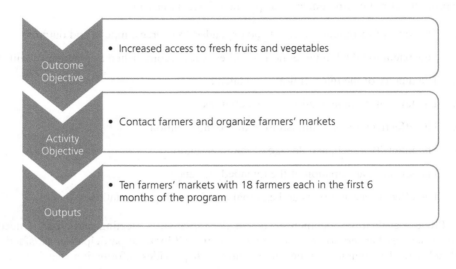

Outcome Objective
- Increased access to fresh fruits and vegetables

Activity Objective
- Contact farmers and organize farmers' markets

Outputs
- Ten farmers' markets with 18 farmers each in the first 6 months of the program

The primary purpose of process evaluation is to determine the hows and whys of a program or policy. Hence, the hows refers to how the program or policy is developed, implemented and operates, whereas the whys try to understand why it does so and what is being done that allows it to produce the changes that occur. The whys get at the resources and activities that allow the program or policy to be implemented and has the effect on the beneficiaries that are expected. The program or policy can only achieve its outcomes if there are activities. There are only activities if there are resources for such activities that explains the why. The program or policy achieves its effects because there are resources devoted to it.

A. The Level of Resources Allocated and Expended (Resources, Inputs, and Outputs)

You can see, I hope, why it is important to assess the resources associated with the logic model because, if there are insufficient or no resources allocated to implementation of the logic model, it stands to reason that the program or policy is likely to fail. Failure of the program then in part is due to a lack of resources and failure to implement the program as intended!

In assessing the resources of a program or policy as in all aspects of the evaluation, the information about the resources budgeted and the resources expended are obtained as part of describing the program. In a skillful organization, the executive director or his/her designee should have this information. The board of directors may also provide this information from existing financial documents and minutes of meetings. Getting financial information is always a little tricky, and the evaluation team must handle this aspect of information retrieval with patience and tact. If the contract for the evaluation required a cost benefit assessment or a comparison between the initiative being evaluated and another to determine which is more cost effective, it would be impossible to do without accurate documentation of financial resources received (grants, donations, and fees) and financial resources expended.

In addition to financial resources, there are human resources that are required, both in quantity and in quality. The number of personnel required to implement a program is determined by the needs of the intervention. One intervention may require 4 well-trained staff members and another may require 20. The goals and objectives of the organization, as well as available financial resources will provide the guidance for this figure. Process evaluation assesses both quality and quantity. For example, in assessing a specialized training on advocacy, it was important to determine the quality of the personnel who were proposed for the training. When their credentials were reviewed, only one person was qualified to be a trainer. The other personnel who were assigned could only assist with the logistics. The trainer had other commitments and there was nobody else. Hence, the workshop could only be offered on alternate weeks.

Assessing quantity of staff is both a matter of documentation as well as determining the extent to which the number of staff is appropriate for the tasks involved. This later information may be assessed from reviewing a task and personnel matrix and making judgments with regard to the match between the task and the personnel based on the experiences of the team. Another means of assessment is in individual or focus group interviews when staff can be asked questions about their work load and ability to meet the objectives and achieve the specified outputs. For example, the project plan may say that 48 workshops be carried out within the year to educate a range of population groups in order to build support for a new policy. Realistically, for 48 workshops to be conducted within a year with an expected participation level of 100 persons per workshop it would require that there are $48 \div 12 = 4$ workshops per month every month of the year. Let's stop for a minute and consider if this is realistic for one person. It may require a team of staff to pull this off. Process evaluation assesses the absolute number of staff who conducted the workshops, the total number of workshops conducted, and it determines if the number assigned to the task is adequate. In this example, with lower numbers of staff than required to ensure that there was a workshop every week, the organization was unable to achieve its activity objective, "by the end of the first year of funding, the staff of the Health for All Coalition will conduct 48 workshops for 100 participants each." The evaluation data showed that instead of a workshop every week, there was a workshop every other week on average and with a lower number of workshops, a lower than expected number of persons trained. To summarize, the lower than anticipated number of trainers affected the number of workshops offered and the number of people trained in advocacy techniques (Table 6.1), which in turn affected the ability of the coalition to achieve its outcome objective to have legislation passed in three years.

There is another set of resources required for this initiative in addition to financial and personnel resources, and those are material resources. The material resources for a training workshop would include such things as adequate space and education and training materials (paper, flip charts, markers, etc.) Process evaluation assesses the

TABLE 6.1. **Activity Objective: Expected Output and Actual Output**

Activity Objective	Expected Output		Actual Output	
	Workshops	Participants	Workshops	Participants
By the end of the first year of funding, the staff of the Health for All Coalition will conduct 48 workshops for 100 participants each.	48	4,800	24	2,200

extent to which these resources are utilized by the training. In the example we just reviewed, the process evaluation conducted answered the following questions:

- What human, financial, and material resources were provided and used?

- Were the resources provided for this program adequate?

- What were the barriers to program implementation?

- What were the costs associated with the initiative? How do these costs compare with costs of similar programs or policy initiatives?

B. The Extent to Which Intervention Activities Were Accomplished as Planned (Fidelity)

Process evaluation is also interested in determining whether the activities identified in the plan were accomplished as intended with fidelity. Fidelity, used as a noun, means "the degree of exactness with which something is copied or reproduced." Synonyms include, accuracy, precision, authenticity, and faithfulness. Drawing on this definition, process evaluation determines with regard to the plan that was developed following the community assessment the extent to which the present logic model matches the initial logic model but more importantly are the specific activities outlined in the plan being implemented as intended with accuracy. So it is not sufficient to determine if the training is being conducted, but whether it is being implemented as stated in the plan. Does it, for example, use the curriculum that was intended by the plan or has it adopted an alternative curriculum for training? If it has adopted a different curriculum, in process evaluation there is a range of additional questions that must be asked; however, the initial finding confirms that the program activity is not being accomplished as planned. As in the previous example, without using the appropriate curriculum, that training may not be adequate or appropriate, leading to ineffective training and ineffective advocates and thereby threatening the coalition's ability to achieve its stated outcomes! The questions that would help us to answer the questions related to fidelity include

- Was the program or policy implemented as planned?

- What training was provided or received?

- What educational and advocacy activities were carried out?

- Were all the components of the plan implemented? If not, why not?

- What was the level of implementation of the initiative?

- To what extent did the activities occur at multiple levels of influence (individual, interpersonal, community, organizational and policy)?

C. The Quality of the Intervention Components

Quality is defined as "the standard of something as measured against other things of a similar kind and degree of excellence of something." In addition, it is defined as, "a distinctive attribute or characteristic possessed by someone or something." Process evaluation is responsible for determining the program quality and worth, as well as disentangling the different components of the initiative to understand which components contribute to the outcomes, which are worth keeping, and which might safely be eliminated to reduce cost but more importantly perhaps to improve the logic of the intervention with regard to outcomes and allow for a more precise understanding of the theory of change. When the standard against which the quality of components is assessed, is the theory of change, the evaluators assess the operational logic model, which is the logic model that stakeholders identify as being how the intervention operates against what the literature and others' experiences suggest is the best approach to dealing with the public health problem. A theory-driven intervention is much more likely to contain components that are known to affect behavioral change. For example, an intervention based on the transtheoretic model will have components that take into consideration the need to identify each participant's stage of change and each person is categorized as being in the precontemplation, contemplation, preparation, action, or maintenance stage. For each of these stages there are components of the intervention that are recommended for moving the person from one stage to another. In stage 1, precontemplation, the focus of the intervention will be providing information in culturally appropriate ways such that the individual is able to make a decision to consider adopting the behavior to reduce their risk factor(s) for the health problem. The activity in this component of the intervention and for these participants is providing information in a variety of formats, which may include using traditional print and audiovisual materials, discussion groups, and counseling or using social media approaches and peer-to-peer interventions. The quality of the component would be assessed based on best practices for assessing information-sharing material and practices. For the group in the action phase and moving into maintenance of the behavior change when skills development and building self-efficacy are critical for behavior, the assessment would focus on the quality of the interventions for achieving this outcome.

There are a number of components in an intervention to get legislation passed to reduce the rates of suicide among adults 18–30 years by limiting their access to prescription drugs. The first part of this might be the development of the policy with components that include research and analysis, solutions identification, community organizing, stakeholder education, and media advocacy. See Table 6.2 for a complete list. A process evaluation may evaluate the process by which legislation

TABLE 6.2. Components in Formulating Policy

Item for Review	Activities	Quality Indicator and Standard
Research and analysis		
Solutions identification		
Community organizing		
Issue framing and messaging		
Public education and information campaigns		
Stakeholder engagement		
Building relationships with policymakers		
Media advocacy		
Education of opinion leaders and policymakers		
Formulation of policy proposal		

was developed. For example the standard of quality of the research and analysis component may include (a) the extent of review of published literature (b) the level of analysis to identify risk factors that are amenable to a change by legislation, and (c) the extent of the problem and the groups most affected. The criteria for the quality indicator could be developed around a rating scale such as "met, partially met, and not met." For example, the standard for review of published literature may be all articles published in the last five years on the topic of interest. For this component, the evaluator determines first the total number of articles on this topic and then, of those, the number published in the last five years and included in the analysis. This quality standard includes the number of reviews as well as the level of competence in the analysis. These together provide an indicator of the quality of the component. Another example from the list of components (see Table 6.2) is *building relationships with policymakers*. This component is critical for passing legislation and criteria against which the quality of the engagement is assessed and may include the number of legislators reached, the type of legislator, the number of sessions with legislators, and the likelihood of a legislator's supporting the bill. In addition to assessing each component independently in a tool such as the one used below, individual interviews and document reviews will provide evidence of implementation.

When training sessions are offered for a range of stakeholders, the quality of the training is an important component to assess. One aspect of the quality of the training addressed earlier is the aspect of the number and credentials of the trainers. However, beyond those two, there is also the quality of the training. Questions may arise based on the type of curriculum used, the appropriateness of the curriculum, the length of the training, and its ability to cover the concepts and provide the skills needed to complete a task. Appropriate evaluation questions may include

■   Were the training sessions developed and implemented based on best adult learning principles?

■   Was the curriculum appropriate for training in advocacy skills?

■   Was the length of the training appropriate?

■   Did the participants show evidence of being able to use the skills they were taught?

There is another component to policy evaluation, however, which is the evaluation of the implementation of the policy. This would follow more closely the evaluation of a program answering similar questions about the implementation of the policy and its associated outcomes. In a process evaluation, the questions, "Was the policy implemented with fidelity?" "Was the intended population reached?" are still relevant approaches.

D. The Level of Implementation of the Activities

The level of implementation of activities is another crucial aspect of assessing the extent to which the activities are being implemented as planned. For example, in an intervention with multiple activities, which synergistically make up what beneficiaries would need to achieve the outcomes, a lower level of implementation than planned or needed of any component would prevent the intervention participants to get to outcomes. One illustration could be in developing a set of activities across the levels of the ecological model where changing behavior relies on the availability of resources and which in turn relies on an enactment of a city ordinance. Without the city ordinance, nothing else can happen, but the level of implementation of activities to get the city ordinance is woefully low. Assessing the level of implementation against the plan would require determining what happened, when and how it happened, and the barriers to implementation.

In another illustration involving the implementation of a social media campaign, the plan may require that media messages go out to previously defined segments of the audience. The assessment of the level of implementation would determine the social media platforms that were used compared to what was available and intended as well as the extent to which multiple audiences were provided access to the information. The barriers to implementation of the various social media may also be assessed.

Relevant process evaluation questions for assessing the level of implementation could include

■   How many of the intended activities were implemented?

■   What materials were developed and distributed?

■ Do preliminary findings indicate that the intervention is likely to produce the anticipated outcomes?

■ What barriers exist to implementation of activities?

■ How were barriers removed/mitigated?

E. The Effectiveness of Administration of the Intervention

The effectiveness of administration of the intervention is influenced by the effectiveness of the organization overall. An assessment of the organization determines the extent to which there are structures that support the administration of the intervention. Assessment of the organization includes reviewing the documents of the organization, assessing staff levels and responsibilities, and determining how well staff administer and deliver the intervention in order that it achieves its intended result. Other indicators include the ability of staff to manage conflict and competing priorities from inside and outside of the organization. For example, if the goal of the intervention is to reduce the incidence of diabetes among individuals within a named jurisdiction, then all the activities of the intervention should be organized and coordinated in order to achieve that goal. Poor administration of the intervention—which may include case management, outreach, clinical interventions, and health promotion to reduce risk factors—will result in higher likelihood of individuals being diagnosed with diabetes.

■ Were resources provided on time and in appropriate amounts project activities?

■ Were activities administered using patient centered models of service?

■ Was there adequate coordination of activities?

■ How effective was the administration in ensuring that all the components of the intervention received a fair share of the resources available?

■ What was the overall performance of the administrators in delivering the services?

■ To what extent did competing priorities undermine the implementation of activities?

F. The Intensity, Reach, and Dosage of the Intervention

Changing behavior requires that individuals have sufficient information to be able to make an informed decision. The amount of information that is required for behavior change is based on the individual's previous exposure to the information as well as their readiness to change. Assessing the intensity of the intervention requires that the evaluator determines the extent to which the intervention provided sufficient information and supports such that behavior change may take place. Intensity, therefore, is assessed by the amount of the intervention delivered. The number of sessions may be an indicator as may be how long the sessions lasted. Dosage is related to intensity and is assessed by how much of the intervention was provided or how much of the intervention was received by the participant. The reach may be assessed by how far the intervention went to get to the population at risk, and it may be assessed by the number of communities reached, and the number of individuals who participated in the intervention. Intensity and dosage determine the likelihood of getting individuals and communities to take action to improve health or conditions for health, whereas reach provides an indicator of how large an area was covered. All have implications for achieving outcomes. Behavior change requires the development of specific skills, and the intensity of the program will determine the likelihood of skills development. Skills required for behavior change include decision-making, communication, assertiveness, time management, planning, and problem solving skills. Evaluation questions may include

- Did participants in the different sessions receive sufficient information to actively participate in decision-making?

- How many communities and individuals did the intervention provide services to?

- What were the intervention components and how often were they delivered?

- Was the training offered to participants sufficient to build communication skills to reduce their risk of infection?

- What is the extent and quality of training in the community to learn skills in planning and problem solving?

The reach of a policy change is by definition much greater, although it is influenced by the extent to which the policy's implementation is monitored and enforced.

G. The Level of Participation of the Intended Audience

Assessing the level of participation of the intended audience fulfills a need to ensure that the program was implemented as planned, but it also assesses issues of social justice. For purposes of replication, it provides documentation about who participated and for whom the intervention was successful. It documents the level of participation of eligible individuals and determines the extent to which those who should benefit from the program have access to it. The Ottawa Charter (1986) reminds us that individuals living in isolated areas and those of low socioeconomic status should have equal access to resources. Process evaluation determines the level of participation of various groups by race, gender, socio-economic status, sexual orientation, and ability. It reminds us that interventions should be designed to ensure that cultural and traditional ways of learning that are familiar to community members are honored.

- What methods were used to recruit participants? When and how many were used?

- Who are the participants in the intervention compared to those who were identified in the plan?

- Were those identified in the plan the population that would most benefit from the intervention activities?

- Who are the participants advocating for, developing, and changing the policy?

H. The Effect of Assumptions and External Factors on Implementation

The assumptions that are made in the development of an intervention must be identified and assessed. Not addressing and mitigating assumptions is the difference between a successful and a failed intervention. In describing the program and the logic model, evaluators must ask stakeholders to describe the assumptions and external factors they identified and mitigated and those that continue to be problematic. Assumptions about participation in interventions is often one evaluators must deal with. The assumption often is, "if we build it, they will come." This is often found not to be the case if assumptions are not addressed in the design of the intervention. When cultural differences are not accepted, interventions may be designed but not acceptable to the population they were intended to serve. Around the world, there are many stories about interventions that have seemed like a good idea to the developers and are being developed in the absence of a well-designed community assessment and local interest.

- What barriers were there to program implementation? How were they addressed?

- What assumptions were made about the intervention's likelihood of success?

- To what extent have these assumptions undermined getting to outcomes?

- What social, economic, or political factors have influenced program implementation?

- How has the intervention been modified to ensure the participation of individuals with cultural beliefs different from your own?

SELECTING QUESTIONS FOR PROCESS EVALUATION

In the first step of the Participatory Model for Evaluation, we described the initiative for evaluation and discussed the importance of a clear description of the initiative. The culmination of this listening activity is a logic model that highlights the program's basic components, the resources, the activities, the immediate results of program implementation (outputs), as well as short-, medium-, and long-term expectations of program effects (outcomes). Process evaluation is concerned only with the columns to the left of the logic model—the resources, activities, and outputs columns. (See Figures 5.6 and 5.8.) In this chapter we frame the evaluation by using these elements since they are the focus of process evaluation.

Ultimately, identifying the evaluation research questions that become the focus of the evaluation requires a series of steps, the first of which is ensuring the participation of stakeholders. The stakeholders may include those who commissioned the study, funders, beneficiaries, and anybody who has an interest in the results of the evaluation. The steps that are required for determining the questions for the evaluation include:

- Assemble stakeholders

- Review work plans and logic models and identify potential questions

- Sort the questions

- Select the evaluation questions

- Prioritize the questions

Assemble Stakeholders

Assembling stakeholders for purposes of identifying evaluation questions gives them the opportunity to participate in the process and select questions to be answered that are of interest and relevance to them and would contribute to their understanding of the program's implementation. It is important to distinguish between those issues that must be explored in depth in the evaluation and those that are less important and may be left out. Since a standard of evaluation is utility, the evaluation process must understand the needs of the stakeholders but especially the client who has commissioned the study and with whom the contract was drawn up. It would be important to understand from their perspectives the need for the evaluation and how the evaluation findings will be used. This provides support for the selection of questions that might otherwise not be incorporated. Stakeholders' expectations of the program may be different from the stated objectives. In a recent evaluation the following questions were identified by a stakeholder:

1.   Are customers purchasing fruits and vegetables more frequently since the intervention has taken place? At the store? In total?

2.   Which food items are selling the most?

3.   Are customers able to purchase a variety of fruits and vegetables that meet their needs and expectations?

These questions led to considering a number of factors about the evaluation, the stage of the initiative, the evaluation design, and the data-collection methodology. However, given the varied interests of stakeholders, funders may ask different questions. Their questions may be more related to the cost of the program compared to other similar programs or the cost-effectiveness of the program being evaluated. The staff who run the day-to-day affairs of the intervention may also have a different set of questions; theirs may be related to how much their work demonstrates reach, intensity, and dose, and the extent to which the intervention is likely to show any effect in 3 years' time when the funding ends and they must justify their existence! The type of intervention will naturally guide the questioning, and the evaluation team must allow time for the priorities and concerns of the stakeholders to be clearly identified and ensure that they remain a part of the process of selecting the questions that the evaluation team will answer.

Review Work Plans and Logic Models

Reviewing work plans and logic models is an important component of the process because understanding the program leads to questions about the intervention's implementation and likely effectiveness. The theory of change represents the structure that is assumed underlies the program's success and is depicted in the logic model. The theory of change shows how and why an initiative works. When the evaluation is complete, it may validate a program's theory such as the health belief model, the theory of planned behavior, and so forth. The components of the logic model may help frame evaluation questions and provide insights into the most appropriate elements to measure. Each box in the logic model provides opportunities for evaluation. Evaluation questions related to inputs allow the evaluation team to assess what resources went into the program as well as what resources were expended, be it a program or a policy (Figure 6.4). Those related to activities will address the number, level, and standard of implementation of activities as well as the likelihood of their achieving the initiative's objectives and the outputs provide evidence that the activities took place.

Outputs provide the first indications that the program is working. They provide the numbers produced but do not tell us if the intervention had an effect on the beneficiaries. For example, in assessing an intervention to end childhood obesity, the fact that 10 new farmers' markets have been created indicates that a program component has been implemented. Assessing that output alone does not tell us the effect of the component on access to healthy foods or on childhood obesity. However, stakeholders may be interested in many of the outputs from their interventions. Outputs are the most-often assessed results of a program's implementation in the early stages, before outcomes and effects of the program can be measured. The logic model framework is used to identify questions that are most appropriate to answer. In addition, a review of the project's work plan that has more detail about intervention activities may be useful in identifying questions (Table 6.3).

In addition to specific objectives that serve as benchmarks and direction for measuring the program's implementation, stakeholders may identify principles against which the initiative can be appraised. These principles may form the basis of the organization's mission and, therefore, they are important to assess. These principles may include social justice and the equitable and ethical distribution of benefits, goods, and services to the beneficiaries.

FIGURE 6.4.   *Logic Model Framework for Process Evaluation*

What is the evaluation question being answered? For example, Was the program to increase policymakers' knowledge about the need to increase access to opportunities for physical activity in a low-income community carried out as planned?

Inputs	Activities	Outputs
What human, financial, or other resources were used for this activity or set of activities?	What activities or set of activities were used to achieve the stated process objective? For example, education sessions conducted to increase knowledge of policymakers about the need to build walking trails to increase access to physical activity in a low-income community that has little access to opportunities for physical activity. Education materials produced?	What evidence is available to show that the activities were implemented? For example, how many education sessions were held for policymakers? How many policymakers attended each session? How many pieces of education material were produced and distributed?

Assumptions: There were trained facilitators and other resources to carry out the activities and policymakers are willing and able to be engaged in training.

TABLE 6.3.   **Workplan for Identifying Questions for Process Evaluation**

Outcome Objective:														
Activity	Means of verification	Implementation in Year 1												
		1	2	3	4	5	6	7	8	9	10	11	12
Training of Trainers	Workshop reports													
Activity 2	Log sheets													
Activity 3	Data Base													
Activity 4	Meeting Notes													
Activity 5	Outreach													

Sort the Questions

There are many approaches for sorting the research questions. The process that is used may depend on the number of questions that emerge from the brainstorming process. When there is a large number of questions, electronic options for selecting and voting for questions may be the more efficient approach. However, in a small group of stakeholders, each person is given Post-it notes and asked to write down one or two questions that are important for the evaluation to answer once the purpose of the evaluation has been carefully explained. Other information that might be useful as stakeholders contemplate their questions is how much time is available for the evaluation and how the results are likely to be used. Once each person has written their questions, the facilitator presents each question to the group and sorts the questions into themes that are predetermined or emerge with the process. These could include (a) assessment of financial, human, and material resources; (b) assessment of the process of implementation; (c) assessment of administration of the initiative; (d) identification of initiative components and the contribution to the initiative; (e) management information systems and data collection processes; and (f) the effectiveness of the intervention for getting to outcomes. Once the questions have been sorted, the group is ready for the next step, which is prioritizing the questions for evaluation. An alternative version of this participatory approach has individuals voting for the questions during the process. A modified *nominal group technique* described by Delbecq and Gustafson (1975) is as follows:

1. Each member of the stakeholder group makes a list of evaluation questions he or she would like answered.

2. The facilitator asks members of the group in turn to provide one question each to a "master list" on a flip chart or a board that is visible to the whole group. As an evaluation question is added, a show of hands provides a count of how many people included a similar question in their lists. This number is recorded next to the question on the flip chart. The questions on the participants' lists are canceled as they are accounted for on the master list.

3. The process continues until all members have contributed all the items on their lists that are different from previous questions and all the questions have been crossed off their lists.

4. The facilitator reviews the master list with the group and, with the consensus of the group, eliminates or merges questions that appear similar and that ask fundamentally the same question.

The final list sets the stage for deciding on the final set of questions. If the evaluation is to be useful and the results utilized, questions that are of primary importance to the person(s) requesting the evaluation must be answered.

Select the Evaluation Questions

The evaluation question drives the research design and the data-collection methods. Without an evaluation question, there is no evaluation! The list of questions can be put up on flip charts arranged around the room or written up on a board as they are being submitted. The questions for evaluation are influenced by

- Relevance of the questions to program development and replication

- Expertise of the evaluation team and resources available for the evaluation

- Time frame required for the evaluation

- Access to data

Questions are often generated from the brainstorming sessions as has already been described, and although these questions are generally the first set of questions considered, there may well be some overlap with questions identified later. Previously developed activity objectives that describe the specific activities that will take place as well as the outputs are also important for the evaluation as they form the expectations of the program and the starting point for determining if the program was implemented as planned, as well as if the implementation resulted in the expected outcomes of products, services, or participation. For example, "Staff of the Health for All Coalition will organize 20 advocacy events for 100 persons each by the third quarter after implementation." This activity objective reframed into an evaluation question says, "How many advocacy events did the staff of the Health for All Coalition organize and how many persons participated?"

Questions may be selected also based on their relevance to program development and replication. The questions selected based on this purpose may be less inclined to focus on how many events took place and more on how well the events were implemented and how effective they are for producing outcomes. The expertise of the team influences the questions selected based on their knowledge of the purpose, the time frame, the budget, and how any questions fit into a matrix of questions. Their overall purpose would be to make sure they fulfill the requirements of the contract and they have the best view of the overall intent of the evaluation. Their previous experience will guide them to select questions that serve their purpose.

An important consideration is the hierarchy of questions and how answering one question may allow you to make the assumption that the previous question need not be answered.

The selection of the question also depends on the stage of the program. For example, if an important question to answer is one about utilization and there are insufficient resources to answer a question on access, one makes the assumption that if utilization has taken place then there must have been access. In this case, only utilization need be measured. Another example is, more mature programs are expected to have resolved issues around recruitment, whereas assessing the effectiveness of the intervention would be a more appropriate use of resources.

In addition, the number of questions that can be answered is influenced by the time allowed for the evaluation. For example, if the evaluation team is contracted at the very beginning of the intervention, the time frame it has for answering questions is very different than it would be if they get called in three years into the intervention. At this point, there are also questions for which there may not be data, so in addition to the time element, the availability of data or the evaluation team's ability to collect data may be limited, thereby also limiting which questions can form part of the evaluation plan. Once a list of questions has been generated and those that cannot be included in the evaluation are excluded, the next phase is prioritizing questions based on preselected criteria and a process that allows for discussion of the strengths and weaknesses of each question for fulfilling the overall purpose.

When the purpose of the evaluation is to replicate a program, it is important that the questions that are asked help the team to understand what resources were provided and consumed by the intervention, what components and steps led to the success or failure of the initiative, what outputs were observed as a result of the implementation, and the strengths and weaknesses of the intervention. These questions form the basis for understanding the program's structure and its functional elements that make them relevant for process evaluation. The strengths and weaknesses help the program staff to build on the strengths and address the weaknesses to strengthen the theory of action or, if required, to reassess the need for the weak link. It provides insights into the likelihood of the intervention being able to achieve its stated outcomes.

Prioritize the Questions

The list generated by the stakeholders and edited by the evaluation team, with concurrence from stakeholders, is ready to prioritize the questions so that the most important and relevant questions are answered while taking into consideration the expertise of the team and the resources available for the evaluation.

Once the questions have been selected for further consideration in this multistep process, each question may be subjected to a two-by-two table that forces the stakeholders and evaluation team to make decisions based on the impact the question is likely to make in the context of the selected goal of the evaluation (see Figure 6.5). For example, if the goal of the evaluation is program implementation and development, then the questions that have priority will be those that focus on assessing implementation. Among those questions is the one that is asked about its ability to contribute to decision-making.

Each selected evaluation question is reviewed and placed in the appropriate box. If the evaluation team considers that the question will have a high impact in its ability to contribute to the decision-making process and to improve evaluation knowledge at the same time, the question is put into the quadrant labeled "best choice." Another question that might

FIGURE 6.5.   *Two-by-Two Table*

Ability to improve evaluation knowledge

	High	Low
High Ability to contribute to the decision- making process	Best Choice	Good Choice
Low	Okay Choice	Poor Choice

have a high impact in contributing to decision-making but does not improve evaluation knowledge overall goes in the "good choice" box. A question that contributes neither to decision-making nor improved evaluation knowledge may be placed in the "poor choice" box. This process continues until all the questions are placed.

Once this process is complete and the results of the two-by-two table are reviewed, the questions in the "best choice" and "good choice" quadrants are the most valuable because evaluation is primarily about the initiative being assessed and it must contribute to decision-making. Research-oriented evaluations may want to answer questions in the "okay choice" quadrant, since the evaluators may have slightly different purposes and may well find that answering those questions provides useful information and expands evaluation knowledge even though they may have less direct impact on the implementation of the initiative. Questions that fall into the "poor choice" quadrant may not warrant time or resources as they neither improve knowledge overall nor contribute to decision-making. The contract for the evaluation, its purpose, and resources will dictate the direction of the evaluation. In the final analysis, it is important to be careful and deliberate in selecting questions to maximize the use of resources and reduce the likelihood of overwhelming the evaluation.

RESOURCES FOR EVALUATION

An important consideration in the evaluation is the expertise of the evaluation team. Their expertise will help direct the stakeholders in a process that ensures the most important questions are answered. The evaluation team also has the advantage of knowing which questions are likely to provide the best information taking into consideration previous evaluations, their knowledge of the literature, their comfort with addressing questions of a quantitative or qualitative nature, the time frame for the evaluation, and the level of resources to which they will have access.

Resources available for evaluation will vary from one evaluation to another and will dictate how comprehensive or how restrictive the evaluation will be. Often in public health, resources allocated to evaluation are limited and make a comprehensive evaluation almost impossible. As a result, the evaluation team must determine which questions are critical to answer, a decision that may come after the last encounter with stakeholders. It is important, however, to provide a plan to the stakeholder and the rationale for the selection of the final set of questions. In some cases, answering one question rather than two on the same theme is sufficient and this selection is easily justified. A review of the final plan and confirmation of the questions and the approach to the evaluation may help ensure buy in and utilization of the results. Resources such as personnel to work with the evaluation team to provide the data, a management information system, and databases that provide the information are required for showing the program was implemented as planned. Process evaluation determines implementation so it relies on data that is collected continuously. The timeline for evaluation is also an important resource. Often evaluators are called in long after the intervention has been implemented and no baseline data has been collected, limiting the effectiveness of a process evaluation. So, when the evaluation team is engaged and for how long they are engaged influences the cost of the evaluation and which questions are relevant and, therefore, are more likely to get answered. The existence of data collected becomes a critical consideration in decision-making.

MEASURING RESOURCES, PROCESSES, AND OUTPUTS

A source of confusion for beginning evaluators is the difference between outputs and outcomes. It is important to be able to distinguish between them. Outputs only represent what was done, for example, the number of people trained, number of materials produced, number of sessions offered, number of lights installed, and so forth. Outputs differ from outcomes, which assess whether the activities made a difference. Although it is helpful to say that 50 people participated in the training, it is more important to be able to assess how those people who participated benefited (outcome); whether they learned anything or improved their attitudes or skills.

The outputs of the initiative are the products of the initiative, so to assess the products we have to know what the initiative was intended to produce. We get this information from the description of the program and from a well-developed and complete logic model from talking to stakeholders. During the planning phase, too, objectives provide direction for the program. These objectives known as activity or process objectives are SMART objectives that provide a focus for an objectives-based evaluation. For example, by January 2019, 250 youth ages 18 to 25 will have participated in a well-supervised advocacy training. In assessing the outputs from this activity, the evaluators would assess the number and demographics of those who actually participated and the number and quality of the training sessions they were exposed to. Their satisfaction with the training may also be assessed. It does not tell us what benefit the youth got from being trained. Information on expected outputs may also be contained in other project documents.

Indicators for assessing resources and processes are the quantitative or qualitative variables that allow the changes that occur as a result of an intervention to be measured. Indicators show whether the intended results are achieved. They are objectively verifiable and can be assessed repeatedly. Quantitative indicators measure changes in numerical values; qualitative indicators measure changes that are less well defined but that are agreed to by the stakeholders as measures of success. Indicators are the standards against which performance of the initiative is measured. In conducting a process evaluation, the resources may be measured using a question such as, "What funding, personnel, space, or materials were provided for the initiative?" and is answered by using different indicators, one representing each of the variables. The issue of funding may be assessed by reviewing grants received (indicator), and personnel are assessed not just by the number of staff hired but also what training they have received (Table 6.4). Because a large part of the responsibility in process evaluation is process monitoring and documenting the initiative's day-to-day activities and expenditures in a consistent manner, data may be collected by visiting and observing activities and reviewing documents like work plans and minutes from meetings (Stufflebeam & Shinkfield, 2007). In addition, indications that the event occurred can be found in logs, surveys, individual interviews, and focus groups, as well as discussions with program staff and beneficiaries.

TABLE 6.4. Logic Model Components: Questions, Indicators, and Data Sources

Logic Model Component	Appropriate Question	Indicator	Data Source
Resources	What funding, personnel, space, or materials were provided for the initiative?	Grant funding received	Minutes and audit reports
		Staff hired	HR dept. documentation
		Office and training space	Minutes and legal dept.
		Information brochures obtained from a local vendor	Accounts records; minutes
Activities	What training activities were carried out and how many people participated?	Individuals participated in 2-hour training sessions	Training logs; instructor notes
	Who were the participants in the training?	Policymakers trained	Reports of training; participants logs
	Were barriers to program implementation addressed?	Venue size	Physical plant record; minutes of meetings
	How satisfied were participants with the training sessions they received?	Satisfaction index	Satisfaction survey

Let's look at another example related to policy development. One question the evaluation team may be required to answer is, "What educational activities were carried out to inform the legislators of the need for new legislation?" This question is related to policy development and one of the activities that underlie the process. In policy development, a crucial component is educating legislators so they are familiar with the need for the legislation and there is sufficient advocacy to achieve a majority when the legislation is presented for a vote. This process could entail many years of hard work by coalitions, nonprofit organizations, the media, and individuals. It could include workshops organized for individual legislators, groups of legislators, a series of individual meetings, marches, testimonies, and so forth before a legislation is written and even more meetings and training sessions, as well as discussions in subcommittees, before it gets to the floor. The purpose of process evaluation in answering this question is to understand what happened, how it happened, who it happened for, who was involved, and the strengths and weaknesses of the process.

TOOLS FOR PROCESS EVALUATION

Program evaluation requires that the tools for process evaluation are designed before the intervention starts so that there is a systematic and thorough data collection plan and data is collected when the first contact is made. In the case of this question, "What educational activities were carried out to inform the legislators of the need for new legislation?" educational activities may include materials that were printed, formal and informal in-house and outreach activities that were conducted, media messages and activities, text and e-mail messages, and other educational activities, including the use of social media platforms. Each activity constitutes an indicator. So, for example, in wanting to assess the different activities, you could have the following question, "What activities did the organization engage in to educate policy leaders on the need for the legislation?" The specific items would be derived from the plan devised by the organization and any additional activities the evaluation team determined had taken place during the period under review. Activities would include those listed earlier, in-house and outreach educational workshops and seminars, media messages and interviews, text and e-mail messages. The types and numbers of activities undertaken would be needed to answer the question. To expand our understanding of the initiative's likely impact, the number of legislators reached would also be helpful.

In this case, the tools for answering the evaluation question and collecting this information include reports and notes that contain information, such as dates, venues, participants at different educational sessions (names and contact information); copies of materials distributed; transcripts of media and other educational events; meeting and other notes; and databases that were compiled with this information on an ongoing basis. The tools for process evaluation require systematic and sustained data management systems that can be searched to answer specific questions and allow for continuous monitoring.

Logs are used to enter data to track participation and the level of exposure and they help in the assessment of reach and dosage in determining the extent to which the information is likely to result in change in knowledge, attitude, and subsequent behavior. Surveys are also useful for collecting data to answer process evaluation questions. In a recent process evaluation of the context of policy change, respondents were asked to complete a table that

TABLE 6.5. Assessing the Context for Policy Change Using a Table Format in a Survey

Instructions: Complete the following table using the scale indicating support for policy change.

1 = never supportive/barrier

2 = almost never supportive

3 = somewhat supportive

4 = supportive most of the time

5 = supportive all of the time

6 = I do not know

	1	2	3	4	5	6
Administrative/organizational support						
Alliances with critical partners						
Community support						
Media advocacy						
Organizational capacity						
Peer and family support						
Political climate						
Support from policymakers						
Other (specify)						

included items assessing the different levels of support for policy change from for example, community, media, family, and policymaker support. See Table 6.5.

Other tools, such as individual interviews, audio, and photographic research tools may be more applicable for answering a question. The approach that is used to collect the data is always dependent on the type of question and the most effective means of answering it. Data can be reported to reflect changes in implementation and changes in participation over time. For example, in assessing the change of participation in coalition leadership meetings, attendance was observed four times in a 1-year time frame for each of three groups. The presentation of the data in line graphs provided a visual and helped the stakeholders understand how the levels of participation changed during the year. During the second

FIGURE 6.6. *Changes in an Indicator Across Four Observations of Three Samples*

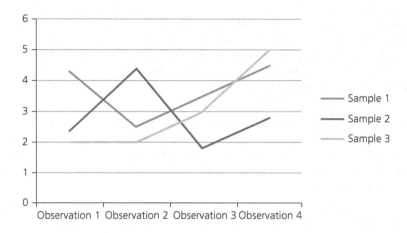

observation, two of the groups realized their numbers were dropping and increased their outreach to members through newsletters, phone calls, and getting them more involved in the coalition. The third group observed a dip in the third quarter and also increased its level of activity, which resulted in increased participation (Figure 6.6).

Process evaluation relies on a combination of qualitative and quantitative approaches, so having expertise in both research approaches is useful. A mixed methods design leads to being able to triangulate the results and increase confidence in the findings. For example, in assessing satisfaction, a survey might ask the question, "how satisfied were you with the advocacy training that was offered during the policy development process?" There might be a range of responses from not at all satisfied to very satisfied. There may be 25 percent of respondents who said they were not satisfied, but from the survey there would be no way to know without having additional questions what that response actually meant. The same question asked in a focus group or in an individual interview format might have a follow up probe like, please explain. The focus group would them generate responses such as, "the venue was not appropriate," "the trainers were not well trained in advocacy techniques," and "we did not have access to technology that would help us understand better," providing a range of ideas for improving the training program in the future. Using the survey data, we got a percent of people who were not satisfied, and using the qualitative data we got the reasons why they were not satisfied. A useful addition to a survey is an open ended question that allows the respondent to provide the why. Having a multidisciplinary team allows a diverse approach to the process.

ETHICAL AND CULTURAL CONSIDERATIONS

During the process of designing and implementing a process evaluation, the evaluation team must ensure that no harm is caused to the program beneficiaries, other stakeholders, or the larger community. In addition, evaluators should ensure that the evaluation is culturally responsive using approaches that emphasize stakeholder involvement and organizational experience. They must adhere to the standards for evaluation (Chapter 4) so that evaluations are conducted and reported in ways that the results are likely to be used (utility); efficient in their use of resources (feasible); respect human dignity; be ethical and fair (propriety); and use accurate and systematic processes for collecting, analyzing, and reporting data (accuracy). In addition there are ethical principles related to the conduct of the research in evaluation. I remind you of them here since it is important that evaluation teams maintain the integrity of the evaluation process.

These principles are as follows:

1. *Systematic inquiry:* Evaluators conduct systematic, data-based inquiries. They adhere to the highest technical standards; explore the shortcomings and strengths of evaluation questions and approaches; communicate the approaches, methods, and limitations of the evaluation accurately; and allow others to be able to understand, interpret, and critique their work.

2. *Competence:* Evaluators provide competent performance to stakeholders. They ensure that the evaluation team possesses the knowledge, skills, and experience required; that it demonstrates cultural competence; practices within its limits; and continuously provides the highest level of performance.

3. *Integrity/honesty:* Evaluators display honesty and integrity in their own behavior and attempt to ensure the honesty of the entire evaluation process. They negotiate honestly, disclose any conflicts of interest and values and any sources of financial support. They disclose changes to the evaluation, resolve any concerns, accurately represent their findings, and attempt to prevent any misuse of those findings.

4. *Respect for people:* Evaluators respect the security, dignity, and worth of respondents, program participants, clients, and other stakeholders. They understand the context of the evaluation, abide by ethical standards, conduct the evaluation and communicate results in a way that respects the stakeholders' dignity and worth, fosters social equity, and takes into account all persons.

5. *Responsibilities for general and public welfare:* Evaluators articulate and take into account the diversity of general and public values that may be related to the evaluation. They include relevant perspectives, consider also the side effects, and allow stakeholders to present the results in appropriate forms that respect confidentiality, take into account the public interest, and consider the welfare of society as a whole (American Evaluation Association, 2008, pp. 233–234).

(The full text of the American Evaluation Association Guiding Principles for Evaluators is available at http://www.eval.org)

As discussed in Chapter 1, it is also important to ensure that the evaluation research process is culturally sensitive and takes into consideration in the planning and execution of evaluation that the cultures of the organization and the clients they serve in the design of the study. It means that members of the team have to be willing to become culturally competent and learn about the culture, what is appropriate to do and say, and what is not.

It means paying attention to the way questions are asked, the selection of data sources, the data collection methods, the way results are interpreted, and the way they are communicated including what recommendations are appropriate to make.

Evaluating programs or policies requires a team approach as well as engaging multiple stakeholders who have varying roles and experiences with the program or policy being evaluated. It is important that cultural competency is a fundamental principle of doing business. It ensures that evaluation teams are more likely to achieve the goals of the evaluation while creating an environment of trust and equity. It requires that the evaluation team understands

- The realities of the communities in which evaluation is conducted

- The need to identify influential power structures and groups that can be allies

- How to identify and work with cultural tensions of subgroups

- The skills necessary for working in a variety of cultural contexts

- How to use culturally acceptable language, communication, and negotiation skills

BACKGROUND

An experienced evaluation team from the state university was asked to conduct an evaluation of the health ministry at the Wesleyan Church. The congregation had a well-developed ministry that provided services to their members primarily in and around the urban community for five years but had never had their initiatives evaluated. The Church needed to write grants since their reach had expanded well beyond the congregation to serve the larger community, but also over time many of the members of the church had moved further away but still relied on the health ministry to keep them healthy. Since its roots were in public health, they mostly provided preventive services educating the community about risk factors for common health problems and worked with the local council to improve access to healthy nutrition and opportunities for exercise through passing community-wide policies. The purpose of the process evaluation was to assess the components of the intervention and determine which components were likely to be retained. They wanted to be sure that going forward their initiatives would be theory based and have the best chance of improving the health of the community. The evaluation team was asked to assess the quality of their program and make recommendations for program improvement but especially to help them make a case for funding to expand their program to include youth at risk. The primary stakeholders were the pastors and other church leadership and the parishioners. The health ministry had a separate organizational structure with a deacon as the coordinator. The deacon had

(Continued)

(*Continued*)

a team of providers all of whom had some training in health or public health and gave their time voluntarily. The deacon had a public health degree and was anxious to make sure he was providing evidence-based interventions. His team relied on him for guidance.

They had recently conducted a community assessment making sure to include not just the members of the congregation but members of the larger community since they understood that they had to expand their services to include them. Given the expertise of the team and the local resources at their disposal they were able to conduct a very comprehensive assessment to determine what the health issues were that needed to be addressed and who was most affected. They found that the older adults had many risk factors for chronic disease and the communities that seemed to have the fewest resources were the ones that also appeared to have the heaviest burden of disease. One of the questions they asked them was on a survey that was distributed to all the adults. The question came from the Behavioral Risk Factor Surveillance Survey (BRFSS) since they wanted to be able to compare their results with other data they found in the literature. The question asked whether they had ever been told by a doctor that they had a certain condition, and other questions asked about their nutrition, physical activity, and other behaviors. The youth completed a survey that asked questions about their risk behavior. In addition, they conducted focus groups with members of the community. They had focus groups with just men, just women, and just youth (women and men separately) so they were free to discuss issues that concerned them the most without feeling shy. In addition, they conducted observation studies when they went around the community and using their GIS technology took coordinates for all the health-food options, places where community members could exercise, and places they felt would add to their understanding of the context of the community, the things they would have to pay attention to. The map they drew of the community assets as well as its problems turned out to be really helpful in describing the community. To their surprise they discovered that although they had come to realize the extent of chronic disease among the older adults, they had not appreciated the level of risk behaviors among the youth population as well as the lack of resources available and accessible to them. They were suddenly faced with a dilemma. How were they going to expand their services to be sure to protect this urban community? That was when the idea of writing a grant and getting help came to them. They were committed and had been doing good work, but they also understood that they needed to make their case. This case included evaluating what they had already been doing and showing in the application how they could expand their ministry to address this emerging need. It made sense to them since their goal was "To prevent the occurrence of preventable disease and disability."

Description of the Program

The intervention that the Wesleyan Church had offered the community was based roughly on the health-belief model. They had developed programs that mainly focused on addressing issues of susceptibility, seriousness, benefits, and barriers to common health problems. They had helped them identify cues to their taking action and had worked with many to build the skills and the confidence necessary to eat healthy and be physically active. They had undertaken many forms of outreach and distributed information materials and, when necessary, doctors and nurses on the health team went out and saw patients. In collaboration with the local hospital they had also offered members of the congregation and the surrounding communities, opportunities to screen for breast and prostate cancer, diabetes, and high blood pressure at least twice a year. The mission of the organization was to provide preventive services to ensure that members of community were able to manage their health and live healthy and productive lives. They recognized the importance of a healthy environment so they had components that focused on this aspect also. The evaluation team was eager to see how all this came together and assembled as many of the stakeholders as they could on a day when they were available. Tuesday evenings were the only night that everybody could make it to meetings, so sessions were scheduled for four consecutive weeks to get a complete picture of the organization's programs, draw the logic model, and identify questions for the evaluation. The completed logic model looked very much like logic models the team had developed in the past (see Figure 6.7). It provided a very high level view of the programs that the health ministry implemented.

The evaluation team worked with the stakeholders to brainstorm questions that were of interest to them, but more importantly they were asked to consider the purpose of the evaluation. The purpose of the evaluation was to assess the interventions and determine if they are likely to achieve the outcomes that the logic model suggested. Since the emphasis of this evaluation is to conduct a process evaluation, the first two columns were the focus of the evaluation. The two columns for which questions were identified were the Inputs/Resources and the Strategies for achieving the outcomes they specified. Six questions emerged from the brainstorming, sorting, and prioritizing process.

Process Evaluation Questions and Research Design

The evaluation questions selected were:

1. How effective was the administration in ensuring that all the components of the intervention received a fair share of the resources available?
2. What educational and advocacy activities were carried out?

(Continued)

(*Continued*)

FIGURE 6.7. *Logic Model for the Wesleyan Church Public Health Ministry*

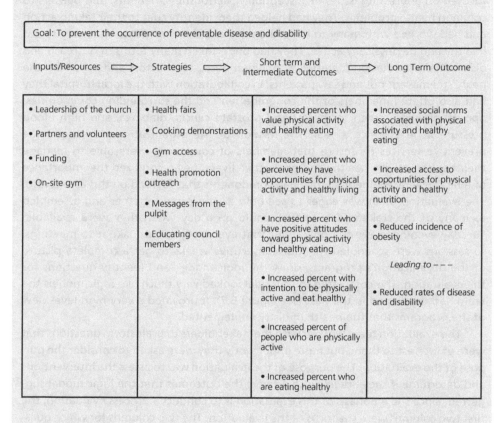

Goal: To prevent the occurrence of preventable disease and disability

Inputs/Resources ⟹ Strategies ⟹ Short term and Intermediate Outcomes ⟹ Long Term Outcome

Inputs/Resources	Strategies	Short term and Intermediate Outcomes	Long Term Outcome
• Leadership of the church • Partners and volunteers • Funding • On-site gym	• Health fairs • Cooking demonstrations • Gym access • Health promotion outreach • Messages from the pulpit • Educating council members	• Increased percent who value physical activity and healthy eating • Increased percent who perceive they have opportunities for physical activity and healthy living • Increased percent who have positive attitudes toward physical activity and healthy eating • Increased percent with intention to be physically active and eat healthy • Increased percent of people who are physically active • Increased percent who are eating healthy	• Increased social norms associated with physical activity and healthy eating • Increased access to opportunities for physical activity and healthy nutrition • Reduced incidence of obesity *Leading to - - -* • Reduced rates of disease and disability

3. What materials were distributed?

4. Do preliminary findings indicate that the intervention is likely to produce the anticipated outcomes?

5. How did the level of implementation of activities affect the logic model and the intervention's likelihood of getting to outcomes?

6. What social, economic, or political factors influenced program implementation?

In support of these evaluation questions, the evaluation team reviewed the activity objectives previously developed by the program and found that many of the activity objectives provided the who, what, when, and how of the interventions as well as the targets that would allow the evaluation team to answer their overarching questions. The activity objectives provided information about who was responsible for the activity, what the activity was, when it took place, and how often.

Evaluation Studies

The next step for the evaluation team was to design the plan for the evaluation. They needed to be clear about what constituted the evaluation given that they had the evaluation questions. They identified the specific process evaluation objectives (SPO) and developed a table to summarize the information they had from the documents they reviewed (see Table 6.6). The team realized that the intervention has already

TABLE 6.6. **Log Frame**

Title	Process Evaluation of the Wesleyan Church Health Ministry
Project Goal	To prevent the occurrence of preventable disease and disability.
Beneficiaries Sample Size	Members of the church family as well as members of the larger community. The church has a congregation of about 600 and the population of the community was 50,000.
Specific Process Objective (SPO)	SPO1 Members of the health ministry will undertake outreach activities to reach a total of 1000 parishioners' and community members with health information and skills training during the first three years of the intervention. SPO2 By the end of the fifth year of the intervention, the leadership team of the church and the Health Ministry team will provide training for 50 policymakers. SPO3: The leadership of the Church will ensure that adequate resources are provided to each component of the intervention during each year of the intervention.

	Outputs	Indicators	Means of Verification	Risks and Assumptions
SO1	1000	Signed documentation from parishioners and community members who received any services	Follow-up interviews, survey questions	Signatures may not be obtained; outreach activities may be prevented by social, physical, or political barriers

(Continued)

(*Continued*)

TABLE 6.6. (*Continued*)

	Outputs	Indicators	Means of Verification	Risks and Assumptions
SO2	50	Trained policymakers	Documentation of the training	Documentation is not collected systematically; training was interrupted by competing priorities
SO3	Satisfied staff	Reports of adequate funding based on budgeted needs	Key informant interviews; focus groups; document reviews	Staff not willing to talk about financial matters

been in existence for five years and the objectives had not been reviewed, but they were a good starting point.

The evaluation team wanted to be sure to include members of the church as well as the larger community, so they asked for volunteers to join them. Many had participated in the process of selecting the questions so they were somewhat familiar with the participatory nature of the team and how much they wanted to be sure to reflect the culture of the community in their work. Four people volunteered. Having members of the church on board also meant that they would learn how to navigate any sensitive issues. They each had skills that the evaluation team would find useful but the team had a week of training just to be sure everybody was familiar with the expectations and they could develop the details of the plan together. The new additions to the team would be very instrumental in the recruitment of study participants. One of the women who joined the team had been a member of a research team previously and has very strong data analysis skills, so the team was especially delighted to have her on board. The expertise on the original team was mostly qualitative although they did have one statistician.

The plan the team developed started with the results of the community assessment and a description of the different components of the intervention. The research questions were included followed by a description of how the research questions will be answered and a time line for the evaluation. The information from the plan is summarized below. Evaluation questions were aligned with available

TABLE 6.7. **Alignment of Evaluation Research Questions (EQ) With Specific Project Objectives (SPO)**

Evaluation Question	Corresponding Specific Project Objective
EQ 1. How effective was the administration in ensuring that all the components of the intervention received a fair share of the resources available?	SPO3: The leadership of the Church will ensure that adequate resources are provided to each component of the intervention during each year of the intervention.
EQ 2. What educational and advocacy activities were carried out?	SPO1: Members of the Health Ministry will undertake outreach activities to reach a total of 1000 parishioners' and community members with health information and skills training during the first three years of the intervention. SPO2: By the end of the fourth year of the intervention, the leadership team of the church and the Health Ministry team will provide training for 50 policymakers.
EQ 3. What materials were distributed?	SPO1: Members of the Health Ministry will undertake outreach activities to reach a total of 1000 parishioners' and community members with health information during the first three years of the intervention.

specific project objectives (Table 6.7.), which already had standards associated with them (Table 6.6, Log Frame).

Additional questions for the team were:

1. Do preliminary findings indicate that the intervention is likely to produce the anticipated outcomes?
2. How did the level of implementation of activities affect the logic model and the intervention's likelihood of getting to outcomes?
3. What social, economic, or political factors influenced program implementation?

The team thought long and hard about how to answer each of the questions and as a result devised a sampling plan and later the data collection tools.

(Continued)

(Continued)

TABLE 6.8. Process Evaluation Work Plan With Funding From July Year 1 to March Year 3

Evaluation Tasks	Q3—Y 1 Jul–Sep	Q4—Y 1 Oct–Dec	Q1—Y 2 Jan–Mar	Q2—Y 2 Apr–Jun	Q3—Y 2 Jul–Sep	Q4—Y 2 Oct–Dec	Q1—Y 3 Jan–Mar
Data collection mechanisms and management information systems developed	X						
Base-line data collected and analyzed		X					
Community survey (b)			X				
Beneficiary survey			X				
Review of log books and other records			X	X	X		
Focus group interviews					X	X	X
Key informant interviews and data analysis					X	X	X
Follow up survey planned (Baseline survey rpt)							X
Data analysis and report writing			X		X		X

They would rely on the information the Health Ministry had collected to help them answer some of the questions. The following list is an overview of what the evaluation team intended to do accompanied by a work plan (see Table 6.8).

- Sample (type, number)
  - The sample included members of the leadership (n = 5), members of the Health Ministry team (n = 10), beneficiaries of the intervention (n = 100), and members of the larger community (n = 150)
- Data collection tools (qualitative or quantitative) were to be developed
  - Community-wide surveys
  - (a) Assessed community health and associated risk factors (baseline and follow up)

(b) Assessed the community's perception of the outreach, materials, quality of the intervention components, satisfaction with the intervention (staff, timing, reach, dose); effectiveness

- Beneficiary survey
  Assessed perceptions of the outreach, materials, quality of the intervention components, satisfaction with the intervention (staff, timing, reach and dose); factors that influenced program implementation and participation; effectiveness
- Key informant interviews with church and intervention leadership
  Assessed resource allocations; implementation of the intervention; satisfaction; barriers and factors that influenced implementation; effectiveness
- Focus groups with members of the Health Ministry team
  Assessed implementation of the intervention; satisfaction; barriers and factors that influenced implementation
- Document reviews
  Assessed distribution of information, reach, dose, quality of staff, efficiency; beneficiary participation

Evaluation Results

Evaluation questions 1–3 were quite easy to answer. The information was collected and the data was easy to interpret. For example, question 1, "How effective was the administration in ensuring that all the components of the intervention received a fair share of the resources available?" relied on information that had already been documented. Confirmation of the findings was from the key informant interviews with members of the senior leadership. The focus-group discussions with staff were able to assess the effectiveness of resource distribution. All the data together gave a complete picture of how resources were allocated and distributed, which every interviewee described as fair. In the other three questions (4–6) however, the answer to those questions required a little more thoughtful discussion by the team. For example, in answering 5, "How did the level of implementation of activities affect the logic model and the intervention's likelihood of getting to outcomes?" the team had to consider a number of things. First, what did the logic model look like and what was its intention? Second, did the logic model they were able to create after they understood the program and collected the data mirror the initial model? If not, why not and what had changed. Third, how did the difference in the logic model affect the intervention getting to outcomes? They had to address the why not, and level of implementation (quality and quantity) of the different components as well as the barriers to implementation to provide a balanced picture. So although the answer to the question, "How did the level of implementation of activities affect

(Continued)

(*Continued*)

the logic model and the intervention's likelihood of getting to outcomes?" reflected a lower level of activity than would be required to achieve the outcomes that were specified, in identifying the barriers they were able to make realistic recommendations to the Health Ministry. Addressing the barriers would strengthen the program and allow them to consider the expansion to include youth. You will notice that in this process evaluation, baseline data was collected. This is to understand and describe present conditions among the target community but also to support a planned outcome evaluation in the future.

SUMMARY

- Process evaluation assesses the implementation of the intervention and asks the question, "Was the program implemented as intended by the plan?" It assesses the intervention at the level of resources put into and expended, activities undertaken, and outputs.

- Process evaluation assesses the reach, dose, quality, and quantity of the intervention and its benefits for beneficiaries.

- Evaluation questions are best selected through a participatory process involving the evaluators and the stakeholders. Utilizing a two-by-two table allows the group to arrive at a set of appropriate evaluation questions.

- Evaluators must be culturally competent and conduct ethical evaluations

FIGURE 6.8. *Valuable Take-Aways*

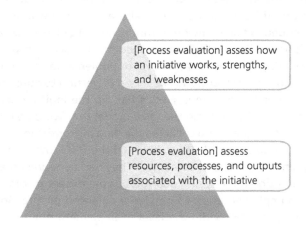

[Process evaluation] assess how an initiative works, strengths, and weaknesses

[Process evaluation] assess resources, processes, and outputs associated with the initiative

DISCUSSION QUESTIONS AND ACTIVITIES

1. Think of a concept you would like to understand. Fully conceptualize it and identify the variables that you would need to assess to get at this concept. Conduct a literature review of the concept. How has it been assessed by other researchers? What was missing/different in your conceptualization? Was the difference likely to have been influenced by culture?

2. Draw a logic model of a program or policy of your choice. Identify questions that would be appropriate for process evaluation. Draw a table showing the question, the indicator, and the data source.

3. Review the mini-case study and design an evaluation plan to answer question 4, "What data would you collect and what methods would you use? What findings would you expect to be able to use to answer the question?"

KEY TERMS

ethical
cultural
implementation
indicator

process evaluation
logic model
stakeholders
special project objectives

CHAPTER

7

DESIGNING THE EVALUATION

PART 2B: OUTCOME EVALUATION

LEARNING OBJECTIVES

- Describe how to choose an outcome evaluation question.
- Describe how to measure concepts and constructs.
- Describe evaluation research designs.
- List and describe the threats to internal and external validity.

An outcome was defined by Rossi, Lipsey and Freeman (2004) as "the state of the target population or the social conditions that a program is expected to have changed" (p. 204).

Unlike a process evaluation, which assesses the implementation of the initiative, outcome evaluation assesses its effects. In program and policy development, objectives are written to guide the implementation of the program or policy and are benchmarks of progress, showing the effect of the initiative on the goals of the initiative and the organization's mission. They are essentially the intermediary between the intervention and the goal. Outcome objectives reflect expected changes at the different domains of influence (individual, interpersonal, organization, community, and public policy).

In the first step of the participatory model for evaluation (designing the evaluation) stakeholders identify evaluation questions to determine the effects of the intervention on the beneficiaries of the intervention, whether it is a program or a policy initiative. Outcome evaluation differs from its counterpart, impact evaluation, in that impact evaluation assesses broad population level changes in quality of life that occur at the local, state, and national levels. An impact evaluation may ask questions about whether programs that were instituted in this community as a whole make a difference in the incidence, prevalence, or rates of disease, or if the quality of life of the residents of a particular jurisdiction improved. The reader is referred to other texts for detailed explanations about conducting impact evaluations. This book adopts the "objective focused evaluation," and the outcome objectives form the basis for the evaluation. Other questions may be added as required to fulfill the needs of the contract and the desire of the stakeholders or the evaluation team.

THE RELATIONSHIP BETWEEN PROCESS AND OUTCOME EVALUATION

A process evaluation component is sometimes included in an outcome evaluation to provide the additional perspectives the evaluation team might need to understand not just the effect of the initiative but its implementation. A process evaluation provides additional insights and is especially helpful if the initiative does not show the expected effect and the evaluators have to explain what reasons might explain the results. Having process evaluation data would also help in developing recommendations for program improvement. However, a process evaluation would only be feasible if it had been planned during program planning and implemented during the program. In the absence of implementing data collection and data management systems, important data for process and outcome evaluation may not be available. Collecting data for the purposes of conducting a process evaluation is best practice in program implementation.

Purposes of Outcome Evaluation

Outcomes are the effects of an intervention, be it a policy or a program. The intervention may occur at multiple levels resulting in changes at multiple levels of influence—individual, interpersonal, community, organizational, and public policy. The purpose of an outcome evaluation is to assess the changes that occur as a result of an intervention. Changes may be anticipated when outcomes are framed as SMART objectives, which are aligned with the public health goal during the early stages of program planning. Alternatively, changes may occur that were not previously anticipated but for which new objectives can be written. In an objective-based approach to the evaluation, the objectives become the standard against which the program or policy is assessed. Outcome evaluations may include questions about associated costs and benefits when an objective about cost benefit would not have formed part of the planning phase for the program or policy.

The evaluation question drives the design of the research study and the specific data-collection methods. Without an evaluation question, there really is no evaluation! The evaluation question provides the direction for the evaluation.

Evaluation questions must

- Be clear and specify what is to be assessed

- Be linked directly to the program or policy being implemented

- Be related to objective(s) identified during the development of the program or policy or identify additional changes of interest to the stakeholders

- Be linked to indicators that allow for direct or indirect measurement

- Incorporate the needs and expectations of stakeholders

The logic model may be used as the starting point for identifying evaluation questions, as illustrated in Figure 7.1. The assembled evaluation team and other stakeholders make their way across the logic model from left to right. In the column(s) identified by outcome objectives, the question asked is, "What do we want to know?" The evaluation team and the stakeholders may want to assess the effects of the program on the participants. They may have questions such as, "What changes occurred in the participants or beneficiaries?" or "Were beneficiaries of the initiative more successful than those who did not benefit from the program or policy?" or more specifically, for example, "What effect did the enactment of the policy have on underage drinking?"

The evaluation questions may be influenced by a number of factors. These include

A. The concerns and priorities of the stakeholders

B. The components of the logic model

C. The initiative's previously developed outcome objectives

D. The expertise of the evaluation team

E. The resources available for the evaluation

A. The Concerns and Priorities of the Stakeholders

Stakeholders' expectations of the program may be different from the stated objectives. Stakeholders may require information for decisions about expanding or replicating the program, which may be different from other stakeholders whose interest may be solely in the program's performance for specific age groups or related to certain objectives. In a recent evaluation, the following questions were identified by a stakeholder:

1. What changes occurred in regular physical activity for children 12–18 years?

2. What was the change in obesity rates among children 12–18 years?

FIGURE 7.1. *Logic-Model Framework for Identifying Evaluation Questions*

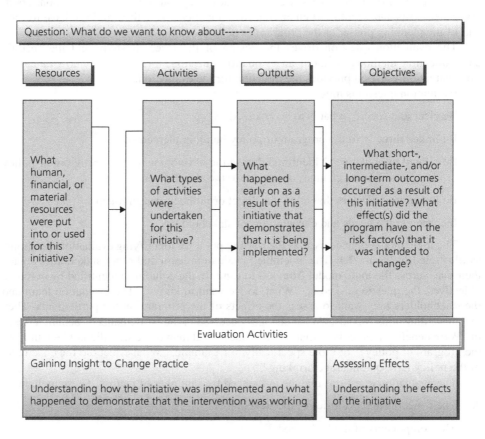

Regardless of the source of the questions, they lead to considering a number of factors about the evaluation, including the stage of development of the initiative, the evaluation design, and the data-collection methodology.

B. Components of the Logic Model

The components of the logic model may help frame evaluation questions. The logic model is an excellent tool for thinking through the most appropriate elements to measure. Each box in the logic model provides opportunities for evaluation. Evaluation questions related to inputs allow the evaluation team to assess what resources went into the program as well as what resources were expended as a result of the program. This is valuable information in the conduct of a cost-benefit analysis or for purposes of accounting or replication, although it may not always be done if the focus of evaluation is limited to understanding the effects of the interventions on the beneficiaries.

The initiative's short-, medium-, and long-term outcomes form critical components of the evaluation. Outcome questions are concerned not with whether the program is working but with whether it made a difference (see Figure 7.2).

C. The Initiatives Previously Identified Outcome Objectives

The objectives adopted during the development phase of the program or policy define the expected outcomes and are the basis for developing the evaluation plan and assessing the effectiveness of a mature program. The evaluation assesses objectives such as, "By the end of the 6-month intervention, 20% of the participants joining in the school's physical activity intervention plan will report cycling at least 30 minutes per day." In addition to objectives that serve as benchmarks for the program, stakeholders may identify principles against which the initiative can be appraised. These principles may include social justice and the equitable and ethical distribution of benefits, goods, and services.

FIGURE 7.2. *Logic Model–Inspired Questions*

What is the evaluation question being answered? What effect did the policy to have 30 minutes of exercise daily in schools have on youth 12–18 years?			
Resources	**Activities**	**Outputs**	**Outcome Evaluation Questions**
What human, financial, or other resources were used for activities or set of activities undertaken to achieve the stated outcomes?	What activities or set of activities were used to achieve the stated outcome objectives? For example, • Media programming and interviews • Outreach education and distribution of information materials • Training policy makers • Policy analysis • Policy advocacy activities	What evidence is available to show that the activities were implemented? For example, How many education sessions were held? How many policymakers participated? How many e-mails and text messages were sent out?	What evidence is available to show that short-term objectives were met, for example, increased knowledge about the topic of interest across multiple stakeholders? What evidence is available to show that intermediate objectives were met, e.g., changes in attitudes, social norms, policies, environment? What evidence is available to show increased exercise in schools to 30 minutes was implemented and sustained: lower drug use, fewer injuries, behaviors adopted?
Assumptions: There were resources available to carry out the activities and policymakers are willing and able implement this policy across the entire school district.			

D. The Expertise of the Evaluation Team

Evaluators with a high level of expertise and experience may provide additional insights into the program that lead to added ways of thinking about the evaluation. The expertise of the evaluator and the evaluation team determine the most appropriate evaluation design for conducting the study although the evaluation question drives the process.

E. Resources Available for the Evaluation

The financial, human, and material resources available for evaluation will, to some extent, determine the evaluation questions and hence the evaluation design. An experimental design requiring a control group or a quasi-experimental design requiring a comparison group will require many more resources than a simple pre/post or post only assessment of outcomes. The financial resources that drive the design will be based on the contract negotiations and how much is available for the evaluation. An outcome evaluation requiring that the evaluation team is in place from the beginning of the project will also likely cost more than an evaluation team that is brought in later in program implementation. The financial resources available will drive the kind of tools that are selected to answer the evaluation question, as will the selection of the questions themselves. It is generally expected that 10% of the total budget for the program or policy should be devoted to the evaluation. This is rarely the case.

SORTING AND SELECTING EVALUATION QUESTIONS

Once the questions have been identified from the logic model, and from existing documents from stakeholders' concerns and interests, there are many approaches for sorting them and selecting those that are most suitable for the evaluation. The process that is used may depend on the number of questions that emerge from the brainstorming process. When there is a large number of questions, electronic options for selecting and voting for questions may be the more efficient approach. However, in a small group of stakeholders, each person is given Post-it notes and asked to write down one or two questions that are important for the evaluation to answer once the purpose of the evaluation has been carefully explained. Other information that might be useful as stakeholders contemplate their questions is how much time is available for the evaluation and how the results are likely to be used. Once each person has written their questions, the facilitator presents each question to the group and sorts the questions into themes that are predetermined or emerge with the process. These could include:

1. Short-, intermediate-, or long-term outcome objectives at the individual level

2. Short-, intermediate-, or long-term outcome objectives at the interpersonal level

3. Short-, intermediate-, or long-term outcome objectives at the community level

4. Short-, intermediate-, or long-term outcome objectives at the organizational level

5. Short-, intermediate-, or long-term outcome objectives at the policy level

6. Questions requiring cost benefit analyses

7. The effectiveness of the intervention overall

Once the questions have been sorted, the group is ready for the next step, which is prioritizing the questions for evaluation. An alternative version of this participatory approach has individuals voting for the questions during the process. A modified *nominal group technique* described by Delbecq, Van de Ven, and Gustafson (1975) is as follows:

1. Each member of the stakeholder group makes a list of evaluation questions he or she would like answered.

2. The facilitator asks members of the group in turn to provide one question each to a "master list" on a flip chart or a board that is visible to the whole group. As an evaluation question is added, a show of hands provides a count of how many people included a similar question in their lists. This number is recorded next to the question on the flip chart. The questions on the participants' lists are canceled as they are accounted for on the master list.

3. The process continues until all members have contributed all the items on their lists that are different from previous questions and all the questions have been crossed off their list.

4. The facilitator reviews the master list with the group and, with the consensus of the group, eliminates or merges questions that appear similar and that ask fundamentally the same question.

The final list sets the stage for deciding on the final set of questions. A traditional two-by-two table can be used to sort the questions and identify priorities (see Figure 7.3). If the evaluation is to be useful and the results utilized, questions that are of primary importance to the person(s) requesting the evaluation must be answered.

Once this selection process is complete, a review of the questions that meet the criteria for the evaluation will determine the focus of the evaluation. Any questions that do not meet this criteria are excluded. An outcome evaluation is appropriate if the selection process led to the identification of questions about the effectiveness of a program. An outcome evaluation measures the extent to which the initiative made a difference to those who were exposed

FIGURE 7.3.   *Two-by-Two Table*

Ability to improve evaluation knowledge

	High	Low
High (Ability to contribute to the decision-making process)	Best Choice	Good Choice
Low	Okay Choice	Poor Choice

to it. It assesses the results of efforts to address the concerns and risk factors identified in the needs assessment and focuses on improving the health condition.

Outcome evaluation questions may include

- Did participants' level of knowledge or awareness change with regard to the program focus?

- What percentage of participants increased their use of a product or technology for the prevention of a disease or disability?

- What percentage of participants reduced their exposure to disease or disability?

- Did the reduction of pollutants in the air reduce the rates of asthma among children one to five years old?

- Did a policy that was aimed at reducing the incidence of violence in a local community have any effect on violence among youth 18 to 25 years old?

- Did an intervention to reduce violence against the elderly result in fewer seniors with life-threatening injuries over a 12-month period?

- What were the costs of the initiative relative to the benefits?

As described previously in this chapter, a two-by-two table may be used to identify the questions that are important for the evaluation.

Indicators

Indicators are the quantitative or qualitative variables that allow the changes that occur as a result of an intervention to be measured. They are used to provide the answers to the questions. Indicators show whether the intended results are achieved. They are objectively verifiable and can be assessed repeatedly. In asking the question, "Did participants' level of knowledge or skills change based on the program or policy?" Indicators of change would be their knowledge and skills. Quantitative indicators measure changes in numerical values; qualitative indicators measure changes that are less well defined but that are agreed to by the stakeholders as measures of success of the intervention. Indicators are the standards against which performance of the initiative is measured. Numerical indicators that show change has occurred from a baseline measurement can be plotted in a bar graph or shown in a pie chart as in Figure 7.4.

Often proxy measures are used as indicators rather than a direct indicator when one is not available. It is important that proxy measures have been validated previously. Indicators have to be related to the objective and must be sensitive enough to show a change in status. Let us consider this example. Assessing social vulnerability requires the use of many different indicators as was shown in the study by Cutter, Mitchel, and Scott (2000). One indicator of social vulnerability is the structural condition in which people live, and the researchers use the number of mobile homes as an indicator since mobile homes are more vulnerable to natural disasters and, therefore, increase social vulnerability. Another example could be using the nutritional status of children as an indicator of adequate food consumption.

Carrying out an effective outcome evaluation requires that baseline data are collected prior to implementing the initiative or in assessing environmental conditions that may change in a disaster. An outcome evaluation requires knowledge of how to reach the

FIGURE 7.4. *Changes in Conditions from the First to the Fourth Quarter*

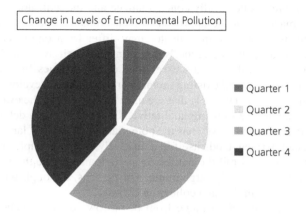

Change in Levels of Environmental Pollution

■ Quarter 1
  Quarter 2
■ Quarter 3
■ Quarter 4

population, or the object of the evaluation, the resources for carrying out the evaluation, the expertise available, and a time line.

Measuring Concepts and Constructs

Outcome evaluation often uses surveys, individual interviews, focus groups, and observation techniques or combinations to assess concepts and constructs that can be difficult to measure. Measuring concepts and constructs may require multiple indicators. For example measuring happiness requires more than one indictor because happiness is multidimensional and reflects a state of well-being and contentment. Therefore, measuring it would require assessing both well-being and contentment and, therefore, using multiple indicators. The process of specifying the indicator involves fully expanding the concepts and then deciding on the best means for determining their existence within the sample being studied.

Either qualitative or quantitative data-collection approaches can be used. For example, access to services could be measured at one or more domains:

■ Individual level (knowledge, attitude, practices)

■ Interpersonal level (peer or family influences)

■ Community level (jobs and transportation and their influence on utilization)

■ Organizational level (organizational norms, practices, policies and services that influence an individual's ability to access and utilize services within the institution)

■ Public-policy level (laws and jurisdiction-wide policies that influence utilization of services by members of the community)

The approach that is adopted in the measurement of access to healthcare or other services allows for different conclusions to be drawn. Incorporating more than one domain allows for a comprehensive view of issues and the root causes that affect access; measuring access only at the individual level leads to a more restricted view, and hence there are fewer indicators to measure. By contrast, measuring access at the multiple domains requires a larger number of indicators, but would provide a more accurate assessment.

Once the measure has been fully conceptualized and the indicator has been specified, decisions can be made about the approach to measurement. The conceptualization of a measurement and the choice of an indicator may differ from one researcher to another and is often influenced by the researcher's discipline and their available knowledge about the concept. A team of evaluators discusses measurement issues for the evaluation and relies on both their expertise and existing research and practice to develop valid and reliable data-collection instruments. The tools that are used for answering the evaluation questions vary from being quantitative to being qualitative. The tool will also determine the size of the sample. A self-completed survey has the potential to collect very large amounts of data while a face to face interview lends itself to a relatively smaller sample size. Focus groups of 6–8 per group may also limit the number of participants although over time it may be possible to interview a relatively large number of persons, although with a considerable amount of hours invested in the data collection exercise.

The tools for data collection range from being low-cost approaches requiring little expertise to being fairly high-cost and requiring some expertise either at the data collection stage or during data analysis (see Table 7.1).

TABLE 7.1. **Tools for Outcome Evaluation (What you use to answer the questions)**

Data Collection Tool	Level of Expertise Required	Cost
Self-administered surveys	Expertise to develop, little to gather, expertise to analyze	Moderate
Face-to-face interviews	Skill to gather and considerable skill to code and analyze	Expensive
Archival data	Little skill to gather but some skills to analyze	Inexpensive
Observation	Considerable skill to gather, code, and analyze data	Inexpensive but can be time-consuming
Participant observation	Skill to gather and skill to analyze	Inexpensive but can be time-consuming
Record reviews	Little skill to gather but some skills to analyze	Inexpensive
Open-ended questions on survey	Little skill to collect and analyze	Moderate
Focus-group interviews	Considerable skill to gather, code, and analyze data	Depends on who does it; in-house is less expensive

TABLE 7.2. **Assessing Effectiveness of Policy Change from the Perspective of Stakeholders**

Scale

1 = I don't know

2 = very effective

3 = somewhat ineffective

4 = somewhat effective

5 = very effective

	1	2	3	4	5
In changing social norms					
In increasing access to opportunities for physical activity					
In increasing access to opportunities for healthy nutrition					
In strengthening organizational capacity					
Other outcome (Specify): _____					

In a recent study assessing the implementation of new policies, stakeholders who were involved in the program were asked to provide their perceptions on the effectiveness of the policies in a face-to-face interview survey style data collection tool. Respondents were asked to complete the table by selecting their most appropriate response in assessing the effectiveness of a range of outcomes resulting from policy change using the scale (1–5) provided. See Table 7.2.

Of course assessing the true impact of the policy would require a very different approach, one that measures the effect of the policy on the specific problem it set out to address and not assessing their perceptions of the change, although one might argue that perceptions are real! Often determining such outcomes requires the use of experimental or quasi-experimental evaluation research designs.

Evaluation Research Designs

To determine outcomes and test the efficacy of an intervention, a rigorous research design using a control or comparison group may be required to produce defensible conclusions.

In answering questions related to causation and testing the underlying assumption that the initiative caused the outcome, the beneficiaries of the program are compared with themselves before and after the program or to a similar sample of individuals who did not participate in the initiative.

Assessing outcomes may include assessing knowledge, attitudes, behaviors, frequency, and the existence or nonexistence of an indicator. Or it may involve using biological or chemical markers in the participants or the environment to determine, for example, whether a test result changes from negative to positive, whether blood pressure rises or falls, whether hemoglobin A1c levels have changed, or if levels of pollution or chemicals that provide evidence of drug taking have altered over time.

Determining whether the initiative made an actual difference for the population requires the use of experimental or quasi-experimental evaluation designs. In an experimental research design, groups are created by randomly assigning individuals to the intervention or the control group. Given the need in public health to consider social justice concerns in its research, the formation of groups is not often based on random assignment. In general, public health has opted to design studies that create comparison groups, with the comparison group sometimes being offered the intervention in a delayed intervention model. However, this is not to say randomization is never used in public health. Randomization may be used to select the cohorts that get the intervention, but within the cohort, all individuals will have access to the intervention. For example in a study within a large school district, classrooms or schools may be randomly selected to participate in a physical activity and nutrition intervention, but all students in the classroom or school selected for the intervention will be exposed to the intervention. Those not selected to receive the intervention will form the comparison classrooms or schools. The effect of the intervention is assessed comparing the classrooms or schools that received the intervention with the ones that did not receive the intervention. An alternative approach is matching selected variables on those who received the intervention versus those who did not receive the intervention and is another approach to determining the likely effect of an intervention.

Many evaluations rely on less rigorous designs that have neither a baseline nor a comparison or control group and as a result their findings are less defensible. These are often called *observational* or *nonexperimental* designs. These evaluations are less time consuming, require fewer resources, and require less expertise than more rigorous designs, but without a baseline, a comparison group, or a control group little can be said about the effectiveness of the intervention. In the simplest designs, the intervention is tested in a single after-intervention-only assessment with one data point. An improved design to assess the effect of the initiative is comparing the population sample before and after the initiative in a single-sample pre/post test design. This chapter provides a brief overview of the commonly used designs for conducting less involved and less complicated evaluations. Detailed explanations of evaluation design may be found in other texts (for example, Cook & Campbell, 1979).

Single-Sample Designs   A single sample design relies on showing changes that occur as a result of the intervention in one group with nothing to compare that group with. In a single-sample design, there is no control or comparison group, and measurements are taken only of the group that is exposed to or that experiences the initiative or the treatment. Measurements may be taken either after the exposure in a post-only design or before and after in the improved pre/post design. The assessments may be conducted using either qualitative or quantitative measures, but research designs are more often associated with quantitative studies. The designs are represented by notations that show the intervention as X and the measurement of the change that is observed or measured as O.

Post-only: $X O_1$

Pre/post: $O_1 X O_2$

The pre/post design allows a comparison of baseline data to post intervention data with the assumption that only the initiative could have changed the outcome. If O_1 is significantly different from O_2 and there were not likely to have been any other influences on the beneficiaries of the intervention, the initiative might have produced the change. These are designs that may be familiar, and you have probably used them to evaluate workshops and training, but they are usually ineffective for determining whether the intervention caused any significant outcomes especially in uncontrolled environments. If, however, the evaluation is carefully designed to assess what could only have been learned in the workshop or training, there may be some reason to believe that the training caused the change in knowledge that was shown to occur at the end of the training.

A post-only design, however, leaves no confidence at all that the training changed the participants since you have no idea what the participants knew before the training. Therefore, a pre/post design will always be preferable to a post-only design as long as the same instrument is used before and after the training to assess any changes. Reasons that these designs do not provide confidence in the intervention causing the results will be discussed later in this chapter.

In general, the design used to assess the outcome is dependent on the research question, the most appropriate approach to answer the question, and the expertise and preferences of the evaluator and the evaluation team. The other factor that determines whether a pre/post design can be used is the ability to collect the data before and after the intervention.

Let us look at a specific example. The research question is, "Did the participants in the one-day workshop on policy advocacy improve their knowledge of strategies for improving children's utilization of dental care?" Using the pre/post design, this question can be answered by conducting a survey before and after the policy workshop using a combination of quantitative and qualitative measures. Questions in the survey should be limited to information provided during the workshop in order to determine whether the changes in scores were a result of participating in the workshop and relate to the content provided in the workshop. The difference between the baseline data (O_1) and the post-test data (O_2) is the change that occurred in the knowledge scores of participants (Figure 7.5).

In a very controlled environment, it is relatively easy to tell that participants increased their learning between coming into the workshop and completing the workshop; particularly if the workshop only lasted one day. However, imagine trying to use the single pre/post design in a community intervention and an uncontrolled environment; it would be impossible to draw any meaningful conclusions in such an uncontrolled environment. There are ways to design a study that increases confidence in the results.

FIGURE 7.5.   *Pre (O₁) and Post (O₂) Test Scores*

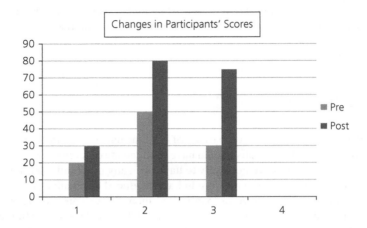

Interrupted Time-Series Design   A single-group design with multiple measures is an improvement over the single-group design just described. The interrupted time-series design takes the measurements over an extended period to determine whether intervention effects are sustained. Using a time-series design may involve the use of historical or secondary data for some or all of the measurement points. A significant limitation of these simple designs is that they do little to address threats to internal validity, as discussed later in this chapter. If the multiple measures depict a sustained change following the intervention (x) there may be some confidence in knowing that the intervention had an effect. A modification of the design may be possible in cases where withdrawing the treatment (intervention) could result in a drop of the variable of interest to preintervention levels. This is not a very useful option in public health because changes based on evidence-based and sustained interventions are unlikely to revert to preintervention levels or to show significant differences, although there may be some loss of the effect of the change over time. The importance of monitoring the implementation of the intervention and the measurement of the variables are critical.

Post-only : $X\,O_1O_2O_3O_4O_5$

Pre/post : $O_1O_2O_3O_4O_5\,X\,O_6O_7O_8O_9O_{10}$

Adding a Control or Comparison Group
Comparison-Group Designs   In order to improve our confidence in the assessment of changes in the intervention group, a control or comparison group is added to the design of the study. Adding a control or comparison group improves the single-sample design since the group that gets the intervention is being compared with a group that does not get the intervention. Using a control group rather than a comparison group improves that confidence further as the control group participants and the intervention group participants are randomly assigned to the groups, increasing the likelihood of having individual

characteristics distributed equally across the groups. The researchers must strive to ensure that the comparison group is as similar as possible to the group that gets the intervention. In either case, it is important to determine the characteristics of the final sample to determine their equivalence. Measurements are taken of the individual, group, or community exposed to the intervention and the control or comparison individual, group, or community at the same time. These designs address many but not all of the threats to internal validity, as described later in this chapter. The following diagram reflects the changes to the design notation.

	Post-only	**Pre/post**
Intervention group	$X\,O_1$	$O_1\,X\,O_2$
Comparison group	O_1	$O_1\quad O_2$

Note that the comparison group does not receive the intervention (X).

To give an example, let us assume Alethea's team is assessing a policy-information workshop at a public health facility that has 60 staff members. Two groups of 20 receive the training. The first group can use the second group as its comparison group, with the second group receiving the intervention later. A third group of 20, who are not exposed to the contents of the workshop, can serve as the comparison group for the second group. The third group may attend training after the first two workshops are completed, but because that group is not part of the research study, it does not need a comparison group, and the only data that needs to be collected from them is as a comparison group for group number 2. Providing the exact same training, or a modified version of the training to the third group is dependent on resources, but doing so addresses the social justice standard of fairness.

Interrupted Time-Series Designs With a Control or Comparison Group A control or comparison group can be incorporated into a interrupted time-series, pre/post design. As described earlier, the groups must be similar. Note also that the comparison group does not receive the intervention.

	Post-only	**Pre/post**
Intervention group	$X\,O_1\,O_2\,O_3\,O_4\,O_5$	$O_1\,O_2\,O_3\,O_4\,O_5\,X\,O_6\,O_7\,O_8\,O_9\,O_{10}$
Comparison group	$O_1\,O_2\,O_3\,O_4\,O_5$	$O_1\,O_2\,O_3\,O_4\,O_5\quad O_6\,O_7\,O_8\,O_9\,O_{10}$

Although a control group is critical for improving the confidence in a causal relationship, there are also challenges to using a control group.

- It is costly to set up and administer, doubling the cost of the study.

- It is often difficult to find individuals who have not been exposed to a similar intervention to the project intervention.

- There may be challenges with selecting what to control and what not to control.

- Selecting the control site may be fraught with difficulty when locating a site that is similar to the intervention site in environmental, social, and political factors.

- Without incentives, participants in the control group may drop out of the study since they are not receiving the intervention and are less inclined to complete surveys and participate in other necessary measurement of the outcomes being assessed in the intervention group.

Efficiency Assessments

Cost-benefit or cost-effectiveness analyses of a public health initiative assess the efficiency of a program. Such analyses complement outcome assessments and can be used only after the program's outcomes are attained. Cost-benefit analysis requires recording all direct and indirect costs of inputs as well as estimates of all tangible and intangible benefits of the initiative. All the costs and benefits are specified in monetary terms, although doing so can prove difficult. Imagine trying to give a value to the multiple tangible and intangible benefits of a child-care program!

Data for assessing the efficiency of an initiative must be gathered from all units participating in the initiative. These cost-related data can be gathered from organizational records and receipts from staff, volunteers, and other stakeholders.

■ Administrative expenditures include salaries, benefits, incentives, and travel expenses of personnel; costs for office space, utilities, office equipment and supplies; costs of running the office, for example, photocopying expenses; office-maintenance costs, such as outlays for cleaning, repairs, insurance, and equipment.

■ Direct costs associated with initiative implementation include participant stipends; transportation reimbursements; costs for child care; cost of supplies, such as games, food, books; rent for space/venue; cost of amenities; cost of equipment; costs associated with instituting a program or policy; costs to the beneficiaries of the initiative of participating in the intervention or of adopting a policy. Costs may also be incurred by community advisory committees.

■ Unintended costs associated with initiative implementation are the unexpected costs engendered by a new initiative (program or policy).

■ Building and renovation costs incurred through retro fitting or developing new structures and spaces.

The benefits-related data may be more difficult to obtain than the cost data. They include such items as the value of play areas for children, lives saved, reduced injury, improved health status, or quality of life. Benefits may also be the cost savings that accrue in the long term.

Cost-benefit and cost-effectiveness analyses require skills that may not be available on the evaluation team. Accounting and economics experts may be needed to support this kind of evaluation. Should this type of evaluation be required, the team will need to include these individuals as part of the team from the beginning or have them contribute to the team's work as needed in a consultancy capacity, which may itself be cost saving.

Key Issues in Outcome Evaluation

There are two key issues that may affect the answer to the overarching question, "Did the initiative make a difference?" In an outcome evaluation, issues of process would generally not be assessed; however, if the evaluator had some doubts about the likely outcome of the outcome evaluation and wanted to be sure that the team had some answers to help provide recommendations to stakeholders, conducting even a minimal process evaluation might be helpful. I refer the reader to the previous chapter for a fuller explanation of those issues that affect conclusions in process evaluation. In this chapter I identify issues unique to outcome evaluation. The issues are:

- Internal validity

- External validity

- Control and comparison groups

- Sampling

Internal Validity *Internal validity* is the extent to which an effect that is observed was caused by a systematically planned intervention (Cook & Campbell, 1979) and does not occur in the absence of the intervention.

In assessing the outcomes of an intervention in an experimental or quasi-experimental evaluation research design, we would like to conclude that the result that occurs in the intervention group does not appear in the control or comparison group. We assume that the difference is real and is not due to random or systematic error. When we draw this conclusion correctly, we can claim that the intervention caused the outcomes we observed.

However, when we draw this conclusion erroneously and conclude that the intervention had an impact on the intervention group and not the control or comparison group when, in fact, the intervention group and the control group did not differ, then we have a *Type I error*. When we draw the conclusion, also erroneously, that the intervention had no impact when in fact it did and the results for the intervention group should have been different from the results for the control or comparison group, then we have a *Type II error*.

It is important to consider the multiple factors that may influence the evaluator's ability to conclude that the intervention resulted in the observed changes. The factors that prevent or limit an evaluator's confidence that the initiative caused the effect (outcome) are referred to as threats to (internal) validity. The most frequent threats to validity, which are discussed in detail by Cook and Campbell (1979), are summarized here.

Attrition A loss of participants in the intervention group that is different from the loss that occurs in the initially similar control or comparison group results in having different kinds and different numbers of people in the posttest phase. The end result may be another threat, selection.

History Events that take place outside the intervention may affect the measurement of changes that are due to the program. Such events may result in an inflation of posttest scores unaccounted for by the intervention. It is important that events that occur during the intervention that might affect both the intervention group and the control or comparison group must be carefully monitored. This threat may be especially a problem when the control and intervention groups are affected differently?

Instrumentation Changes occur to the reliability and validity of measurement tools used to assess the effect of the program.

Maturation Changes in the study participants that are due to natural and physiological development that take place over time and are not necessarily caused by the program. Such natural changes occur in children and in the elderly.

Regression When study participants are selected on the basis of high or low baseline scores, the results of the testing will show they regress toward the population mean. High scorers will show lower scores in the posttest, and low scorers will show higher scores giving inaccurate measures of the impact of the intervention if present.

Selection Differences in the intervention and the comparison group occur when people self-select into the groups or when people drop out of the groups disproportionately. The result is that those who stay may be likely to succeed with or without the program, giving an inaccurate assessment of the effectiveness of the intervention on groups of individuals with mixed abilities and interests.

Statistical Conclusion In the analysis of the data, for example, when the sample size is too small to show the effect of the intervention or the measurement instruments are unstable and unlikely to measure true changes because of high standard-error estimates. Other statistical-conclusion threats include violated assumptions of statistical tests and the likelihood of concluding that there is covariance when there is not, as in Type 1 errors. "Fishing" occurs when multiple comparisons are run during a statistical analysis without recognizing that the results may be significantly different just by chance.

Testing Changes that occur to the study participants when a test that is given before the intervention affects the results of the posttest when the same test is given again after the intervention in pre/post designs. The threat may be due to participants' familiarity with the test items and their responses are based on what they remember.

The evaluation designs that contain single-sample pre/post measurements and those utilizing comparison groups address the threats to validity to a lesser or greater extent. A design that incorporates a randomly assigned control group addresses most of the threats to validity. The one it does not address is selection. One approach to addressing this threat is through the use of incentives or the delayed intervention design. In providing an incentive to participants it encourages their ongoing participation and reduces the likelihood of their dropping out of the study. A delayed intervention may also serve as an incentive if the participants perceive a real benefit in participating.

Overall, the single-group post-only design is the least likely to minimize threats to internal validity, whereas evaluation designs using randomly assigned control and intervention groups, units, and communities are the most likely to minimize these threats, and, therefore, they allow the most certainty that the intervention caused the changes that occurred in the beneficiaries. In a quasi-experimental design, many of the threats to validity are addressed also, but they may require additional measures to ensure the same level of confidence that randomly assigned control groups provide. Measures include using matching and randomly selected groups and units (not individuals) in the evaluation design.

Additional threats to internal validity take place that are not minimized by using randomly assigned control and intervention groups:

■ *Diffusion* or *imitation* occurs when the information intended for the treatment/intervention group is obtained by the control group resulting in a mimicking of the intervention; the difference between the treatment and control group is thereby narrowed.

- *Compensatory equalization* occurs when the control group is provided with or obtains an alternative intervention that influences the outcomes of interest; the narrowing of the differences between the treatment group and the control group reduce the evaluators' ability to draw the appropriate conclusions about the intervention.

- *Compensatory rivalry* occurs when the control group works hard to rival the intervention group to improve their outcomes; such rivalry minimizes the differences between groups and may result in erroneous conclusions. (Cook & Campbell, 1979).

External Validity *External validity* is the extent to which an observed effect (outcome) can be generalized to other times, settings, and populations (Cook & Campbell, 1979). The larger and more heterogeneous the sample that participates in an intervention that was found to cause the outcome of interest, the more likely it is that the outcome is generalizable. Generalizability is influenced by the sample that is selected for the study. If the sample that participates in the intervention is representative of the population, then the result is assumed to be generalizable to the larger population. A related issue is attrition, which results in the difference in the final samples due to disproportionate losses in either the intervention or the control group. The effect in either case is a more homogenous and biased sample than would otherwise exist, which may not be representative of the larger population.

Even if there is no selection bias, generalizing to another population, place, and time may not always be possible as circumstances, contexts, and populations change over time. These changes may result in considerable shifts in population demographics and assets. It would be important to carefully select the population to which the intervention and indeed the measurement tools are most likely to apply.

Control or Comparison Groups In the use of control or comparison groups, it is important that they are formed appropriately. Control groups are formed by random assignment for the purposes of ensuring that the sample that is drawn and used for the study is representative of the population. In the design of a study testing an intervention group against a control, both groups must be drawn using an approach that gives each person in the population an equal chance of being selected into either the group receiving the intervention or the group receiving the alternative intervention or no intervention at all. When this principle is violated and the groups are not selected by randomly assigning individuals to each group, the groups may not be equivalent and there is a risk of selection bias, with one group being significantly different from the other. On the other hand, a comparison group is formed with the intent of ensuring that the groups are comparable at the beginning of the study. The groups are formed based on preselected variables of interest on which the groups are compared. In both situations, a significant difference in the groups on variables that would affect the outcome of the study will result in inappropriate conclusions being drawn about the study and the evaluators concluding that the intervention made a difference when it might not have done so.

Sampling Any form of research requires sampling of the study population; however, there are many different means by which to obtain a sample of the study population. Some samples are probability samples, and others are nonprobability samples. In quantitative (survey) research it is often important to be able to generalize to the larger population, whereas samples in qualitative research are more likely to be purposeful. In program evaluation, however, although the evaluator is less likely to want to generalize to the larger population, it is nonetheless important to test a sample that is at least representative of the population that was exposed to the intervention. Probability sampling lends itself to four different approaches: random, stratified, cluster, and systematic sampling. In random sampling, each person has an equal chance of being selected; however, stratified random sampling allows for more accurate sampling because the selection of the sample is made within a stratum. In cluster sampling, intact groups—for example members of a class—are randomly selected and the final sample consists of everybody in the classroom. Systematic sampling utilizes a strategy where every nth person is selected from a list of members of the population, without an equal chance of being selected.

Nonrandom approaches result in convenience, purposive, or quota sampling. Convenience samples rely on persons who are available to participate in the study, whereas purposive and quota sampling are based on identifying characteristics relevant to the research.

Qualitative research primarily identifies individuals who have knowledge or characteristics that are required for the study. Purposeful selection of the sample may be based on specific characteristics or the need to develop a theory or concept.

A more expanded discussion of sampling is provided in Chapter 8.

Ethical and Cultural Considerations

During the process of designing and implementing an outcome evaluation, the evaluation team must ensure that no harm is caused to the program beneficiaries, other stakeholders, or the larger community. In addition, evaluators should ensure that the evaluation is culturally responsive using approaches that emphasize stakeholder involvement and organizational experience. The standards of utility, feasibility, accuracy, and propriety apply in outcome evaluation as they do in process evaluation. In addition, there are ethical principles related to the conduct of the research in evaluation. I remind you of them here because it is important that evaluation teams maintain the integrity of the evaluation process.

Evaluating programs or policies requires a team approach as well as engaging multiple stakeholders who have varying roles and experiences with the program or policy being evaluated. It is important that cultural competency is a fundamental principle of doing business. It ensures that evaluation teams are more likely to achieve the goals of the evaluation while creating an environment of trust and equity. It requires that the evaluation team understands

- The realities of the communities in which evaluation is conducted

- The need to identify influential power structures and groups that can be allies

- How to identify and work with cultural tensions of subgroups

- The skills necessary for working in a variety of cultural contexts

- How to use culturally acceptable language, communication, and negotiation skills
- Reciprocity
- Issues of confidentiality

SUMMARY

- Evaluation questions are best selected through a participatory process involving the evaluators and the stakeholders. Utilizing a two-by-two table allows the group to arrive at a set of appropriate evaluation questions.

- Outcome evaluation questions ask whether the program achieved its stated objectives at individual, interpersonal, organization, community, or policy levels.

- In assessing efficiency, the perspectives from which the costs and benefits may be assessed are participants, program sponsors, and overall costs to society, the societal costs being the most difficult to value monetarily.

- In determining outcomes and the effectiveness of an intervention, a rigorous research design using a control or comparison group may be required to produce defensible conclusions.

- Internal validity describes a causal relationship; external validity describes the generalizability of the intervention across time, people, and places. A Type I error occurs when it is erroneously assumed that the intervention caused the outcome. A Type II error occurs when it is erroneously found that the intervention did not have an effect on the outcome.

FIGURE 7.6.   *Valuable Take-Aways*

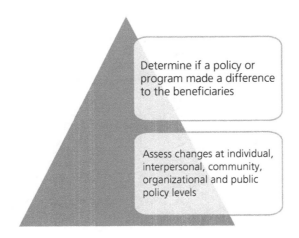

DISCUSSION QUESTIONS AND ACTIVITIES

1. Identify a program of your choice and develop a logic model. Write 10 questions that correspond to the outcome column of the logic model. Prioritize the questions based on the type of evaluation being conducted, stage of the intervention, importance to the contract, and level of resources available. Select two questions for your evaluation and an appropriate evaluation design for answering the question. How will you address any threats to validity?

2. Think of a concept you would like to understand. Fully conceptualize it and identify the variables that you would need to assess to get at this concept. Conduct a literature review of the concept. How has it been assessed by other researchers?

3. Enumerate the threats to internal validity. To what extent do the different evaluation designs minimize these threats?

KEY TERMS

attrition threats to internal validity
experimental design
external validity
fidelity
history threats to internal validity
implementation
indicator
instrumentation threats to internal validity
internal validity
maturation threats to internal validity

observational/nonexperimental design
outcome evaluation
process evaluation
quasi-experimental design
regression threats to internal validity
selection
statistical-conclusion threats to internal validity
testing threats to internal validity
Type I error
Type II error

CHAPTER

8

COLLECTING THE DATA

QUANTITATIVE

LEARNING OBJECTIVES

- Identify and describe data-collection approaches for quantitative research.
- Explain how to ascertain reliability and validity in quantitative research.
- Describe the functions of an Institutional Review Board.

The second step of the participatory model for evaluation is to collect the data (see Figure 8.1). This chapter focuses on collecting quantitative data to answer the research questions in either process or outcome evaluation.

Answering the research question uses one of a variety of approaches, all of which require the collection of data. Data collection for outcome evaluation requires a number of specific and deliberate data-collection steps and activities at the beginning, during, and at the end of the initiative; such data collection may involve quantitative approaches alone or in combination with qualitative approaches. Mixed-methods approaches combine qualitative and quantitative data in a systematic and synergistic way to answer the research question on hand or they can be used in sequence with qualitative approaches used to collect data for the development of an instrument or to explain or interpret findings. Likewise for process evaluation, data collection needs to be planned and executed early in the life of the intervention. This chapter focuses on quantitative approaches for answering the research question and the next chapter discusses qualitative approaches.

QUANTITATIVE DATA

Surveys are not the only approach for collecting quantitative data, although they are used primarily for assessing changes in social, behavioral, and psychological factors. Other forms of quantitative data include weight and height, which may be used as an independent measure for the purposes of calculating BMI and, therefore, determining if an intervention has had an effect on obesity rates. Anthropometric tools for measuring size and proportions of the body are often engaged in nutrition and physical activity interventions. Other

FIGURE 8.1. *The Participatory Framework for Evaluation: Collect the Data*

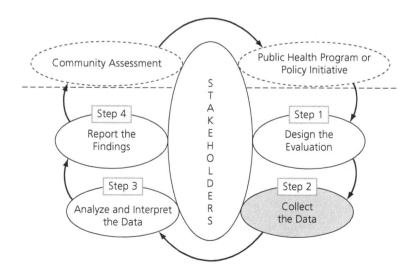

measures are used in public health in collaboration with laboratory and clinical services to provide quantitative and what are often referred to as objective measures. Determining the effect of programs may include assessments of blood pressure, hemoglobin A1C3 levels in the control of diabetes, alcohol and drug levels in the blood, and so on. Quantitative measures may also be attained, for example, in the measurement of water and air quality using specially designed laboratory based quantitative instruments that produce numerical data which can be plotted or used in calculations to assess changes following a public health intervention. In the assessment of overall jurisdiction-wide changes, surveillance data for determining the combined impact of community-wide initiatives will require the collection of quantitative morbidity and mortality health outcomes data assessed in rates per 1,000 or 100,000 depending on the indicator. For example, the number of low-birth-weight infants or infant or maternal deaths.

In assessing community health, a useful tool for understanding how individuals are influenced by others is network analysis (Keane, 2014). For example, during the recent Ebola virus epidemic in West Africa it was important to understand individual's behavior and how interactions took place at the family level during traditional ways of caring for the sick as well as at the community level during burials. Both these practices resulted in the spread of disease across town, district, and regional boundaries as a result of extensive social networks. Quantitative data are required to assess changes in networks during health promotion interventions using network analysis tools, but the reader is referred to other texts for these approaches and to other methods of measuring quantitative outcomes.

This chapter focuses on the use of surveys, which are the most often used quantitative assessment for measuring changes at individual, interpersonal, organizational, or community levels although they produce primarily individual level data.

FACTORS INFLUENCING DATA COLLECTION

The most appropriate data collection approach is the method that provides the best information to answer the question given the resources that are available and the needs of the project. The data collection for a quasi-experimental or experimental design necessitates different expertise, training, and approaches than the data collection for a single sample pre/posttest study. The quality of the data is entirely dependent on the ability, experience, and ingenuity of the researchers to collect the data. A number of factors influence the credibility of the data that are collected, which include whether appropriate methods are used, the suitability of the source from which the data was collected, the use of theoretical frameworks for developing the data-collection instruments, the quality and the quantity of the data collected, and access to appropriate and effective staff and logistical support.

Appropriate of the Methods

There are multiple approaches for collecting data, and the type of question that is asked and how the data will be analyzed determine the appropriateness of the method. For example, if the question is asked, "How many policy makers participated in the advocacy activity that was held on the Hill over the last five years?" the first thing we notice from this question is that it requires a number for its answer. To get the answer to this question, the researcher would be required to review existing documents or reports that recorded attendance at each of the advocacy activities over the past 5 years. Once this data is identified, a total number of participants is recorded. However, another question, "What changes in attitude occurred among participants in the Healthy Now program?" requires that attitude is assessed before and after the intervention. This data may be obtained using a self-report/interview or computer assisted survey approach for collecting the data. Likewise the most appropriate method for determining BMI would not be a survey. The researcher would take measurements of height and weight in order to calculate BMI.

There are limitations sometimes in the use of appropriate methods. For example, it may be most appropriate to use a survey to collect data; however, the approach to collecting the data may have to be modified based on the characteristics of the population from whom the data are to be obtained. For example, collecting data from individuals who do not read in any language may require face-to-face interviews rather than a self-administered written survey. This changes a number of factors associated with the research, including the number of researchers required to collect the data, the level of training necessary, and the logistics of collecting the data.

Suitability of the Source

In survey research, the source of the information is important for ensuring the credibility of the data and the quality of the findings. For example, it would be important to interview an individual who lives within a culture about the culture rather than someone who has heard things about the culture, watched shows on television, or spent only a short amount of time within the culture. The likelihood of a person from the culture being more authentic and understanding the culture and the interpretations of its practices is high. It is not to say that somebody who has spent a very long time studying a culture is not authentic, but the level of authenticity must always be questioned in the context of the research. The individual's position within the culture or within the context of the research question must be defined. The question must be asked, does the individual represent the culture or the phenomena of interest or have firsthand experience, or is the individual a key informant. Does the person speak from experience or does the individual simply offer an opinion, a key informant. It is important to recognize the difference and ensure that the data, the analysis, and the results reflect the difference in order to ensure that the conclusions are valid.

Since surveys rely on individuals' real or perceived notions of a particular variable, the quality of the data is determined by their understanding of the variable and the extent to which that understanding influences the response. In a cross-cultural study or a study that includes individuals from different cultures, their understanding of a phenomenon or variable may be limited. For example, in some languages words may not exist that adequately describe a phenomenon that may exist in the English lexicon; therefore, there may not be a word that can be used in a direct translation. The explanation of the concept, however, that may be required may not accurately reflect the phenomenon of interest affecting the validity of the research. Care must be taken in ensuring appropriate translations of the survey as well as back translations to ensure accuracy.

Theoretical Frameworks

In the community assessment and again in the development of public health interventions, we discussed the use of theoretical frameworks. The tools used in community assessments include surveys and if the intervention is to have theoretical underpinning, the data that are used for the baseline and subsequent assessment of changes to risk and protective factors must also follow a theory. In using a theory, the assessment of changes would be based on specific known constructs, which, when influenced by the intervention, would show a change status. For example, if the intervention is based on the theory of planned behavior (Ajzen & Fishbien, 1980), the constructs of the theory that would form the basis for the pre- and post-intervention assessment are:

- Attitude toward the behavior (behavioral beliefs and evaluation of behavioral outcomes)

- Subjective norm (normative beliefs and motivation to comply)

- Perceived behavioral control (control beliefs and perceived power)

- Behavioral intention

- Behavior (of interest)

Other theories that can be adopted for use in community assessments and the development of interventions include, for example, the health-belief model, the social cognitive theory, the transtheoretical model, organizational theory, and theory of diffusion of innovation. Using the constructs of the theory as intended ensures a full conceptualization of the concepts that are likely to achieve the behavior change. However, based on some cultural contexts these theories may be missing important constructs; consider how they might influence your research. The use of theory brings with it expectations of understanding how the theories are used in survey development and may limit the number of questions that are included in the study since there is a definable structure on which the subsequent intervention is likely to be based.

Quality and the Quantity of the Data Collected

The quality of the conclusions of an evaluation study is determined in part by the ability to collect data that is both valid and reliable. The quality of the data is affected by the authenticity of the source as described earlier. Culture and cultural values may affect the data in cases where the culture prefers not to discuss its beliefs and practices to outsiders. Any data that is gathered by an outsider will almost certainly not contain the necessary depth of understanding. This has been found to be true of indigenous cultures and African populations. For example, among many African populations there is the practice of initiation and individuals aspire to be a part of the group through engaging in associated rituals. While there are some practices of the culture that are good and need to be supported, there are a few that may be detrimental to health. In either case, those practices are rarely discussed outside the cultural group. Individuals often do not want to divulge aspects of their culture that they consider to be private and therefore may not provide complete information.

Educational levels and preferences may also affect the type and quality of data that can be collected. For example, individuals with low educational levels may not have the conceptual understanding and the understanding of disease patterns that are evident with individuals with higher levels of education. In practical terms, in the context of data collection, it means that where a seven-point Likert scale is feasible for individuals who are able to make clear distinctions between points, individuals with low levels of education may be less able to be as discerning forcing the use of different response categories and limiting the type of analysis that is possible. For example, instead of using a 5-point agreement scale the researcher may be forced to use a format which allows for a yes/no or a simpler agree/disagree response instead. Although race and ethnicity are not determinants of educational levels, individuals' experience of the educational system results in lower levels of educational attainment and affects the quality of the data. Individuals who participate in public health studies may be fluent in English yet may not be able to complete a survey based on high-level concepts and constructs. When individuals are fluent in both spoken and written language, data are improved if the survey is provided in that language, most often their mother tongue. For example, if individuals are fluent in Spanish, the surveys should be developed in Spanish or translated into Spanish before they are administered. The reading level of instruments for the general public must be kept a sixth-grade level or less.

The age of the individuals may influence quality and quantity in that younger and much older individuals may not be able to provide accurate information based on the lack of experience or their inability to remember or make sense of the world around them. Different approaches for data collection for different ages can be used—for example using smiley faces for assessing changes in circumstances or conditions may be useful for children and older adults. Age may also affect sight, and asking an individual with poor eyesight to complete a survey may result in items being rated inaccurately. Often, individuals with poor eyesight will not report this disability for fear of losing any incentives associated with the study.

Issues of accessibility and availability of resources associated with data collection will also affect the quality of the data and the conclusions since, for example, a lack of accessibility to computers for a proportion of the intended population sample may result in a biased sample if the mode of data collection is on-line. If the original sample size was 1,000 and the assumption was made that each person has access to a computer terminal, but only 50% actually do have access, the sample size drops by 50%. Rapidly changing technology also affects who can be reached for survey research. For many individuals, cell phones have replaced the use of land lines, yet directories do not exist for cell phones and the location of the individual may bear no relation to where a potential respondent is when the phone is answered. For example, a sampling frame requires that all individuals live in Kentucky, yet an individual with a Kentucky cell phone area code may live in Florida. Unless the question is asked about where the person lives, the assumption is that they live in Kentucky and the answers relate to Kentucky, compromising the quality of the data. If the inclusion criteria specify that individuals who currently live in Kentucky are those who should be interviewed, individuals who live in other states should not be included as respondents. Questions should be included in the initial screening that excludes individuals who do not fit the criteria.

Individuals have the right to refuse to participate in our research, but when they do, it may bias our sample, or reduce the number of individuals who are eligible to participate in the study to levels that may affect the final sample and bias the conclusions. If for example, individuals who were not satisfied with the program refused to participate in the study leaving only individuals who are satisfied, the conclusions that might be drawn from this sample may be that the program was very successful; this does not take into consideration those for whom it was not successful. This biased outcome may result in the program being considered effective and replicated with much less chance of success. Those who did not participate may have provided perspectives that would have been useful for program replication.

It should be clear by now that the quality of the data influences the validity of the conclusions. We have discussed individual-level factors that might affect data collection, but additional factors occur at the organizational level that also affect quality and quantity of data.

Appropriate and Effective Staff Support

Achieving valid and reliable outcomes in evaluation requires a process that considers how staffing also affects data collection. The use of staff who are not trained in research and data collection approaches specifically undermines the quality of the data. Training for staff who are inclined to collect good quality of data is vital. For example, poorly trained staff may subject the study to occurrences of instrumentation—a threat to internal validity—and if the individual is unable to build adequate rapport and trust, collection of good data from the respondent may also be unlikely.

Another aspect of trust building is in interactions between the interviewer and the respondent in the conduct of culturally sensitive interviews. It is important that individuals with responsibility for collecting data in cross-cultural settings are adequately trained in cross-cultural interviewing to improve their capabilities to conduct culturally sensitive interviews. Examples of cross-cultural and potentially sensitive interactions and interviews are likely to occur with men who have sex with men, individuals with drug taking habits, individuals from minority ethnic cultures such as Hispanics, African Americans, indigenous peoples, subpopulations from Africa, Asia, Europe, and Middle East who may have escaped persecution in their home countries and are seeking refuge in another country. Suggestions for successful cross-cultural interviewing can be found at http://calswec.berkeley .edu/files/uploads/doc/CalSWEC/CrossCulturalInterview_BulletList.do

Additional tips for cross-cultural interviewing are listed below:

- Take time at the beginning of the interview to provide thorough information about the scope of the interview and the role of the interviewer. Take extra care to explain the duties of the social worker and the child welfare agency if conducting interviews related to child welfare because these concepts may be unfamiliar. If law enforcement is involved in the interview, be sure to explain why they are involved and what their role will be.

- Continue to check in with the interviewee throughout the interview, providing explanations when needed and ensuring the interviewee understands the process as it evolves.

- Leave time in the interview for the interviewee to ask questions and allow for a period of silence to give the interviewee time to formulate their answers.

- Reassure interviewees that you won't be shocked or upset by what they have to say.

- Assure confidentiality.

Other staff support that is required for good quality data includes logistical support for project management, scheduling interviews and other data collection, and ensuring that adequate and appropriate resources are available at the site of data collection. Resources include data collection tools, consent forms, audio, video and computer equipment for data entry and data analysis, forms and logs for field notes, incentives, signature, demographic, and sign-in sheets, transportation, child care and meals, if provided.

USING SURVEYS

Surveys are the most often used data-collection tool for quantitative research designed to collect information from those who experience or have a personal insight into the issue being assessed. Surveys may be used to collect information in a community assessment, as baseline data before or at the start of an initiative, and in assessing the process or outcomes of an intervention. Like all other measurement tools, they can be used in any of the evaluation research designs. Often they are used when there is no specific research design.

The survey tool is made up of a group or sequence of questions designed to elicit information about a subject from individuals who may be members of the community and affected by the problem. Key informants, who see the problem from their own vantage point but have considerable insight, may also be surveyed. These may include providers of the services and community and organization leaders.

Using surveys as a data-collection method has several advantages and disadvantages:

■ Constructing items for a valid and reliable survey can be a difficult and time-consuming exercise, but once the items are developed, they may be used over and over again for similar projects.

■ Surveys are relatively easy to administer; they collect a large amount of data in a relatively short period of time.

■ Surveys can be evaluated for reliability and validity.

■ Surveys lend themselves easily to communitywide data-collection efforts.

■ Written surveys can be administered in groups or individually, by mail, face-to-face, by telephone or electronically.

■ Surveys are generally less expensive to administer than other research instruments. There are several considerations in opting to conduct surveys:

■ Surveys collect large amounts of data but often leave the researcher asking, "Why?" or "So what?"

■ Surveys have to be just the right length, long enough to measure the concepts accurately and ensure stability of the measure, but short enough to be completed fully and not burden the respondent unduly.

■ The time or expertise it takes to develop a reliable and valid survey may not be available.

■ Survey data collection can take a long time to complete because respondents may not respond to a request to complete it face-to-face, open their mail for a mail-in survey, answer the telephone, or respond to an email request. Getting the survey completed may take several attempts at contacting the potential respondents through reminder post cards or multiple phone calls and emails spread over an extended period.

Surveys require a considerable amount of skill to develop and analyze. One of my students had this to say about the process: "Although it could take multiple hours and many drafts [to develop] your survey or questionnaire, it is best to put the time in[to] creating it, … this will make the remainder of the process go a lot smoother." In designing a questionnaire, it is important that consideration is also given to the formatting and quality of the survey. Surveys should be written with plenty of white space and in an easy to read format, they should be printed on good-quality standard-length paper so they fit easily onto a clip board when they are being used for field research. Surveys should be printed on one side only to avoid the likelihood of the respondent not answering whole sections of the survey, and they should contain headings to allow easy and clear transitions between sections.

Maximizing the potential for the survey to provide the best information requires engaging diverse stakeholders in the development process, conceptualization of the survey, identification of specific survey areas and items, selection of survey language and wording, and the approaches to survey administration (Israel et al., 2005, p. 108).

In addition, a variety of activities can improve survey research, including:

- Using expert panels to assure appropriate and complete understanding of the concepts being measured

- Using a pilot test with the potential study population to ensure understanding of the survey items

- Incorporating tests of validity and reliability

- Providing appropriate and adequate training to the people collecting the data

- Partnering with trained and experienced statisticians or biostatisticians to determine appropriate response categories for the anticipated data analysis

If resources are available and it is appropriate to develop web-based surveys, a variety of survey-development tools are available to support this process. These online tools include SurveyMonkey® and Zommerang.® The online tools provide easy-to-follow directions and formatting options. In addition, for computer-distributed surveys, they may also offer appropriate distribution options. Once the surveys are completed and returned, the tools offer data-analysis options and the opportunity to download the participant data into other data-analysis software such as Microsoft Excel® and SPSS®, a statistical data-mining and analysis software for analyzing quantitative data. KoBoToolbox a more recent addition, is a free and open source iOS or Android devise based tool for collecting survey data on and off line.

Before a survey can be taken, it must reach the study population. It is important that the distribution method is sensitive to the cultural norms of the population and appropriate for the setting and the study. Participants for a survey may be available in one place, or they may need to be individually recruited. Advertisements to recruit participants may be placed in flyers and other media. People can also be invited to complete a survey contained within an envelope, placed on a web site, attached to an email, or through a telephone call. Recruitment scripts that are included with the surveys distributed by mail, read over the phone, or included in an online solicitation must be developed and approved by a local Institutional Review Board.

Staff must be hired and trained to conduct telephone or face-to-face interviews for data collection. In an empowerment model, such training leaves communities with skills they can use long after the evaluation. Training may include improving facilitation and listening skills but always includes familiarization with the interview guide so that there is little or no change in its delivery from one interview to the next. Consistent delivery of questions in facilitator-mediated data collection increases reliability and minimizes the threat to validity caused by instrumentation.

Administering Surveys

Surveys may be completed by self-administration, in face-to-face or telephone interviews, through online distribution either directly on the web through a link provided by the researcher or via email. Questionnaires are most valuable for collecting data from a large number of people. Considerations in the selection of the method include the type of information required, the population to be surveyed, and the financial and human resources, and time available.

The type of information that is required often determines the approach to survey administration. The more sensitive the information, the less likely some individuals are to want to discuss it with another person, so an interviewer-facilitated survey may be less successful than a self-administered survey. Face-to-face interviews may be appropriate with less-sensitive questions. Obtaining information through interviews requires the interviewer to be tactful and to build rapport with the interviewee. Using a conversational tone may help in building rapport and eliciting trustworthy information.

Both open-ended and closed-ended questions may be used in surveys completed face-to-face or by telephone; getting information from open-ended questions is less successful in a self-administered format. Telephone interviews tend to have less missing data and fewer "don't know" responses than self-administered surveys (Feveile, Olsen, & Hugh, 2007), although building rapport for a good telephone interview may be difficult. A face-to-face interview will likely produce more valid information than a self-completed survey in populations with low reading levels. It is important to do a check and ask yourself, "Did the respondent understand the question?" "Will the respondent know the answer?" "Will the respondent tell me the answer?" Yes to each of these questions will increase the likelihood of having a successful interview and collecting valid data whether you are using a face-to-face interview or self-administered survey format.

The resources available for the distribution of surveys or to conduct interviewer-facilitated surveys may control the approach that is selected. Face-to-face meetings require additional time, training, and travel. Mail-distributed surveys incur postage costs for initial and follow-up reminder post cards or letters. Although the cost of distributing surveys by email is low, the likelihood of having wrong email addresses is high and when an email address is no longer in use, the email will not be delivered to the appropriate person. Utilizing telephones may require high tolls for long-distance calls. Even when resources are available, the population that the survey is intended to reach may be a limiting factor. Participants who do not have telephones cannot be reached with a survey using this technology, and likewise a web-based survey cannot reach somebody who neither has nor uses a computer.

The channel that is used for survey distribution influences the response rate and how quickly the study can be completed. Mail-distributed surveys may not be opened or the call may not be responded to by the person for whom it is intended. With the extensive use of cell phones and the precipitous decline in the use of land lines, researchers are forced to address the challenges in using cell phones for data collection. One of the biggest challenges is the frequent changes in cell phone companies to get more competitive rates with the resultant change in telephone numbers.

Ensuring That Data Are Valid and Reliable

When survey instruments are developed, they are subjected to a variety of procedures to increase both their validity and reliability and reduce error. Error in the data may occur for example if you ask a question for which the respondent does not know the answer but feels he/she has to answer the question. Alternatively, a question is asked about an event or occurrence that relies on the respondent's memory of long ago. The response error in a long recall period is not due to a lapse in memory usually, but an error in guessing what the "correct" answer should be. The significance of the event, its frequency, and the time since the event will influence recall, so keep the recall period as short as possible and focus on significant events or occurrences that the respondent is likely to remember. Validity and reliability are standards for measurements, and they dictate collection processes. Validity is the extent to which a measure assesses the underlying concept that it claims to measure, while reliability refers to the consistency of the measure when it is applied repeatedly. Although reliability and validity are assessed separately, there is a relationship between the two that is worth remembering. For an instrument to be reliable, it must also be valid, but it can be valid without being reliable.

Reliability When an instrument is developed, it is assessed for its stability in order to determine the level of random error that may interfere with true measurement of the variable. Any error variability causes an underestimation or overestimation of the true measurement, making the assessment unreliable. This variability is measured using a reliability coefficient that is at 1.0 when no error exists. A range of approaches can be used to assess the extent to which there is variability in the collection and interpretation of the data. Intrarater reliability assesses the extent to which the individual changes with each successive assessment. Interrater reliability measures the differences between two persons assessing the same situation or the same data. Cohen's kappa (Cohen, 1960) is the statistical test generally used to assess reliability using nominal or ordinal data. *Internal consistency* is a measure of correlations across given items in a test (Carmines & Zeller, 1979). Cronbach's alpha assesses the correlation among the total number of items on the scale and the extent to which they assess the same underlying concept (Windsor, Clark, Boyd, & Goodman, 2004). An instrument with a high internal-consistency coefficient has an alpha ≤ 1.0. An acceptable range for psychometric analysis of an instrument is ≥ 0.65 to ≤ 0.90. *Test-retest* assessment measures reliability by using the same test and administering it two different times with the same sample. To increase the validity of this test, the repeat test must be conducted within a short period of time and must record a Cohen's kappa of ≥ 0.80 (Windsor et al., 2004).

Validity Validity concerns the degree to which scores that are achieved reflect the underlying construct. Three types of validity are generally associated with instrument development: construct validity, content validity, and criterion validity (Carmines & Zeller, 1979). *Construct validity* is the extent to which the measure is theoretically sound and correlates with the theorized construct. It measures phenomena that can be observed that reflect the underlying concepts. *Content validity* assesses the extent to which the items in an instrument are well defined and represent all the facets of a given construct. Experts may be used during the instrument-development phase to assess the accuracy of the items that are selected to measure the variable of interest. A literature review or qualitative research may also provide information to improve conceptualization and understanding of the variables and their impact on the measurement. *Criterion validity* describes the concurrence of the item or scale with a previously assigned "gold standard" that confirms its predictive value (Carmines & Zeller, 1979).

Sample Selection and Sample Size

An accurate definition of the target population and of the inclusion and exclusion criteria for the study participants are critical in any research study. The sample consists of population units, things, organizations, geographical areas, and so forth that have the characteristics of interest to the researcher. It differs from one research study to another and is directly related to the evaluation question. For instance, a study of the relationship between childhood obesity and the intake of vegetables will likely focus on children ages 3 to 12, while a study of substance abuse and teen driving may focus on youth 15 to 21 years old. Sampling is the process of selecting a small set/group of units from the target population.

There are two main types of sampling: random/probability and nonrandom/nonprobability.

Random Sampling Methods *Probability sampling* involves random selection of the participants in the study. It is achieved by selecting names or numbers at random from a list of all potential participants with each having an equal chance to participate. In addition it lends itself to four different approaches, random, cluster, stratified, and systematic sampling.

Random selection methods are used when the resulting sample has to be representative of the population and conclusions are drawn about the whole population based on the results of the sample. In random sampling, each person has an equal chance of being selected; it is used primarily in quantitative studies, such as surveys, because it enables the researcher to generalize the results to the population as a whole. A sampling frame is required that allows for a random selection of participants who are representative of the underlying population being studied.

Cluster sampling may be used to select a group or participants from a group or entity such as a business, a school, a faith community, a census tract, or a neighborhood. The entire group or location can be selected, or a randomly selected number of participants may be selected to represent the group or the entity. In cluster sampling, intact groups—for example members of a class—are randomly selected and the final sample consists of everybody in the classroom.

Systematic sampling is an alternative strategy to probability sampling. It is achieved by selecting names or numbers from a list such as a voting register or a phone book at the same regular interval. Systematic sampling utilizes a strategy where every *n*th person is selected from a list of members of the population, without an equal chance of being selected.

Stratification sampling is achieved when the members from a population group of interest are subdivided into strata and systematically sampled from a list of the population of interest. The sample that is selected is proportional to the size of the population type in the general population. Stratified random sampling allows for more accurate sampling because the selection of the sample is made within a stratum.

Nonrandom Sampling Methods *Nonrandom* methods are used primarily when the goal is to explore and reach an understanding about issues that pertain to a specific group of people. Although these methods are convenient for obtaining a sample for study, they rely on having captive audiences or on the particular characteristics of the population. For instance, it is impossible to randomly select a sample from a hidden or hard-to-reach population, such as illegal immigrants, drug addicts, and runaway youth. Although the bias in selection of participants is much higher when using nonrandom sampling techniques, the method can still lead to valid statistical conclusions. Nonrandom sampling includes convenience, purposive, and snowball sampling. They do not provide samples that are representative of the underlying population and therefore results from them are not generalizable to the population at large.

Sample Size The sample size for data collection is determined by the research approach, the population selected, the needs of the study, the type of analysis required, the resources and expertise available, and the cost. The size of a random sample or the number of units on which data have to be collected is computed based on several types of information:

- The size of the population.

- The amount of error that can be tolerated. This is generally 5%, yielding a 95% confidence that the study results are accurate.

- The effect size, or the degree to which the groups in the study differ in the characteristics of interest in the study—for example, how much heavier kids are who do not have at least one intake of vegetables a day compared to those who do.

The larger the sample the more representative it will be and the more power it will have for making accurate and reliable interpretations of the data; but the cost will be higher also. Sample size is generally computed to give the researcher a minimum of 80% power to detect a difference between groups, should the difference exist.

In general, the more heterogeneous the population, the larger the sample size required for quantitative-research analysis. The sample size is also determined by the number of variables in the study and the number of subgroup analyses that are proposed. If, for example, a survey was conducted as part of a study about workplace injuries at a treatment plant, a larger sample size would be required to understand the factors leading to the injuries if the analysis were conducted to provide subgroup analysis by gender, age, race, or type of occupation.

The sample size for a research study may be calculated based on a formula from a table or calculated using computer programs such as STATA, SAS, or EpiInfo (Shi, 2008). There are also on-line calculators that require a minimum amount of information for the calculation. Detailed discussion of this topic may be found in other texts.

DESIGNING SURVEY INSTRUMENTS

Survey-Development Process

Before developing a survey, the first consideration is "What is the research question and what information does this survey have to elicit?" If the answer is not available in existing data and a new survey has to be developed, then the next question becomes, "Is there a survey available that can be adopted or adapted?" Answering the second question requires doing a literature search for peer reviewed articles that contain surveys or results of surveys, consulting with colleagues in the same or a similar field, or scanning the internet. In program evaluation, finding the right survey can be difficult because initiatives are unique and have different characteristics, and the needs of the evaluation can be different each time.

Identifying the questions that are suitable for developing a survey to assess a particular outcome may be possible. Survey items with appropriate indicators may be found through a literature search. In cases where there is little information about the phenomenon, brainstorming with experts in the field or conducting focus-group interviews with a sample of the population may provide useful insights. Indicators provide the evidence that a change has occurred. Examples of indicators include:

- The percentage of participants reporting an increase in the number of minutes per day of exercise

- The percentage of respondents registering under a newly implemented expansion of eligibility for health insurance

- The reduction in the number of homeless individuals

- The change in air or water quality

Identifying existing reliable and valid instruments that serve the purposes of the study or compiling a new instrument using existing valid and reliable items from a variety of sources may be quicker than developing an instrument from scratch. Modified or new instruments should be validated with a sample similar to the study population in a pilot test. In developing an instrument, it is essential to keep in mind the potential respondents for the survey, the questions and question formats, and data-analysis needs.

Potential Respondents

The persons required to complete a survey are a key consideration. They will determine the language and the reading level of the survey tools. Surveys to solicit information from Spanish-only speakers will have to be written in Spanish or translated into Spanish. By the same token, if reading levels are low, the survey must be developed at a third- to sixth-grade level in the appropriate language. Particular attention is given to developing surveys for children and adults who function at a lower cognitive level and who have less developed conceptual skills; they require more concrete questions and simplified response categories. For example, children may be more familiar with and respond better to a scale represented by pictures rather than numbers or categories.

The Flesch-Kincaid Grade-Level Readability Formula developed by Rudolph Flesch and John Kincaid may be used to assess the reading level of surveys. It is built into Microsoft Word® and can be accessed through the spelling and grammar function. Survey developers must balance their need to know against the real-life experiences of the respondents and keep surveys short.

Question Formats

Survey instruments may contain closed-ended, open-ended, or multiple-choice questions or questions that provide 3- to 5-point Likert scales for respondent feedback. Surveys may also ask respondents to match, rank, or compare a set of options.

Babbie (1990) points out that the response categories of closed-ended questions should be exhaustive, including all the possible responses, and should be mutually exclusive. However, because it is often not possible to meet these criteria, respondents can be given the option of writing in their own response by using the "other" category. These answers are coded before data entry to allow for appropriate analysis.

A survey instrument with closed-ended questions expects responses such as yes/no, ranking responses, and other numerical formats. The type of questions also determines the level of understandability of the items and, therefore, influences the response. Giving a yes/no response may be easier for a low-level reader than selecting a response on a 5-point scale of "very unfavorable to very favorable." However, a survey with only yes/no responses provides limited understanding of underlying concepts and restricts the variability in the items. In addition, it limits the level of data analysis that can be conducted. It is important to field-test the instrument with persons similar to those in the final audience to determine how well the items are understood and how well they produce the appropriate responses. Table 8.1 provides some sample questions with corresponding response formats.

A useful addition to closed-ended questions in traditional surveys is the use of open-ended questions. Respondents are asked to provide their own answers to the questions. For example, respondents may be asked to explain a response they gave to a closed-ended question. They may be asked a new question such as "What did you experience when you visited the site of the earthquake?" Lines or a text box are provided for answers. Using open-ended questions as part of a survey provides for deeper understanding of the phenomenon, which is usually not achieved from typical survey research. Answers to open-ended questions may be coded before data entry to allow them to be converted to quantitative data.

Steps in Creating a Survey Instrument

When the research question is fully conceptualized through a review of the literature, an expert review panel, or by conducting focus groups with the intended audience for the survey, you are ready to frame the specific survey questions. The survey questions are developed to reflect the information that is being sought. They have content validity. It is instructive to have content experts review the questions to ensure that they reflect the concepts

TABLE 8.1. **Questions and Response Formats**

Questions	Possible Response Types
Do you know about the recent changes in the policy to increase eligibility?	Yes/no
What is your opinion about the following statement: Changes in the policy improved access to health care for residents of my county.	Five-point scale of strongly disagree to strongly agree
The clinic that was opened in your community recently offers the following services [list of services].	Check all that you might use
What is your opinion about the services provided in the newly opened clinic?	Five-point scale of very unfavorable to very favorable
How old are you?	Age in years
Has having the clinic changed the lives of residents of this community?	Yes/No

that are being measured; additional feedback from a statistician can ensure that appropriate response formats are used to allow for the analysis. When evaluators decide to develop their own instrument, they can do so by following these steps:

Step 1: State the evaluation research question and define the indicators that reflect the construct of interest.

Step 2: Frame appropriate questions making them as clear and as simple as possible. Assess only one concept per question.

Step 3: Order the questions into an instrument that flows smoothly from beginning to end. Consult a statistician as needed to confirm the appropriateness of the response categories for the proposed data analysis.

Step 4: Review the instrument for construct and content validity. Does it ask the question it intends to ask, and does it measure the construct fully? Have an expert panel review the instrument.

Step 5: Check the instrument's readability using the Flesch-Kincaid Grade-Level Readability Formula built into Microsoft Word® if required to determine the reading level.

Step 6: Pilot-test the formatted draft instrument with individuals or groups similar to the study population.

Step 7: Edit the survey instrument as needed.

Step 8: Prepare the final instrument for use in an easy to read, logical format complete with clear instructions for how the survey is to be completed.

Using existing valid and reliable surveys or drawing ideas from them saves time. If you take this route, be sure to get permission to use the material or include a reference if it is a publicly available survey.

In the design of surveys, Dillman (2000) suggests that difficult and sensitive questions and demographic questions be left to the end. Once the draft survey is reviewed by an expert panel, it is ready for a pilot test. The extensive use of electronic communication such as e-mail and web-based tools makes reviewing by an expert panel and editing questions a more practical and less time-consuming process than it once was.

Additional guidelines for survey development include:

- Make items clear, precise, and short so the respondent knows exactly what question you are asking.

- Avoid using items that contain more than one question.

- Ask only questions that are important to the respondents and that are relevant to answering the research question.

- Avoid asking questions in the negative, using words such as *not*.

- Ensure that concepts are clearly defined.

- Ensure that questions allow for a normal distribution of responses or a fifty/fifty distribution in the case of dichotomous answers.

- Use as large a number of answer categories as possible to provide variability in the responses. In low literacy populations, however, maintaining fewer response categories is preferable.

- Avoid asking questions that result in the respondent's answering the question in a particular way, either negatively or positively to reduce bias and error in measurement (Babbie, 1990).

PILOT TESTING

Pilot testing an instrument is a chance to determine whether it works under real-life conditions and whether it works well in the population for which it is intended. Conduct the pilot test with a representative number of participants drawn from the same sampling frame as the one used for the study. Participants in the pilot test must be similar to the study participants. Babbie (1990, p. 227) refers to pilot testing as "a miniaturized walk through of the final survey design."

A pilot test provides an opportunity to determine whether the instrument is culturally appropriate, is written at the appropriate reading level, is short enough so as not to burden the respondent, and is written so that the questions are interpreted by the respondents in ways the researchers intended. In addition, it provides information on the questions that respondents choose not to answer and alternative response categories. Conducting the pilot test also provides opportunities to test the flow of the questions and to time the entire procedure, including administering the consent form. It provides data for instrument validity and reliability tests and is a way to solicit feedback. When the pilot test is complete, the surveys are revised and edited as necessary and they are ready to be rolled out.

Another value in conducting a pilot study beyond field testing the survey is to field-test the entire process and test the prediction that the intervention caused the outcome that is observed (hypothesis) (Babbie, 1990).

TRIANGULATION

Evaluators should not be confined to using only one method if the research can be appropriately conducted using a combination of approaches. Using a mixed-method approach and multiple sources of data or varying data-collection methods to cross-check and substantiate findings and increase validity in evaluation research is known as *triangulation*.

Primary and secondary data can be used to answer the same research question; they provide complementary or differing perspectives. Primary-data sources include:

- People directly affected by the problem
- People implementing initiatives and services to address the problem
- People knowledgeable about the problem
- People observing the behaviors or conditions that influence the problem
- Influential members of society such as policymakers and community leaders

Secondary-data sources include existing local, state, and national databases that provide behavioral, environmental, and health statistics (Shi, 2008).

In addition to using a variety of sources of data, a mix of qualitative and quantitative data-collection approaches, and different theoretical frameworks may be used to achieve triangulation. A matrix may be used to think through the selection of the most appropriate approaches. The final selection can be based on considerations of appropriateness, expertise, and resources. The planning process can help delineate these factors for decision-making.

Data-Analysis Needs

The question format determines the types of data analysis that can be carried out. *Nominal-level data* are the lowest level and allow for a distinction in mutually exclusive categories such as gender (male/female) or place of residence (house, apartment, trailer home, boathouse). When just two categories are given (yes/no), the values are dichotomous. Nominal data are used to calculate percentages. *Ordinal-level data* allow rank ordering within the categories and are represented by a number or a scale with no meaning other than the indication of a rank order. Nominal data are used to calculate percentages and can also be used to calculate means. *Interval-level data* have more meaning than ordinal data because the distances between the points have real meaning on a numerical scale. A commonly used example is the temperature scale, where the difference between 80 degrees and 90 degrees is the same 10 degrees as the difference between 60 degrees and 70 degrees. *Ratio-level data* provide a true zero; length, height, and age are good examples (Babbie, 1990). Like interval data, means and standard deviations can be calculated from this category of data and used to summarize the data.

Because the type of data collected determines the type of analysis that can be undertaken, the questions must be designed to ensure that the appropriate level of data is collected. For example, if you are interested in having means, then the data must be ordinal, interval, or ratio data. Once the instrument is developed and those data are collected, only limited analyses may be possible if an inappropriate level of data has been used. For this reason, it is important to consult a statistician at the beginning rather than at the end of survey development.

INSTITUTIONAL REVIEW AND ETHICS BOARDS

During the data-collection process, the rights of individuals must be respected and their welfare must be protected. It is also important to protect privacy and confidentiality in data collection and in reporting the results.

Protecting the rights of an individual requires that researchers do not coerce anyone to participate in a study. In addition, participants have the right to know and understand all the research procedures. If they consent to participate, they must be treated in a caring, considerate, and respectful way. All their interactions must be kept confidential, and their data must remain anonymous unless they have been notified otherwise.

Specifically, the American Evaluation Association (2008, p. 234) identifies respect for people as a guiding principle for evaluation practice. "Evaluators respect the security, dignity, and self-worth of respondents, program participants, clients, and other evaluation stakeholders and thus should abide by current professional ethics, standards, and regulations regarding confidentiality, informed consent, and potential risk and harms to participants."

An Institutional Review Board or Ethics Board as it is sometimes called internationally is made up of a panel of individuals who represent both the research institution and the community. The Board reviews research proposals, provides guidelines about informed-consent documents, and ensures that the research does not have the potential to harm research subjects. Requests for IRB review must contain the full research proposal, data-collection instruments, consent forms, recruitment materials and information provided to the study participants.

Consent forms contain a description of the research study and information about risks, the voluntary nature of the study, and the confidentiality of patient information. They specify the benefits of participating and contact information for an independent institutional representative whom the study participants can contact if necessary. Informed-consent forms must be read by or read to the participant and signed by both the participant and the researcher. Consenting to participation in a research study is also required to be culturally appropriate. Alternative approaches must be sought when necessary. Information provided to the participant in the consent form includes how confidentiality and anonymity of respondents' identity and responses will be maintained.

Informed-consent forms should be written in simple easy-to-understand vocabulary suitable for a sixth-grade level of education and include the following elements:

■   The purposes of the research

■   The expected duration of the subject's participation

■   How often the subject can expect to participate in the study

■   The number of people in the study

■   A description of the procedures

■   A description of any foreseeable risks or discomforts to the subject

■   A description of the benefits

■   An assurance that records will be confidential except where they are required by law. Anonymity of the records help to increase confidentiality

■   A statement that participation is voluntary

■   A description of the compensation provided

■   Researcher's contact information

Members of research teams are required to complete training on the protection of human subjects and to be familiar with the Health Insurance Portability Act guidelines. See Institutional Review Board or Ethics guidelines for your institution for further information.

In some evaluation research studies the Institutional Review Board may approve the use of a preamble in place of a consent form for data collection in noninvasive interview/survey research. The preamble contains information about the nature of the study and risks and benefits associated with the study. The respondent still has the option to refuse to complete all or part of the survey.

THE DATA COLLECTION TEAM

Survey data may be collected using a variety of devises and approaches. When the approach for data collection is a team of researchers going out into the field to administer surveys, the quality of the data depends on the quality of the data collection process. It relies heavily on the quality of the evaluation team's experience and attention to detail. It requires that the team remains motivated throughout the process and field staff have adequate supervision based on a set of standards that will ensure the data collected is both reliable and valid.

The selection of additional fieldworkers, whose primary responsibility is to collect the data, must be undertaken carefully to ensure that they have the experience and integrity required of the research. The size of the team of fieldworkers will depend very much on the number of surveys to be collected, the expanse of the area over which the data are being collected, and the kinds of expertise they have from previous fieldwork. Fieldwork will benefit from having researchers with the following experience and qualities:

■   Have previously participated in similar data collection and understand the demands of the research and especially of the repetitive nature of the process.

- A level of education and experience commensurate with the requirements of the research. For example, if surveys are to be conducted among senior staff, the level of education of the researcher should be such that the researcher is able to hold a conversation and build rapport with the interviewee.

- The capacity to build rapport and encourage participation, which is easier when there is familiarity with the language and culture of respondents.

- Diligent and motivated to do the best research possible under often difficult conditions (especially globally).

- Trustworthy.

The training of the field staff before they go out to collect survey data is critical because it is important that they are familiar with (a) the instrument and how to administer it, (b) the goals of the study, and (c) the data collection geographic area and the cultural context. An important aspect of training is role-playing the survey administration to ensure consistency of understanding and delivery across the team.

Successful data collection, especially of a large number of field staff, is achieved with appropriate supervision. Supervision is required to ensure field staff have a point of contact that can address any problems that occur during data collection, maintain work allocation schedules, ensure quality control of the data being collected and the appropriate completion of surveys, provide technical assistance where required, and maintain the morale of the research team. Another role may be to go back to previous respondents and complete any incomplete surveys; although this would not be a very good use of their time, or be appropriate in many cases. Incomplete surveys could affect the sample size, data analysis, and any conclusions from the study.

The supervisor should identify any problems with data collection early and make adjustments to the process where necessary and ensure the appropriate distribution of surveys or availability of logistics. The team leader or the project manager may take on this role, but in very large projects where a large area is covered, it may be necessary to identify others who also have these supervisory responsibilities.

MANAGING AND STORING DATA

All data that are collected as part of the research study must be kept in a secure password-controlled location accessible only to members of the evaluation team. Access may be restricted to those working directly on the data analysis and have a need to access the data. Signed consent forms and data must be kept separately, and no attempt should be made to link personal identifiers with the data in a study that promised anonymity and was approved by the Institutional Review Board or Ethics Board under these conditions.

STAKEHOLDER INVOLVEMENT

Applying the Community-Based Participatory Research principles to quantitative data collection requires paying particular attention to the participation of stakeholders in the conceptualization, development, and implementation of the methods (Keiffer et al., 2005; Schulz et al., 2005).

Stakeholders provide insight into ensuring the data collected are both reliable and valid. They provide information on the methods that are most appropriate for their community. They may facilitate the data-collection process and collect the data. Stakeholder participation is critical for ensuring that the sample population is knowledgeable about the study and is willing to participate. In small communities, previous knowledge of a research activity will often facilitate or hinder data collection. Information about the evaluation can be provided in community meetings, in print, and in electronic media. It is important that the potential respondents understand the value of participating in the study.

In community-based participatory research, members of the community may be trained to collect the data. In many communities this may be advantageous because they already have knowledge of the community and an understanding of the issues.

As in all well-designed research studies, it is important to minimize the risk of bias in the data collection and the threat to validity known as instrumentation, so adequate training of enumerators and facilitators is critical. It is also important to understand that members of the community may not be the most appropriate people to collect sensitive and personal information. A balance must be struck between using members of the community and collecting valid and reliable data. In some cases using outsiders as data collectors may be preferable. A conversation with the stakeholders may help clarify any issues that arise in the process of data collection.

SUMMARY

- The validity of the evaluation relies on the sample characteristics, the research methodology itself, and its cultural appropriateness.

- Answering the question involves using an appropriate mix of data that are gathered from and about the people who benefit, who provide the goods and services, or who are somehow influenced or affected by the initiative.

- The selection of the method for data collection and data analysis depends on the research approach that is adopted, the expertise and skills of the evaluator, the resources available for the evaluation, and the costs.

- Surveys developed to collect quantitative data for evaluation may be administered by a variety of methods that must be sensitive to the context, the population, the type of data, and the type of analysis needed.

- Quantitative and qualitative data are both appropriate methods for collecting data to answer an evaluation question; together they provide scope and depth to the findings. Using both primary and secondary data is also useful in providing complementary or differing perspectives.

- Consent forms contain a description of the research study and information about risks, the voluntary nature of the study, and the confidentiality of patient information. They specify benefits of participating and contact information for an independent institutional representative whom the study participant can get in touch with if necessary.

- Data collection requires attention to detail, as well as qualities such as previous experience, trustworthiness, capacity to build rapport, and alignment with the language and culture of the interviewee.

FIGURE 8.2. *Valuable Take-Aways*

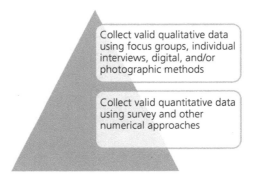

Collect valid qualitative data using focus groups, individual interviews, digital, and/or photographic methods

Collect valid quantitative data using survey and other numerical approaches

DISCUSSION QUESTIONS AND ACTIVITIES

1. Conduct a literature review to identify an instrument that has been validated. What is the underlying construct that is being measured? What do the authors describe as the process for determining reliability? What reliability is reported?

2. You are asked to assess the changes that occur following an initiative in your community. Describe the methods you would use and the approaches you would take to ensure a valid and reliable process for data collection and interpreting the data.

3. Identify a concept of your choice. What variables would fully describe the concept? Identify three of the most important indicators for measuring the concept, and write three to five questions for each indicator. Develop your questions into a formatted questionnaire. Administer the questionnaire to a few of your friends or colleagues. Ask them to provide feedback on content, flow, and understanding. What important lessons did you learn from this process?

KEY TERMS

consent form
data collection team
Institutional Review Board
interval-level data
nominal-level data
ordinal-level data
pilot testing
population sampling
qualitative data

qualitative research
quantitative data
quantitative research
ratio-level data
reliability
surveys
triangulation
validity

CHAPTER

9

COLLECTING THE DATA

QUALITATIVE

LEARNING OBJECTIVES

- Describe data collection in qualitative research.
- Describe reliability and validity in qualitative research.

Qualitative research involves the collection of data that produces results that do not lend themselves to statistical analysis or summarization using numerical data. It involves the collection of data in its most natural form with a view to illuminating and, where appropriate, extrapolating to similar situations and conditions. Qualitative-research methods can be used in program evaluation as the precursor to the development of a survey, to understand the extent to which programs are needed as well as implemented, or to determine whether the intervention activities caused a change in program participants. Qualitative-research methods can be used to understand the context of the initiative and to identify the theory on which the program was developed. Qualitative-research approaches increase the participation of those who are less powerful in the community and give them a voice and especially increase participation of those who are primarily auditory, and nonreaders and writers of the language being used for the survey.

Qualitative research relies on one or a combination of approaches and tools. The selection of the approach or the tool depends on the type of study, what you need to know, and often on the perspective or the training and orientation of the researcher. Creswell (2007, p. 1) describes how a project changed considerably with the input of an ethnographic perspective from a cultural anthropologist.

In public health program evaluation, although all qualitative-research approaches are used to a greater or lesser degree, the tools that have largely been adopted are case reviews, focus-group discussions, individual interviews, participant and nonparticipant observation (drawing on the art and science of ethnography), record reviews, inventories, and diary studies. Community-Based Participatory Research methods such as photovoice and digital storytelling have been adopted as well. This chapter reviews qualitative approaches with interview, document-review, observational, case-review, digital, and Geographic Information System (GIS) formats.

QUALITATIVE DATA

The primary value of using qualitative data-collection approaches rather than quantitative data-collection approaches in evaluation is the difference in the role the interviewer plays in soliciting information when interviewing techniques are used. In qualitative interviewing the interviewer is also an instrument of the study, making adjustments for understanding, clarifying, and probing, whereas in quantitative interviewing, the interview is strictly scripted and consists primarily of closed-ended questions. In qualitative data collection, interviewers ask open-ended questions that allow for elaboration of the responses and require the interviewer to master the skills of asking questions, listening carefully, and interpreting the responses to the questions.

Giacomini and Cook (2000) identify the essential aspects of qualitative research as appropriate participant selection and comprehensive, appropriate data collection that is corroborated by multiple sources. Corroboration by multiple sources of data and multiple methods of data collection and data analysis is referred to as *triangulation*. The methods that are selected for triangulation are dependent on the nature of the study and the criteria associated with the research.

The main disadvantages of qualitative data are in the small sample size, and the analysis of large volumes of interview data that have to be transcribed and coded for themes and patterns.

ENSURING VALIDITY AND RELIABILITY

An important consideration in the collection of qualitative data is its validity and reliability. Validity is equated with credibility and with the extent to which the approach is appropriate for answering the research question (Fern, 2001) and the extent to which the data measure the concepts that they are intended to measure. It assumes that the concepts are appropriately defined based on an accurate understanding of the context and that the findings and conclusions are consistent with the data that are collected and are believable by the stakeholders, who consider them to be accurate (Ulin, Robinson, & Tolley, 2005, p. 25). Alternative terms are that the data be *trustworthy* and *dependable* (Ulin et al., 2005). Conclusions drawn from the data may be invalid if there is bias in the theoretical frameworks, the preconceptions of the researcher, or in the selection of particular parts of the data for emphasis when the results are compiled. An important aspect of evaluation that allows for diverse and culturally appropriate interpretations and increased validity is the emphasis on stakeholder involvement in the entire process (Nelson-Barber, LeFrance, Trumbull, & Aburto, 2005).

Additional considerations for increasing validity include:

- Collecting data rich enough to provide a complete picture

- Soliciting feedback from the respondents about the data and the conclusions that are drawn from the data

- Searching for differing opinions and evidence as well as negative cases to reduce the effects of selection bias

- Triangulating data sources, settings, and methods thus reducing the chance of a systematic bias in the method and assuring the generalizability of the conclusions

- Comparing intervention and comparison/control groups in a quasi-experimental/experimental design and across different settings (Maxwell, 2005)

Reliability in qualitative research is associated with dependability and the extent to which the data-collection approaches are thorough and follow recognized rules and conventions.

Questions associated with reliability include:

- Are the research purpose and design logically connected to the data gathered?

- Are the results complemented by data from other sources?

- Are the interviews conducted by trained interviewers using uniform approaches specified by protocols? (Ulin et al., 2005)

If data are dependable, the relationship between the data and the findings across multiple methods and over time will remain stable. Qualitative research requires that the researcher remain objective and report any conflict of values to the evaluation team because they may influence the collection, analysis, and interpretation of the data resulting in a bias.

Morse, Barrett, Mayan, Olson, and Spiers (2002) argue for the use of verification strategies for establishing reliability and validity describing them as providing methodological coherence and a dynamic relationship between sampling, data collection, and analysis and theory development with the researcher's creativity, sensitivity, flexibility and skill being the critical determinant. Data audit trails may be used to assess post hoc the extent to which specified measures to increase reliability and validity are adhered to. Data audits involve the verification of raw data and the results of data reduction strategies from interview data, process, or field notes.

Conducting qualitative research requires the development of a protocol. Protocols ensure consistency across the interviews, increasing the reliability of the findings. The protocol contains the following items:

- The interviewer's opening remarks

- The process for getting informed consent

- The process for conducting the interview

- The process for completing paperwork related to the interview, including a time sheet, perceptions of the interaction, and the degree of reliability of the respondent and the data

Another strategy for ensuring validity and reliability is to conduct pilot testing of a data collection instrument as a chance to determine whether and how it works under real-life conditions. It is a practice run for the real thing! It involves the interviewer or facilitator, a note taker if there is one, and respondents. Participants in the pilot test must be similar to the research-study participants. It provides the evaluation team with an understanding of what issues might arise when the study is implemented and an opportunity for incident free research. Pilot tests ensure culturally appropriate language and images are used and checks are undertaken for understanding. If researchers ask a question and based on their worldview they expect a certain kind of response, but the respondents interpret the word or the question differently from what was intended, the credibility of the data is affected. Determining if this difference exists is the role of the pilot testing phase of an evaluation study.

Conducting the pilot test provides opportunities to test the flow of the questions and to familiarize the interviewer or focus-group facilitator with the research-study process and the questions. In addition, a pilot test may be used to ensure the validity of observation tools. It ensures that questions and observations are appropriate and culturally sensitive. Following the pilot test, the instrument is edited as necessary to change vocabulary, increase the sensitivity of the questions, and improve the flow. Once this process is complete, the instrument is ready to be used and is likely to produce valid and reliable data for analysis.

FIGURE 9.1. *Uses of Focus Groups*

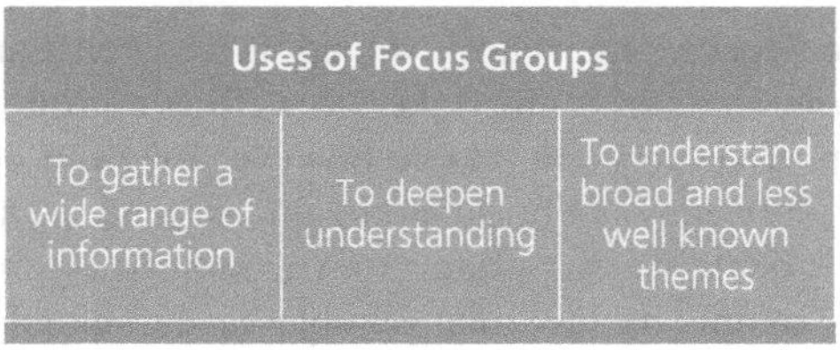

Uses of Focus Groups		
To gather a wide range of information	To deepen understanding	To understand broad and less well known themes

INTERVIEW-FORMAT APPROACHES

Focus-Group Discussions

A focus group is a moderated group interaction used to conduct research that relies on the interaction of participants in the group to produce the data. Focus groups are used for a variety of reasons (see Figure 9.1):

- Gathering information about the range of knowledge, opinions, experiences, attitudes, and beliefs of a group

- Deepening understanding of a phenomenon or a community

- Understanding broad themes

Focus-group interviews can be used at each stage of the evaluation. Participants in a focus group inform the research and provide data on topics of which they have a personal or professional understanding. Telephone and computer-facilitated focus groups have been used by academic researchers to reach dispersed population groups and to provide anonymity to the respondents (Abbatangelo-Gray, Cole, & Kennedy, 2007; Cooper, Jorgensen, & Meritt, 2003).

Six to eight individuals form a purposefully selected group to participate in a focus-group discussion. In some research and across world cultures, gender or other homogeneity in the group is critically important to consider. Fern (2001) suggests that homogeneity is probably more important with regard to socioeconomic status than it is to race/ethnicity. Gender however is an important consideration in Muslim cultures. In some instances, a heterogeneous group may be appropriate, depending on the research questions. Discussion within the group provides the intergroup checking of information, increasing the validity of the data.

Like other research methodologies, focus groups have unique characteristics.

- They provide rich qualitative data that can be used as a precursor to a larger quantitative study or a theory generating study in its own right.

- They can be used to understand a phenomenon of interest more fully than survey techniques.

- Direct quotations from the interview provide powerful imagery for the reader when focus-group data are reported.

- They can be used to augment other research methods.

- They are useful for verifying survey data analysis results

Limitations in using focus groups for evaluation research must also be considered. Focus groups require a moderator, a note taker as well as a group of six to eight people (Figure 9.2). The group of six to eight people however may not be representative of the larger population, and results may not be generalizable beyond the sample and populations similar to the group. Probability sampling from a stratified sample will increase the generalizability of the sample if the final sample is sufficiently heterogeneous even while maintaining in-group homogeneity (Fern, 2001). The number of focus groups can be increased to address issues of representation and provide opportunity for multiple comparisons. Additional limitations include

- The amount of time required to identify, screen, and assemble the group

- The amount of time required to prepare, consent, and conduct the interview could take 2–3 hours

- Their unsuitability for gathering sensitive information when the topic is emotionally charged or likely to lead to contention. For example, focus groups would be unsuitable if the researcher is interested in exploring private and socially sanctioned behaviors of a group.

Other potentially important drawbacks of the focus-group method include the moderator bias in the discussion and the difficulty of separating individual viewpoints from the collective group viewpoint. In a focus group, the perceived lack of confidentiality makes individuals less willing to reveal sensitive information. In some instances, establishing confidentiality of the group's discussions increases group participation and sharing. The moderator discusses with the group the nature of the information that will be discussed and gets buy-in for each

FIGURE 9.2.   *Requirements for a Focus Group Discussion*

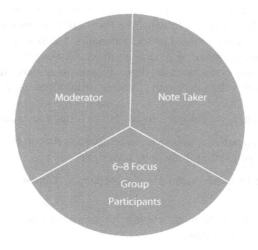

person to maintain confidentiality. This is usually done verbally and may be included as the group establishes other ground rules to govern the discussion. Pledges of confidentiality obtained in this way are, of course, not binding on the group, but may help in providing some assurance to participants that their comments will not be repeated outside the group. The moderator guides the tone of the interaction and the discussion.

The Moderator The role of focus-group moderators is to moderate, not to dominate or to participate in the discussion. Their role is to ask the questions and ensure that everybody participates. It is important that the group discussion not be dominated by any one individual. Not allowing one or two persons to dominate the discussion requires skill and patience.

The moderator may take notes, but having a note taker allows the moderator to focus on moderating the discussion. The note taker not only records statements made by participants but may also keep track of the participants' choice of words, nonverbal communications, expressions of emotion, and the roles played by participants. In discussions that involve sensitive and politically charged topics, paying attention to and recording nonverbal communication among the participants may prove helpful in the analysis and interpretation of the findings. The note taker is responsible to make sure the recording equipment is working throughout the interview.

When conducting a number of focus groups, it is preferable to use the same moderator or to ensure training of all the facilitators in order to control for the influence of the moderator and to improve the reliability of the data. As noted earlier, the researcher's skill in data collection is a critical determinant of the quality of the data.

Recording a focus group discussion minimizes the risk of missing important information and interactions of the group by writing extensive notes. Good digital recorders provide excellent recording quality. The moderator seeks permission to record the focus group during the initial discussions and as part of the informed-consent process. Permission is usually granted if a clear explanation is given such as, "It is important that this interview is recorded so we don't miss anything you say."

Conducting a Focus-Group Discussion The interview starts with an opening question that serves as an icebreaker. It can be as simple as, "Tell me what it is like to live in this neighborhood." The rest of the interview consists of 8 to 10 open-ended questions built around a particular theme and developed to answer the research question. It may consist of probes that allow for an increased understanding of the phenomenon being studied and provides prompts for the researcher. A probe for the previous example could be, "How is it similar to or different from previous neighborhoods you have lived in?" Additional probes to get at what participants are thinking or to expand the discussion include: "Would you explain that further?" "Would you say more about that?" "Tell me more about that." "Explain what you mean by that" (Figure 9.3).

Questions in a focus group must be clear to the participants, must reflect the concept being measured, and be appropriately worded to elicit both depth and breadth in the responses. They must be asked in a logical sequence to allow the respondent to build on a train of thought and go from broad to specific questions. The time taken to develop a well-designed focus group guide is time well spent.

FIGURE 9.3.   *Mini Focus Group Interview*

Moderator: Thank you all for participating in this focus group discussion this evening. The purpose of this discussion is to find out about the new services that were put into your community recently to improve your access to healthcare and education for your children. Do you have any questions for me before we get started? (Answer any questions and move quickly to the discussion.)

Moderator: Tell me what it is like to live in this neighborhood.

Focus Group Participants: Respondents explain what it is like now and some refer to the fact that changes have occurred to improve public health and access to education for the younger children.

Moderator: You have all provided different aspects of the changes that have occurred in your neighborhood; can you tell me when these changes occurred.

Focus Group Participants: Respondents provide a time line starting about 10 years previously when this poor rural community did not have access to health facilities, conditions that would make them healthy, or a school in their community so children would not have to travel so far to get an education.

Moderator: What do you believe brought about the changes that you have just identified?

Focus Group Participants: The group discussed the changes as starting with a needs assessment when the mayor of the town partnered with a college over in the next town. That partnership resulted in an analysis of the needs of this community and a plan to improve living conditions for the 3,000 residents.

Moderator: How is your neighborhood similar to or different from previous neighborhoods you have lived in now these changes have occurred?

Focus Group Participants: One person responds but says very little.

Moderator: Explain what you mean by that.

The following steps are involved in conducting a focus group:

Step 1: Confirm the purpose of the study and the problem it is addressing.

Step 2: Ensure the individual questions are specific to the purpose of the study, are conversational, short, and clear, and contain only one dimension. Use probes to expand the options for questioning.

Step 3: Organize the logistics, including establishing the interview time line, securing a venue, recording equipment and supplies, arranging for participant or community incentives, and developing advertising flyers if appropriate.

Step 4: Recruit and train the moderator and note taker.

Step 5: Contact, screen, and recruit potential study participants by appropriate methods including letters, emails, flyers placed in appropriate venues, and phone calls.

Step 6: Confirm the time and location of the focus group with those recruited and registered to participate.

Step 7: Convene the group and ensure that each person provides informed consent and, where appropriate, permission for the interview to be recorded.

Step 8: Conduct the focus-group interview. Record the interview for later transcription and data analysis.

Step 9: Thank the participants and close the interview.

Detailed guidance for conducting focus groups is provided in Krueger and Casey (2009).

Individual Interviews

The research process within which individual interviews are embedded is not unlike any other research process that involves preparation, data collection, and completion (Figure 9.4). Individual interviews are used to get information about an individual's participation in or exposure to a public health program or about the impact of a policy or about attitudes, feelings, and behaviors related to a public health problem or its resolution. Key informants provide insights about a situation or a population from their own vantage points. They may also provide information about resources and services. They are often community leaders such as heads of agencies or institutions, policymakers, and service providers. Key informants often have a perspective that is different from the perspectives of program participants.

When a member of the community or a program participant is less likely to be invited to participate in a focus group of peers because he or she holds strong views or is likely to polarize the group or the discussion, an individual interview is a great alternative. Individuals who lead departments, organizations, or communities are generally

FIGURE 9.4.   *Research Process for the Interview Instrument*

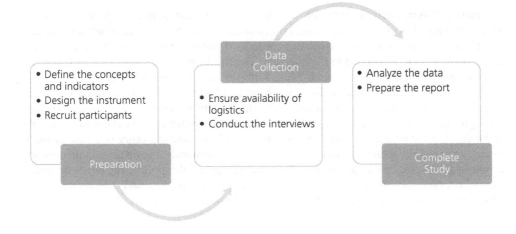

not included in focus groups although a group consisting only of this level of personnel would be appropriate. Unlike questionnaire administration, individual interviews
require a considerable amount of human capital for data collection; they are time consuming and expensive. As with focus groups, the person conducting the interview must
be skilled in order to get the best possible data through direct questioning and probing
when necessary.

Advantages and Limitations   There are advantages and limitations to using individual
interviews for collecting data. Advantages include:

- The interviewer is able to ask additional questions, called *probes*, to improve a response
  or to ask for clarification of an answer much like he/she would do in a focus group.

- Interviewers can elicit sensitive information.

- The views and opinions of nonreaders and those with low literacy levels are easily
  incorporated into the study.

  Limitations include:

- Individual interviews are expensive because of the need to hire interviewers, provide
  travel expenses, and compensate respondents for their time.

- Scheduling interviews may be difficult, and potential respondents may not be easily
  recruited.

- The number of interviews may be small, although data may provide a considerable
  amount of depth and understanding. A small sample size makes it difficult to extrapolate the findings much beyond the sampled population. The number of interviews can
  be increased to improve representation.

- Rapport between the interviewer and the person being interviewed must be achieved
  before an interview because it affects the quality of the data.

- Respondents may choose not to participate in an interview even if the researcher has
  driven for two hours to get there!

Designing the Interview Instrument   Designing the instrument for an individual interview starts with having a clearly defined purpose and research question: What is it that you
want to know? Once the research question is defined, the next task is to define the concepts
and indicators that are related to the question. The third step in this process is to frame the
specific questions that will be asked. These form the basis for the questionnaire.

To give an example: The research question is, "Did the initiatives to improve access
to care make a difference for the residents?" The initiatives are to improve access to care
through two approaches. One, a provision in an existing policy, would allow more people
to be eligible for healthcare based on poverty guidelines, and the other is a new primary
health care facility within 10 miles of 50% of the community's residents. Indicators for
answering the evaluation question include knowledge of the policy, registrations under
the policy, opinions about and use of the new health care facility, and the receipt of services. Alternatively, the questions that need to be answered may be about the theory-based

intervention that was undertaken. In this case, the questioning in the evaluation is guided by the changes that were anticipated based on the theory of change. In the example of access to care, using qualitative research approaches could lead to questions such as

- What do you know about the recent changes in the policy to increase eligibility?

- How do you believe the changes in the policy affect utilization of healthcare by residents of your county?

- What do you know about the exercise facility that was opened in your community recently?

- What is your opinion of the services at the facility?

- How has the new clinic improved access to healthcare for children and the elderly?

- What has changed in the provision of care for refugees since the institution of the new policy?

An alternative approach to asking questions is using a short vignette to present a problem to which the interviewee can respond. When the question, "What do you know about the exercise facility that was opened in your community recently?" is converted to a vignette format it becomes, "There have been many different reactions, both positive and negative, to the recently opened exercise facility in your community. What do you know about the services and how has the new facility changed people's physically active levels in this community?"

Questions must be clear, must reflect the concept being measured accurately, and must be appropriately worded to elicit both depth and breadth in the responses. They must be asked in a logical sequence to allow the respondent to build on a train of thought and go from broad to specific questions. The time taken to develop a well-designed questionnaire for individual interviews is time well spent.

Conducting an Individual Interview Individual interviews can be carried out face-to-face at a time and in a place agreed to by both the interviewer and the respondent; the need for both privacy and safety should be taken into account. Individual interviews are held in neutral locations such as a local library, community center, or any space that is comfortable and that the participant perceives as nonthreatening; private and safe locations allow discussions of especially sensitive topics in an atmosphere of anonymity and confidentiality. Interviews may be conducted in the interviewee's home or office. Conducting a telephone interview eliminates some of the costs in time and travel but has limitations in building rapport with the respondent.

Recording an in-person or a telephone interview minimizes the risk of missing important information and distracting the respondent by writing extensive notes. Good digital recorders provide excellent recording quality. The interviewer seeks permission to record the interview during the initial discussions and makes it part of the informed-consent process. Permission is usually granted if a clear explanation is given such as, "It is important that this interview be recorded so I can listen to you and not be distracted by taking notes, and also to be sure I don't miss anything you say." Videotaping has become popular with qualitative researchers. Although members of some communities may not object to having an audio interview, many will not agree to be videotaped for fear of how the video images may be used in the future. Previous experiences or skepticism about the research method may influence their concerns.

Irrespective of the approach, conducting a good interview takes preparation. Individual interviews require the interviewer to be a skilled listener and communicator and a good researcher. Preparation is required through training and practice. Good researchers are not born, they develop their skills over time with diligence and patience!

Sample Size

The number of focus groups and individual interviews that are conducted may be prescribed by the research questions and by the number of groups and individuals across which the data are to be compared. It may also depend on the likelihood that each successive group or interview will provide the same information. Once the same information is being gathered from different individuals or groups, *saturation* is reached, and the data collection may end (Krueger & Casey, 2000).

A study of attitudes toward healthcare utilization will require more groups or individuals to get at all the phenomena and the variability across subgroups than a research question on adolescent girls' preferences for exercise, for instance. The first question is much broader and covers a wide range of individuals who may have differing attitudes toward healthcare utilization either as consumers or as service providers. The second research question, on adolescent girls, is more focused and conceivably has less variability; therefore, saturation is likely to be reached sooner. Although interviews are generally conducted only once with any one group or individual during a single research study, the same group or individual may be interviewed in follow-up conversations if the phenomena or situation changes or in the conduct of case studies. If a statewide, regional, or national picture is to be obtained from the data, a larger sample size would be appropriate and saturation may be reached later than if the sample were more homogeneous.

Appreciative Inquiry

Appreciative inquiry is a specific use of interviewing skills in evaluation. It is defined as "a group of processes that inquire into, identifies, and further develops the best of 'what is' in organizations in order to create a better future" (Preskill & Catsambas, 2006, p. 1). Appreciative inquiry is implemented in four phases: inquire, imagine, innovate, and implement. The inquire and imagine phases are most applicable to the data-collection phase of evaluation. An individual-, pair-, or group-interview technique is used with a storytelling approach to obtain the following information:

■ Experiences that most represent a participant's pride in being part of the initiative

■ What participants value most about themselves and the program, processes, and successes

■ Three things participants especially wish for the program

■ Recommendations for improving outcomes

In the inquire phase, respondents are asked specifically to think back on their experience and tell a story. Preskill and Catsambas (2006, p. 80) give an example:

Think back on your experience in the workshop and tell me about a moment when you felt that a program or activity was working particularly well, so well that it helped you learn and understand the content in a way that was exciting or inspiring. What was it that made it so effective? What value did you add to the workshop? If the entire workshop were designed to be this clear, interesting, and engaging, what three wishes would you offer the workshop's designers to make this possible?

The stories obtained during this process define success: how well the organization's systems work and how participants experience the initiative. The stories allow for a shared understanding and clarification of the program's culture.

The imagine phase encourages participants to provide information that helps frame the recommendations. The innovate phase produces concrete steps for improving the initiative and shaping systems and relationships differently. The innovate phase moves the initiative toward making changes if necessary. Given the wide range of questions in this approach, it may be used to answer process as well as outcome evaluation questions.

Background

A youth-services-provider organization that has served the community for 50 years has recently realized that it had never really taken the time to understand its program from the perspective of the youth. The organization was situated in the middle of a middle-income neighborhood but it had very little access to community-based resources and no other facilities where young people could be safe after school.

It had provided services to many generations of youth and, because the programs and sports activities were well subscribed, they had not made any changes in the past 10 years. They had historically provided the guys access to training facilities in boxing, basketball, and soccer, but there was little for the girls if they did not want to play basketball or soccer. Very few wanted to box! It was time to evaluate the organization and create a new space for all its youth that was youth centered. After all the youth had changed in the past 10 years, they wanted more input into things that concerned them and they wanted things to be different. The CEO of the organization selected appreciative inquiry as the research approach and called in a team of evaluators. He would use the results of the study and especially the recommendations from the first part of the process and work with the youth to come up with ideas for changes to what was being offered when and how.

The evaluation team discussed the needs of the organization and the approach to the assignment. They discussed the terms of the contract and wanted to be sure

(Continued)

(Continued)

the organization would send out letters inviting the youth to participate. In the end they wanted to have a very balanced report that reflected a cross section of the youth. They needed to be sure they interviewed girls and boys, older and younger youth, as well as staff and outreach workers of the organization. They negotiated the logistics of where they could meet the youth and they assigned a room in the building that ensured that they were in a comfortable and private space. They also decided to give the youth a small token of appreciation for their participation.

In this community, however, paying the youth for participating in a study was frowned upon, and, besides, not all the youth would be participating, so management thought it was unfair to pay a few. The decision was made that they would organize a couple of visioning sessions that all the youth could participate in and for those sessions they would provide their favorite food, pizza! An appeal was made to the local sports store and each young person who participated in the study received a gift certificate for a sporting item of their choice.

With all the decisions made, the evaluation team got to work with firming up their methodology. They decided to try to interview 10 percent of the total number of youth who were currently participating in programs at the center. That meant a sample size of 20 with 5 from each category they identified. Overall there were 10 girls (10–18 years old) and 10 boys (10–18 years old) represented.

	Girls 10–14	Girls 15–18	Boys 10–14	Boys 15–18
Number of participants	5	5	5	5

They wanted to also interview 10 percent of the staff, so that sample size was 6. They selected two persons to be interviewed from each of the major staffing areas in the organization, sports, administration, and custodial services. The team scheduled 26 interviews over the following 6 weeks but they started their interviews with the youth.

Like similar forms of qualitative research, focus groups, and individual interviews, they wanted to be sure the questions were clear and reflected the concept they were trying to measure as well as being able to get both depth and breadth from the responses. They made sure they were written in a logical sequence to allow the respondent to build on a train of thought and go from broad to specific questions. They spent a long time thinking about exactly how to ask the questions, and used a model that the developer of the technique had used in a previous study.

The team asked two major questions and probed when they needed to. They focused on the *inquire* and the *imagine* phases of the process. For the inquire phase, the questions and probes were, "Think back to a time when you were happiest coming to this facility. What made you happy?" "What were you able to do here that you could not do anywhere else?" "What was the organization doing at that time that you liked?" "What things did the organization do that you did not like very much?" For the imagine phase, the questions and probes were, "What do you think are things the organization should do so it is exactly like the time you talked about when you were happiest coming to this facility?" "What changes would you like to see the organization make?" "What recommendations do you have for the CEO?"

The evaluation team collected the data from all the youth and the staff over a period of 6 weeks. They analyzed the data using NVivo® data coding and data analysis software and presented a summary of their findings to a group of the youth to be sure that they had not misinterpreted anything they had said. In effect they wanted the research they had done to be validated. Once the final report was ready it was shared with the appropriate stakeholders which included the youth. The report was presented in meetings that allowed for questions and answers to be sure they understood what had been done by the evaluation team and they could get by-in for the recommendations. One big recommendation was that the youth wanted a major expansion of the services offered and the guys were particularly passionate about the center offering a martial arts program; they wanted so much to address the rising violence in the community and thought that the discipline involved in that program would help. The girls wanted to have opportunities to learn different forms of dancing including Zumba and be able to do more than sports. They envisioned a youth center that allowed them to not only be physically active, but give them a chance to learn how to be well rounded and community minded citizens. The center had its work cut out!

DOCUMENT AND RECORD REVIEW

Document and record review is especially important in process evaluation, when the evaluation questions focus on whether the initiative was implemented as planned and who the participants were. With regard to policy, document and record review could document the process by which the many steps in the development of policy are implemented. An important step in the development and implementation of policy occurs between the stages of the policy passing and its enactment when the guidance is written. Document review will be an appropriate activity to determine the extent to which the guidance has been written and is in line with the appropriate implementation of the policy.

It may also be important in process and outcome evaluations. In the assessment of medical services, for example, medical records may be reviewed to understand the extent of family-support services or in the case of a policy outcome assessment, the extent to which the policy has resulted in public health and child health related improvements.

Documents reviewed for assessing program implementation can include

- The plan for the initiative to determine the extent to which it was implemented as stated

- Existing needs-assessment data and reports to understand the sociocultural, economic, and epidemiological foundations of the program

- Minutes of board, executive committee, and ad hoc committee meetings to understand various aspects of program or policy development and implementation as well as reports of ad hoc meetings that may have been produced

- Meeting, training, and attendance logs of participation in the initiative

- Logs of program implementation and any changes that occurred over time

- Photographs and videos that provide evidence of decisions made, actions taken, and level of beneficiary participation

- Training curricula, teaching, and learning resources for training program beneficiaries and providers

- Guidance for the implementation of policy

In addition, document review would include the materials used during the policy development process such as policy analysis, media reports, newspaper clippings, and other artifacts that show the process of educating the general public and policymakers unfold.

Another important process evaluation activity often undertaken is the review of client files across multiple sectors. Document reviews for example could take place in assessing the need for broader community changes in the conduct of a needs assessment. Documents involved in this review might include economic, financial, health, housing, census, and related documents. More narrowly, hospital case files could be reviewed for patients to determine referral patterns, treatment options given to patients in understanding disparities in healthcare, and issues of health equity.

In a study of patient outcomes, the author reviewed case files that were each given a unique identifier and included the following variables in the analysis: patient case number, age, race/ethnicity, health status on admission, date of admission, date of discharge, treatment provided, referrals if given and reason for the referral, follow-up treatment if provided, readmission if reported, causes, and treatment. This work was based on the recognition that there were disparities in how individuals were treated based on race/ethnicity. Although this process assessed the care given to patients and their implementations, it also assessed referral patterns and outcomes for patients and provided the opportunity to compare patients by race, age, and diagnosis.

As an evaluation tool, document review may also be used in assessing content of materials provided for children and other sectors of the population. For example, assessing media and the extent to which media messages may influence health behaviors and, therefore, health outcomes such as obesity, heart disease, diabetes, and other diet-related health conditions.

Irrespective of the documents that have to be reviewed, like all other research approaches, a protocol improves the likelihood of collecting consistent and valid data.

TABLE 9.1. **Template for Document Review**

Document Title:			
Date of Review:		**Name of Reviewer:**	
Section	**Review Item**	**Meets Review Criteria (Y/N)**	**Comments**
Target of message	Appropriateness of message		
Content of message	Accuracy of message		
	Image associated with message		

The document-review process requires developing a checklist specific to the needs of the project. If the document review, for example, is of the print messages that were used by a range of organizations to promote healthy behaviors, the review criteria with the specified categories would be developed and confirmed. A table similar to Table 9.1 may be helpful in such a review.

OBSERVATIONAL APPROACHES

Observation as a complement to qualitative or quantitative research approaches is an important tool for evaluation. Observations may be made of behaviors, relationships, physical structures, conditions, sociocultural activities, and events. Ulin et al. (2005, p. 72) comment that "observation is the oldest and most basic source of human knowledge, from causal understanding of the everyday world to its use as a systematic tool of social science." Observations are conducted using two approaches, the observer as insider and the observer as outsider. The more-often-used approach in evaluation is the unobtrusive observer as outsider.

This approach is used to understand or determine an outcome through observing its occurrence (Ulin et al., 2005); alternatively, it may be used to assess the implementation of an initiative and provide information during process or outcome evaluation. In answering the research question, "Did the initiatives improve access to services for residents?" the evaluators may choose to observe particular utilization events, such as the reception and treatment of a subgroup of the population that usually experiences discrimination when requiring services. Evaluators may observe clients from their entry into the facility to when they leave, taking note of multiple interactions with all levels of personnel. In this study of patient/provider interactions, for example, it may be helpful to document communication patterns and the extent to which vital information is provided for health promotion and health protection. In a rural community where staffing might be limited, the burden of giving detailed information to each pregnant women on the use of mosquito nets for the prevention of malaria may result in women not getting the information they need and the continuing high rates of morbidity and mortality as a result. In some parts of Africa malaria remains the most important contributor to preventable deaths. It would be helpful for instance to understand barriers to utilization of health care facilities.

■   Observe the length of time that patients are waiting for services could also be a function of access to services. Individuals are essentially denied services if they must wait four or more hours to be seen by a provider as often happens in many parts of the world. Men generally cannot afford this amount of time from work and women must choose between waiting and alternative economic activities or responsibilities associated with their caring responsibilities.

■   Observe the provision of culturally and developmentally appropriate videos and other types of information in libraries, health centers, neighborhood places, and other sites where members of the population could benefit from them. The number, types, and accessibility of similar facilities within the community can also be assessed.

Data quality is improved by developing a carefully validated checklist with appropriate categories and by carefully observing the phenomena under study. The longer the period of observation, the more credible the data because people will eventually return to their natural behaviors. Data may be collected using checklists with space for short comments; the checklists can be on small cards (Ulin et al., 2005) or in a notebook. The development of an observational checklist should include the participation of stakeholders who have the ability to provide unique perspectives on the community and to understand the meaning and relevance of behaviors and conditions for health (Zenk, Schulz, House, Benjamin, & Kannan, 2005). Walking tours to understand issues related to improvements for pedestrians using walkability-assessment tools provide an excellent combination of observation, surveys, and interviewing techniques.

In a study looking at the safety in local parks across two sites (IDN and non-IDN) as part of the Communities Putting Prevention to Work project, communities in the IDN compared to communities on the east side of town, showed higher average scores of incivility in observation studies. In the complementary survey that was conducted during the same period also comparing the two sites, similar differences were observed in individual's perceptions of safety. See Figure 9.5.

Following each data-collection activity, additional observations or interpretations can be added to the data. Observation data are analyzed to reflect both qualitative and quantitative dimensions as appropriate.

Think About It!

For a class project, students in an evaluation class I teach opted to study the relationship between drunk driving and a particular holiday in the year on which large amounts of alcohol are consumed. Students reviewed documents on drunk driving arrests available from the local police and in addition did an observational study outside public houses downtown to assess evidence of sobriety or lack thereof as individuals left. The three students developed an observation sheet and considered carefully how each of the variables they were interested in assessing would be measured consistently across all observations. They worked hard to

FIGURE 9.5.   *Assessing Incivilities in the Park*

Environmental Scan: Incivilities in the Parks

- Avg # Incivilities Per Park, IDN versus Non-IDN

	Avg # Incivilities/Park
IDN (n=19)	2.3
Non-IDN (n=18)	1.5

- Avg # Incivilities by Perception of Safety, IDN versus Non-IDN

		Avg # Incivilities
	IDN (n=8)	1.6
Safe	Non-IDN (n=16)	1.6
	IDN (n=11)	2.8
Unsafe	Non-IDN (n=1)	1.0

improve the validity and reliability of their measure. The day came to test their tools and collect the data. What do you think they learned from their observation study? How accurate do you believe their observation tools were? What conclusions if any, do you think they were able to draw?

CASE REVIEWS

A case review or case study describes the problem and the activities that are being undertaken to alleviate it. It is a focused, in-depth analysis of a program or system. The evaluation looks at the program's geographical location; its cultural, organizational, and historical contexts; and its implementation (Stufflebeam & Shinkfield, 2007). Its primary purpose is to describe the program or situation in specific and illuminative terms. In addition, it makes recommendations for future actions. Case reviews can be used for evaluating initiatives and providing a complete understanding of what happened and why. It focuses on the questions, "What is the program or policy and how was it implemented?" "What is the situation and how does it affect individuals?" Because an individual case review is not generalizable, a group of programs that address a similar problem may be used together to develop a theoretical framework for addressing a problem.

Sources of information for case reviews include agency reports, individual interview and focus-group data, observation, site visits, activity-monitoring reports, and project documents. In addition, case-review evaluation may include digital data-collection approaches such as photovoice and digital storytelling. In many ways a case review combines a number of approaches in order to provide a useful illustration.

In evaluating a community's growth over time or an organization's programs, case studies are valuable although they may be considered time consuming tools.

Case reviews like other data collection approaches for evaluation research present unique challenges, the most important being that the case selected for study is not necessarily typical of all cases similar to it. So for example, a case review of an organization that serves individuals with intellectual disabilities may be very different from another organization that serves individuals with both intellectual and physical disabilities. Although both organizations serve individuals with disability, the specific conditions may result in very different models of care with a different culture. Another concern is the difficulty in ensuring objectivity in the research endeavor since relationships between the researcher and client may develop over time and constrain the interview in ways that result in bias. A third challenge is in the risk of inappropriate interpretations in a cross-cultural setting when the evaluator does not have well-developed skills for working cross-culturally. Poor interviewing skills and trust building may also lead to inadequate or poor quality data.

DIGITAL APPROACHES

Photographic approaches to data collection add an additional set of tools to the evaluator's tool kit. Alternative approaches to interviewing include using photographs and other artifacts to stimulate discussion and to create meaning about the issue. These techniques lend themselves to the active participation of multiple stakeholders (Bender & Harbour, 2001; Wang et al., 1996). Like other qualitative approaches, these methods allow the participation and input of less powerful members of the community.

One approach is to present one or more photographs or other visual aids (Bender & Harbour, 2001) to a group or individual and then facilitate a discussion of what the photograph or artifact means to the participant(s) using a series of reflective questions. In a study currently being undertaken by a colleague and as a result of the recent spate of shootings and violence against black youth, youth in a similarly disenfranchised community are shown photographs of evidence of violence in one community and asked to discuss strategies for reducing the likelihood of such violence in their community. This use of photographs allows images to form the basis for conversation rather than waiting for first-hand evidence in their community. It provides images to which individuals can relate and a forum for discussion and policymaking.

An alternative photovoice technique (Wang et al., 1996) allows community members to be active participants in documenting their observations; in using photography to elicit emotions, feelings, and insight; and in sharing their worldviews. Cameras are given to participants so that they can present their community and environment in visual forms and discuss their findings in their own words. Using this approach stimulates discussion among multiple stakeholders and allows the evaluator to see the images through an alternate set of validating lenses. In an example of this approach, men and women in the North Western Region of Ghana in Kong Village were asked to take photographs of anything that represented the prevention, transmission, or treatment of malaria. Images included different sites of standing water, piles of raw Shea nuts where mosquitoes might breed, and the leaves of the Neem tree that are used to make treatment potions. Residents discussed the role of the chief and other community leaders in reducing the spread of mosquitoes and providing improved access to effective treatments. The university in Ghana, with whom we collaborated during our short 3-week educational and cultural visit planned to develop an intervention with the community to reduce the spread of malaria.

Photographic approaches may be applied in outcome evaluation to demonstrate changes that occur over time in the community from initiatives that leave a visible impact and show distinct physical changes. Before-and-after photographs or video may be used to show changes in lighting to improve individual safety and improvement in the structures in a park or on the roads to increase physical activity. Changes in conditions such as those that preserve or improve the social environment may also be accessible.

Adapting these approaches to evaluation practice allows the evaluation team to

- Identify and discuss the community's concerns before and after an initiative

- Promote critical thinking about issues that are presented in the photographs or are represented by the artifacts

- Understand the values associated with initiatives undertaken in the community

- Discuss the results of an initiative in graphic terms to a mixed stakeholder audience

- Triangulate data in assessing outcomes against the standards of the evaluation

The systematic collection of data requires a set of defined actions that start with the research question and include describing the methodology, identifying the participants in the study, compiling the results of the data collection, and analyzing the data. The participatory nature of digital approaches provides opportunities for discussion of continued action to improve conditions in addition to providing concrete and direct stakeholder input into the evaluation recommendations.

Digital storytelling has gained some recognition in evaluation and complements photovoice in data collection. It may be used to support the photography or may be used alone. In digital storytelling, stories of participants are recorded before and after an intervention or may be used during the community assessment phase of the evaluation process. Like other qualitative methods, the results of a study may not be generalizable unless very careful attention is given to sampling and sample size ensuring both adequate numbers and appropriate nonbiased selection of participants.

GEOGRAPHIC INFORMATION SYSTEMS

Geographic Information Systems (GIS) provide the ability to link foundation database information with health data for public health purposes. Readily available and widely used data sets include detailed street-level information as well as political and administrative information such as zip codes and census tracts. The layering of census data on public health data shows the relationship between socioeconomic factors and disease at the block or census level.

For example, the evaluation team of the federally funded Communities Putting Prevention to Work project conducted in Louisville collected and documented access that residents had to fresh fruits and vegetables over the two-year duration of the grant. GIS mapped the distribution of grocery stores and corner stores and compared the distance from stores with obesity rates across the metro (see Figure 9.6).

FIGURE 9.6. *Distribution of Grocery and Corner Stores*

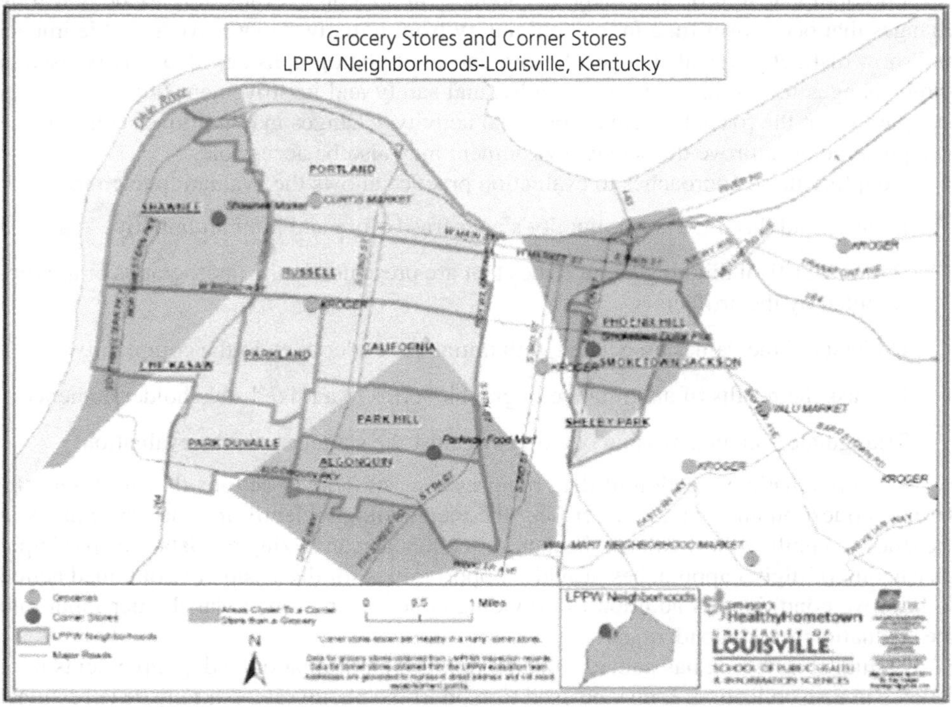

In an earlier study of tuberculosis in the southeastern United States, the disease occurrence as mapped and superimposed on high school completion rates and income levels, demonstrating that the distribution of tuberculosis is related to low high school graduation rates and low levels of income (Harris & López-Defede, 2004). This study combined interviewing, using a semistructured format, and GIS mapping to understand the relationship between the prevalence of tuberculosis and sociodemographic factors that influenced its occurrence.

TRAINING DATA COLLECTORS

Training is important for all qualitative methods to ensure validity and reliability in the data-collection approaches. Conducting qualitative interviews requires that moderators and facilitators be well trained and have an opportunity to practice interviewing and observation skills using the instrument. Training ensures that interviews move smoothly and that questions easily transition from one to the other and the development of keen observation skills to improve reliability. Training sessions are as long or as short as necessary and include

- An introduction to the goals and objectives of the evaluation

- A review of the data-collection techniques

- A review of the data-collection instruments and questions

- Practice in using the interview or observation instrument(s)

- Practice in interviewing, observing, and note taking skills

- Logistics for the interview session, including mechanisms for obtaining consent, recording the session, and identifying and recruiting participants

In this participatory model of evaluation, community members of the team may be data collectors for the first time. In developing the content for the training, consideration must also be given to their needs, but especially to developing listening and summarizing skills. A needs assessment early in the process will provide information for the appropriate training content. The extent of training will likely be determined by the experience of the research team that is assembled.

MANAGING AND STORING QUALITATIVE DATA

Audiotape or digital recordings from focus-group or individual interviews must be transcribed verbatim; notes taken of nonverbal communication during the interview may be written as field notes and incorporated into the final report to provide the context. Transcribing qualitative data is time consuming; if funding permits, this process can be contracted out to a transcription service. The transcription is reviewed by one or more members of the research team against the original recordings to add any words or statements that may have been missed in order to increase the credibility of the study. Often individuals who are able to transcribe are more familiar with medical terminology and less so with public health, so it is important to undertake this final step before coding begins.

If audio equipment is not used and the researcher relies on the interviewer or the facilitator and the note taker to compile the data, it is important that they do so as soon as possible after the data collection to ensure that as little information as possible is lost.

As in other forms of research, all data that are collected as part of the study must be kept in a secure, password-controlled location that is accessible only to members of the evaluation team. Access may be restricted to those working directly on the data analysis and have a need to access the data. Signed consent forms and data must be kept separately, and no attempt should be made to link personal identifiers with the data in a study that promised anonymity and was approved by the Institutional Review Board or Ethics Board under these conditions.

STAKEHOLDER INVOLVEMENT

The data-collection phase is traditionally the phase in which stakeholder involvement is most evident. In the participatory model for evaluation, stakeholders are part of the process and are involved in tasks from identifying the research question to drawing conclusions about the findings. Stakeholders may be trained to collect all forms of qualitative data. Stakeholder involvement supports the selection of culturally appropriate data-collection approaches and the credibility of the findings. They can be instrumental in identifying appropriate study participants for the focus groups, photovoice, and other digital photography approaches and appropriate exemplars for a case study. The community members on the team can be the bridge between the evaluation team and the rest of the community and help provide access and permissions. They can help to identify hard-to-reach groups such as illegal substance users, members of the LGBT community, the homeless, and other disenfranchised groups. They may also be helpful in developing longer term relationships for ongoing cohort or similar studies. In a study of needle abuse among drug users, the first individual who was identified as injecting drugs led to the identification of 60 others who were previously unknown to the public health community. The snowball technique and somebody familiar with the community make an excellent combination for getting a hard-to-reach study population!

THE DATA COLLECTION TEAM

Although there is a range of qualitative data collection approaches, the rigor with which each method is applied will determine the trustworthiness of the data. Unlike survey data collection, qualitative data approaches require fewer researchers in the data collection process, often due to the smaller sample size and the need to develop a level of familiarity with the data that requires more engagement and investment in the process. For example, in a research study into the factors that influenced the spread of tuberculosis, two persons interviewed 50 individuals over a period of 3 months. As the study progressed and interview skills developed, probing got deeper and interviews lasted 45 to 60 minutes with improved quality of the data.

Irrespective of the approach to data collection, the quality of the data depends on the quality of the data collection process. It relies heavily on the quality of researcher's experience and attention to detail. It requires that the interviewer remains motivated throughout the process to ensure the data collected is both dependable and trustworthy.

A large study may require experienced researchers

- Who have previously participated in similar data collection and understand the demands of the research and especially of the repetitive nature of the process.

- With a level of education and experience commensurate with the requirements of the research. For example, if individual interviews are to be conducted among senior staff, the level of education of the researcher should be such that the researcher is able to hold a conversation and build rapport with the interviewee.

- With the capacity to build rapport and encourage participation, which is easier with a familiarity in the language and culture of the respondent. In qualitative research, the ability to build rapport is even more critical than in survey research.

- Who are diligent and motivated to do the best research possible under often difficult conditions; especially in a global context

- Who are trustworthy

The training of the field staff before they go out to collect interview (focus groups and individual) data is critical since it is important that they are familiar with (a) the interview guide and how to administer it; (b) the goals of the study; and (c) the data collection area. An important aspect of training is role playing the survey administration to ensure consistency of understanding across the team. Since interviewing in qualitative research allows more flexibility in questioning, interviewers must understand the goals of the study to be able to adjust and steer the interviewee back on course when they find themselves engaged in a line of questioning that has little to do with the goals of the study.

Successful data collection, especially of a large number of field staff is achieved with appropriate supervision. Supervision is required to ensure field staff members have a point of contact that can address any problems that occur during data collection; maintain work allocation schedules; ensure quality control of the data being collected and the appropriate completion of data; provide technical assistance where required; and maintain the morale of the research team.

The team leader or the project manager may take on the supervisory role and may themselves be collecting the data but in large, time-limited projects in which a large area is covered, it may be necessary to train others as supervisors. In an evaluation study in Sierra Leone which required sampling across a large area in a short time, three tandem teams were created and each team had one person who had overall supervisory responsibility for ensuring the appropriate data collection and security as well as resolving issues. The principal investigator who was also the project manager headed one of the teams and remained in constant cell phone contact with each team.

SUMMARY

■ Qualitative data collection may rely on one or a combination of approaches and tools. The selection of the approach or the tool depends on the type of study, the information that needs to be collected, and, often, on the perspective and/or the training and orientation of the researcher.

■ Qualitative-research tools that have largely been adopted are case studies, focus-group discussions, individual interviews, participant and nonparticipant observation drawing on the art and science of ethnography, and record reviews. Additional Community-Based Participatory Research methods include photovoice and digital storytelling.

■ Validity and reliability are important in qualitative research. *Trustworthy* and *dependable* are terms used to describe validity; reliability is conceptualized as dependability and the extent to which the data are collected by using approaches that are thorough and follow recognized rules and conventions.

■ Basic steps for conducting an interview are developing the instrument, organizing the logistics, and training interviewers, piloting the instrument, contacting potential respondents, and conducting the interview.

■ Data collection requires attention to detail, as well as qualities such as previous experience, trustworthiness, capacity to build rapport and alignment with the language and culture of the interviewee.

FIGURE 9.7. *Valuable Take-Aways*

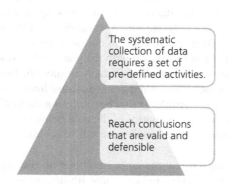

The systematic collection of data requires a set of pre-defined activities.

Reach conclusions that are valid and defensible

DISCUSSION QUESTIONS AND ACTIVITIES

1. Conduct a literature review to identify a qualitative-research study. What was being assessed? What was the process for conducting the research? How was validity assessed or discussed? What limitations of the study did the researchers identify? What limitations were not considered that you think influenced the study?

2. Identify a research question of your choice. What qualitative approach(es) would you use to answer your research question? Develop an instrument with a minimum of 10 questions that allows you to answer your research question. Use the instrument you have developed to interview a few of your friends. What was that experience like? What lessons did you learn?

3. Develop an evaluation plan for assessing the effect of an intervention to improve the living conditions and socioeconomic status of a community of about 50,000 people. Assume that a considerable investment has been made over the past 20 years. What programs would you select to assess? What questions would you ask (process and outcome evaluation); what data would you collect—from whom and over what time frame? Develop a plan for your study including who will collect the data, where the data will be collected, and constraints you might face in undertaking this study. What steps will you take to mitigate some of the difficulties you might face?

KEY TERMS

data collection team
focus group
individual interview
managing and storing data
observation
photographic approaches
photovoice
pilot testing

qualitative research
saturation
stakeholder involvement
stakeholders
training data collectors
trustworthy
validity

CHAPTER

10

ANALYZING AND INTERPRETING QUANTITATIVE AND QUALITATIVE DATA

QUANTITATIVE (PART 1)

LEARNING OBJECTIVES

- Analyze quantitative and qualitative data.
- Interpret quantitative and qualitative data and reach conclusions.

FIGURE 10.1. *The Participatory Framework for Evaluation: Analyze and Interpret the Data*

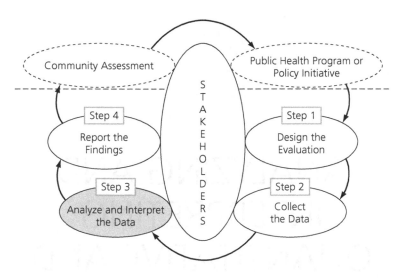

The third step of the participatory model for evaluation is to analyze and interpret the data (Figure 10.1). This chapter discusses how quantitative and qualitative data are analyzed and interpreted to answer the research question. The chapter is divided into two parts. Part 1 focuses on quantitative data, whereas Part 2 deals with qualitative data. Due to the introductory nature of this book, the reader is referred to more advanced texts for detailed discussions of quantitative data analysis techniques and the interpretation of results.

ANALYZING AND REPORTING QUANTITATIVE DATA

Quantitative data analysis is the systematic examination of the evidence that is collected in answering a specific research question. It is the process of sorting and categorizing data using the appropriate tools and approaches. In quantitative data analysis, numerical data is collected and/or the researcher transforms what is collected or observed into numerical data. This chapter discusses the analysis of data from surveys.

The type of data collected during a research study determines the type of analysis that can be undertaken. The data collected in survey research is most often categorized as categorical, dichotomous, or continuous. Categorical data is made up of nominal variables, while dichotomous data indicate the absence or presence of the characteristic being measured. Examples of nominal variables are gender, ethnicity, religion, and so on, while examples of pairs of dichotomous variables are healthy/not healthy, well/not well (sick), male/not male (female), environmental factor or policy present/not present. In this case, "healthy" may be coded as 1 for data entry, whereas "not healthy" is coded as 2. Dichotomous variables like nominal-scale data have limited options in data analysis. Ordinal variables that are used in ranking the indicator provide for more sophisticated analysis than do nominal-scale categorical variables. Continuous data allow for more detailed analysis than either nominal or ordinal data. If required, the flexibility of continuous data allows data to be grouped to produce categories and treated as ordinal data for analysis. For example, 20 children whose heights range from 48 inches to 68 inches can be grouped into two categories. The first group would be children 48 inches to 58 inches, and the second group would be children 59 inches to 68 inches.

Quantitative data can be analyzed in two ways—as descriptive statistics and as inferential statistics. Descriptive statistics describes the sample, whereas inferential statistics attempts to use the sample to make inferences about the larger population.

The initial analysis in a research study produces descriptive statistics, which summarize and describe the data. These measures include

- Frequencies, percentages, and proportions

- Measures of central tendency (mean, mode, and median)

- Measures of dispersion (range, standard deviations, variance)

Frequencies represent the number of times an event occurs or the number of responses, whereas percentages represent the number of occurrences or the number of responses as a proportion of the whole. For example, if 30 people respond to a survey out of a total of 100, the frequency of respondents is 30, the proportion is 0.3, and the percentage is 30%. Each question in the survey, however, may have a different denominator for calculating percentages if all the questions are not answered. If, for example, question 20 was answered by only 60 people, then the denominator for calculating the proportion and hence the percentage is 60.

Means are the most often used measure of central tendency. The mean is the calculated average of the responses. For example, if 30 people have scores ranging from 10 to 30, all the scores are totaled, and the total is divided by 30 to calculate the mean. Means are also used to summarize the responses on rating scales. Modes are the most frequently occurring response, and medians are the middle value of a set of values with an equal number of values falling above and below.

The range is the span between the lowest and the highest scores. The standard deviations represents the variations in the data and the distance that the data point is from the mean. When the standard deviation is calculated a low value indicates that there is little difference between the value and the means of all the values, and a high standard deviation indicates a large difference. When there is no difference, the standard deviation is zero. Variance is the square of the standard deviation.

Analyzing Survey Data

The first step in analyzing survey data is to summarize the data across all the demographic variables and the survey items. In this first step, calculate frequencies, percentages, measures of central tendency, and measures of dispersion. Data analysis can be conducted in the data-analysis software Microsoft Excel®, SPSS®, STATA or other suitable computer software. The greater the variability in the data, the more likely it is that the data can be explained and conclusions can be drawn about the relationship among the variables and about the population as a whole. The statistics calculated will be determined by the type of data you are working with. For example, you could do a mean for age because ages are continuous data, but a mean for gender, which is categorical, would be meaningless. For gender you would be limited to frequency and percentages, so, for example, you could look at the proportion of men compared with the proportion of women in the sample or the proportion of different age groups represented.

The results of the analysis can be presented in a variety of ways, including tables, charts, and graphs. In reporting the data, it is not sufficient to use graphics alone; they must be accompanied by narratives explaining what they mean to the reader. Providing the charts allows readers to also make their own interpretations of the data. Cross-tabulations are a useful way to summarize data in bivariate relationships. They can be used with nominal or ordinal data. When used with nominal data, the statistic associated with them is the Pearson Chi Square and Spearman's Rank Order Correlation when used with ordinal data.

The following four examples illustrate ways of presenting and explaining data.

Example 1: Data presented in a table format (Table 10.1)

Analysis: There were a total of 51 participants in the study, most of whom (75%) were male.

Example 2: Data presented in a single-table format summarizing all the categories in the data (Table 10.2)

Analysis: A total of 160 men aged 31–71 (mean 56.7 years) were included in this study. Most of them (60%) were White, 25% were African American, and 15% were Hispanic of Mexican origin. Most (95%) were satisfied with the program, with a mean satisfaction score of 4.69 on a 5-point scale, and 94% said they would recommend the program to somebody else.

Example 3: Data presented in a bar-chart format (Figure 10.2)

Analysis: Overall, participants were satisfied with all the activities. Mean score for the physical-activity component was 4.5; for nutrition education it was slightly less at 4.0; and participants walking with their peers was 3.6. Although there was no significant difference in satisfaction scores between the nutrition activity and the in-gym activities, there was a significant difference between the in-gym activities and the participants walking with their peers ($p = .02$).

Example 4: Data presented in a pie-chart format (Figure 10.3)

Analysis: There were almost equal numbers of participants in the three offerings of the initiatives.

TABLE 10.1. **Single-Variable Table Format for Presenting Quantitative Data**

Response Category	Frequency (*N*)	Percentage (%)
Male	38	74.5
Female	13	25.5
Total	51	100

TABLE 10.2. **Multiple-Variable Table Format for Presenting Quantitative Data**

Sample Characteristic	Response Category	Number of Participants (*N*=160)	Percentage (%)
Age (years)	Sample mean = 56.7		
Race/Ethnicity	AA/Black	41	26
	Hispanic	24	15
	White	95	59
Satisfaction with the program	Yes	152	95
	No	8	5
Satisfaction with program	Mean score = 4.69		
1 = Not at all satisfied	1	3	2
2 = Somewhat dissatisfied	2	5	3
3 = Neutral	3	0	0
4 = Somewhat satisfied	4	60	38
5 = Very Satisfied	5	92	57
Recommendation to others	Yes	150	94
	No	2	1
	Maybe	8	5

FIGURE 10.2. *Bar-Chart Format for Presenting Quantitative Data*

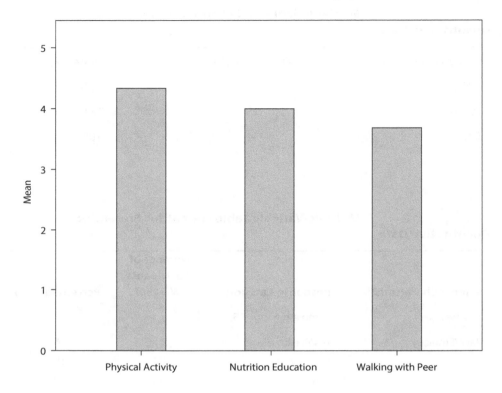

FIGURE 10.3. *Pie-Chart Format for Presenting Quantitative Data*

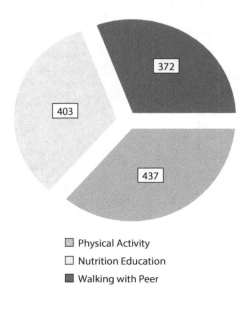

Quasi-Experimental Designs

Analyzing data from quasi-experiments consists primarily of comparing the intervention group with the comparison group against the outcome variable of interest. Inferential statistics describe the analysis that makes inferences about the data and a population from the sample that is studied. Estimation and hypothesis testing are inferential statistics where the null hypothesis determines whether there is a true difference between the two groups being compared (Jekel, Elmore, & Katz, 1996). The p-value provides the confidence in the null hypothesis being correct. If the participants in the sample were not randomly assigned and the assumption cannot be made that the results are generalizable to a larger population, inferential statistics may be inappropriate.

A commonly used test to assess the difference in means before and after evaluation designs is the paired t-test. The t-test is used to compare differences between proportions in a group that has received an intervention compared with a group that did not. A fuller description of these and other statistical tests that may be used in evaluation, including the chi-square test, ANOVA, and bivariate and multivariate analysis, are beyond the scope of this book; the reader is referred to more advanced texts.

REACHING CONCLUSIONS

Interpreting the data to reach appropriate, defensible, and sound conclusions about the evaluation requires that the evaluation is supported by good-quality data and suitable analyses. It means making judgments about the initiative's merits, value, or worth to the program beneficiaries, the program staff, the community, and the funders. Reaching conclusions results in recommendations for decision-making about the initiative's continued implementation and development, replication, funding, or demise. For all these reasons it is important that the results are valid, reliable, and reproducible. However, the data must be reported to reflect practical significance and importance to the stakeholders in the light of their values and standards.

The conclusions are developed based on criteria established at the start of the process and on the standards that were established by the evaluation team and the stakeholders. In an evaluation driven by the objectives established by the program during the planning phase, the analysis of data focuses on answering the question associated with the objective. For example, if one of the objectives is, "by the end of the intervention program 80% of beneficiaries will report a 20% increase in their standard of living," then the focus of the evaluation will be to use previously specified variables for determining a change in the standard of living of program beneficiaries. Proxy measures of earnings, disposable income, and savings could be plotted over time in a longitudinal study design to understand the change in the standard of living. The percentage of individuals whose standard of living has increased by 20% will require a calculation of what percentage each person's standard of living has changed. One both results have been obtained, a conclusion can be drawn as to whether the objective has been met or not.

In order to draw conclusions about the whole program rather than about single interventions, it may be necessary to synthesize the results across a range of different assessments. Going back to the previous example, this program may have had a variety of additional objectives related to activities for which outcomes were defined. All the analyses together will provide the overall understanding of the effect of the program on beneficiaries and determine the program's value or worth.

The aim of the conclusions section of the report is to present a balanced account that discusses the data in the context of the value of the initiative to the different stakeholder audiences. The value of the initiative may be both tangible and intangible and is assessed using multiple criteria that include

- Relevant information about the initiative (description and context)

- Objective, unbiased, and systematic research

- Performance on indicators of merit in process and outcome measures

- Recognized standards and criteria of performance based on comparison groups or other programs or both

- Cost-efficiency criteria

- Policies, regulations, and laws

- Stakeholder and community values and expectations

- Environmental standards

- Standards of social justice and equity

In addition to being assessed against expected outcomes, the data are also assessed for unexpected outcomes that benefit or hurt the community, participants, or nonparticipants. An example of an unexpected outcome could be the effect of a policy change on women that was intended to improve their health. One such policy could be to reduce the use of coal for cooking and, therefore, limit women's exposure to coal dust. However, the policy change may require women to divert needed financial resources to more expensive (if safer) forms of fuel and expose them to additional dangers like the explosion of tank stored gas. It may on the other hand reduce the risk of injury to children.

Learning about the evaluation may be an important aspect of the evaluation team's work. Lessons from conducting the evaluation are identified for each stage in the process; they pertain to the value of the evaluation, the range of experiences in the research approach, participant recruitment, data collection, and research findings. In addition, the assessment covers material, financial, and human resources and expenditures. Assessing failures or shortcomings of the evaluation process and outcomes provides an opportunity to ensure improved future evaluations.

STAKEHOLDER INVOLVEMENT

Members of the community are much less likely to want to be involved in data analysis than in the data-collection phase of the evaluation. However, they can play a number of roles, and their contributions need not be any less than in any other phase of the evaluation. In the spirit of community-based participatory research and empowerment, it is important that data-analysis skills be taught to members of the team to encourage their full participation.

The team may need to bring in new people who are both interested in and have the aptitude to learn the methods; quantitative-data analysis requires background knowledge that usually comes with a higher level of academic preparation and especially in statistical methods. There is always one person who can be identified to participate in this phase of the study so every effort should be made by the evaluation team to find him/her!

Let us review a process for thinking about an evaluation research study. The evaluation team was part of the process from the very beginning and wanted to be sure they were involved in the planning of the intervention to ensure that the evaluation plan would be comprehensive and include both process and outcome measures.

Background

The rates of transmission of sexually transmitted infections were increasing again after a few years of a slow decline in spite of the fact that a range of educational and skill building programs were being offered. In preparation for another intervention, it was decided to conduct an assessment of the most vulnerable population—the population where the rates of infection appeared to be increasing the most. The assessment was designed to provide information on which to base the intervention. The population of interest was a youthful, computer-savvy group that used social networking extensively. Because the intervention was to be implemented via a social-networking mechanism, the computer-based assessment was conducted using the same site. The assumption was that the group that got the survey would be fairly representative of the group that would eventually receive the intervention. The evaluation team had done some research and found that the group on line was fairly stable and individuals who participated regularly were about the same age and gender. They followed the group for about 18 months as participant observers documenting their observations of the group's interactions very carefully using predefined criteria.

Methodology

The evaluation team that came together to undertake this study consisted of specialists in clinical psychology, information technology, quantitative research, drug use, and public health with specializations in health promotion and epidemiology. The team invited a couple of college students to join them so they had a perspective from a similar age group to the study participants. They were invaluable to the team's deliberations.

The researchers designed a survey that consisted of a number of sections, each separated by a short introduction and instructions for how to respond to the items.

(Continued)

(*Continued*)

In some cases, the questions required yes/no responses, whereas in others respondents were asked to answer using a 5- or 7-point Likert scale. The questions they used to compile the survey were culled from similar studies. There was not one study that asked all the questions they wanted to ask in their study. They got permission from the researchers to use their surveys. In some cases they got responses and permission in 2–3 days, and in other cases it took 2–3 weeks. Once the items were selected and the survey compiled, it was sent to ten content experts for review. The review process took about one week. The final survey was pilot tested with a similar group from another chat room on line that one of the students on the team had helped identify. The process overall took a long time, but it finally came to an end and they were delighted with the product. The final questionnaire had 50 carefully selected questions that had been used in previous studies and validated. Putting the new survey together, however, would require that the evaluation team validate their survey since the previous validation would be invalid.

The researchers collected demographic data (age, ethnicity, gender, marital status, state, and county of residence) and asked about alcohol and other drug use, sexual preferences, sexual risk taking behaviors, knowledge, and attitudes about practices related to the transmission and prevention of sexually transmitted diseases and about environmental factors that influenced the culture of drug use. In addition, they asked questions about the practicality of using social-networking sites to conduct an intervention. Once the methodology for the research was clearly defined and the proposal was written, the team submitted a request for the Institutional Review Board (IRB) to review it, provide feedback, and ultimately provide clearance for the study to be undertaken. The IRB conducted an expedited review of the full proposal since the group they were targeting for their study was not considered a vulnerable group and the methodology did not pose any known physical or psychological risks to the potential respondents. However, since this was an online study and that approach is fairly new, they were careful to make sure that protections were going to be put in place to ensure that the identity of the respondents would not be revealed. The researchers assured the Board that the anonymity of the respondents would be protected. In fact, they provided assurances that there would be no trace of their participation in the study. Permission for the study was granted about four weeks after the initial application.

The evaluators distributed the IRB approved survey, the consent form, and a cover letter explaining the intent and nature of the study. The team confirmed the voluntary nature of the study and the confidentiality of the study findings with the assurance that individuals will not be identified in the report of the results. The team provided a link that respondents could click on if they were interested in participating in the study. Within the next few days they received 1,800 responses. Although they did not know exactly how many people frequented the site, they were delighted with such a large sample size. It meant that it would be easier for them to conduct subgroup analysis and some quite sophisticated analysis to answer their research questions.

Data Analysis

The survey within the online data analysis platform generated a combination of categorical and continuous data that were downloaded, transferred into SPSS®, and checked for entry errors. Discrepancies were resolved, and the data were cleaned. The evaluation team calculated frequencies on all categorical variables and the means on all appropriate categories. The chi square was used to test associations of categorical variables. The alpha level for statistical significance was set to 0.05. The evaluators were interested in knowing whether the subgroups within the sample differed in any meaningful way, so they created subsamples and compared them using ANOVA. In one case, they wanted to know if alcohol consumption differed across the sample by age. They were able to do this kind of analysis because of the large sample size. Also, because they had a large sample size, they took the opportunity to validate the survey so they would be confident in using it in the future. The Cronbach's alpha was 0.85.

Describing the Data

The data analysis allowed a description of the sample including a demographic profile and knowledge, attitudes, and practices regarding the transmission and prevention of sexually transmitted diseases. In addition, risk and protective factors, social, economic, cultural, and political determinants of health were assessed. Tables and charts were created to show the characteristics of the respondents and the results of the tests with their corresponding p-values.

The results provided researchers with information about the specific characteristics of subgroups within the sample and significant differences were detected between groups. In addition, the level of risk-taking behaviors that exposed the respondents to sexually transmitted infections were associated with alcohol consumption and drug use, with a difference in the type of risk taking behaviors by age group. Thirty percent of the sample used some form of illegal drug at least once a week in addition to consuming alcohol daily. Interestingly fifty percent of the respondents said they supported drug use and thought it was up to the individual to regulate their use and not the government. Another 30 percent were undecided leaving only 20% who thought that drug use ought to be illegal.

Interpreting the Data

The 18- to 24-year-olds were significantly different in their risk-taking behaviors from the groups that were 25 to 30 and 31 to 35. The group with significantly higher

(Continued)

(Continued)

risk-taking behavior in this study identified as college students although this group was spread across two age groups, 18–24 and 25–30. Overall, they were less inclined toward prevention of sexually transmitted infections and more likely to consume alcohol than those in the older groups. They were much more likely to believe that a cure was available for each of the sexually transmitted infections and less likely to believe they were at risk from their practices. Young people had easy access to drugs fueled by their extensive social networks and the anonymity the Internet provided. They also found out from their study that there was a culture of drug taking and a social norm associated with it that was pervasive.

The team compared their findings with those of other researchers. They reviewed the literature again to be sure they had not missed any recent papers and found that although their study had been conducted online, their results were not significantly different from the results of studies that had been conducted on college campuses. They found it surprising that, unlike previous studies, their study showed no differences among the three ethnic groups that dominated the sample. This was an especially important finding for the researchers and planners because their intervention would be online and they would have much less control over who would take part. They decided to institute a password-secured site for the intervention. They knew that young people shared a lot of information with their friends, including passwords to online programs, so controlling access would be challenging. The team used results about the social, cultural, and political context to guide the development of the intervention and to decide how they would implement and evaluate their work over a 3-year funding period. The team stayed connected through the planning period for the theory based intervention to be sure that the correct evaluation tools were developed and the team was able to conduct both a process evaluation to make sure the intervention was being implemented as planned and an outcome evaluation to be sure the intervention made a difference.

The researchers used the first set of results as their baseline and evaluation tools were developed to collect data half way through and six months following the on-line intervention. The surveys that assessed changes in the participants like the intervention were based on the social cognitive theory, selected constructs from the health-belief model, and the theory of planned behavior. They also took advantage of their extensive use of social networks and social media.

Research Questions:

1. What effect did the Healthy On-Line Youth intervention have on participants in the program?

2. To what extent was the intervention delivered as planned? Who participated?

3. Did 30% of youth who participated report a decrease in risk behaviors immediately following the intervention?

4. What proportion of youth who participated in the intervention indicate they would reduce their drug use?

Purpose of the Evaluation

After a lot of discussion and taking the budget and the timelines into consideration, and knowing that the intervention had been implemented with fidelity, the primary purpose of the evaluation is to answer the outcome questions.

These questions related to a change in risk factors

▪ Did 30% of youth who participated report a decrease in risk behaviors immediately following the intervention?

▪ What percent of youth who participated in the intervention indicated they would reduce their drug use?

Methodology

To measure a change in attitude among the youth and to assess a change in social norms associated with drug use among this population, the following measures were used: a questionnaire that allowed the participants to report directly on their own attitudes as well as report about their attitudes toward others, and specifically those who continued to use or promote the use of drugs. An attitude rating scale was used that provided data on the direction of change in attitude, as well as how strong the attitude was. The 5-point Likert scale that was used ranged from strongly agree (5) to strongly disagree (1) with statements that were presented. Since this same validated scale was used in the baseline measurements, the researchers were able to show a change, which they assumed to be as a result of the intervention. It was one thing to assess attitudes, but what was really important was whether the behavior of the youth changed as a result of the intervention. The researchers asked questions about that also. The risk behaviors they assessed were different types of drug use as well as sexual behaviors, which it seemed, from their earlier research, had a strong influence on drug use. There seemed to be rewards associated with both the use of drugs and sexual risk behaviors. The questionnaire asked questions about both. In addition, the evaluators wanted to know if their knowledge of the risk had changed. They collected demographic information so they were able make intergroup group comparisons. The evaluators compared those who participated in the intervention with those who did not participate. The intervention was set up so those who participated signed up. Those who did not sign up were available to be in the comparison group. There was no way of knowing if they talked to each other and, therefore, whether those who participated had any influence on those who did

(Continued)

(Continued)

not participate. Those in the intervention group were asked to keep any information they got from the intervention private. Maybe the results would help clarify if there was a breach. It was not possible to randomly assign the participants and the comparison group, so they may have set up nonequivalent groups. The evaluators would check to see how similar the groups were each time they analyzed any data.

Results

The results from the analysis showed that those who participated in the study were much less likely to report high-risk behaviors to the same level, and, on the Likert scale, a higher proportion disagreed with the statements that supported drug use and high-risk sexual behaviors. In the data that was collected 6 months following the intervention, attitudes were even stronger and safe behaviors were also reported more consistently. Since the team had concentrated on a smaller group for the intervention than participated in the original assessment, the sample size was smaller and the inter-group comparisons were fewer.

So let us be sure we answered the research questions. They were

- Did 30% of youth who participated report a decrease in risk behaviors immediately following the intervention?
- What percent of youth who participated in the intervention indicated they would reduce their drug use?

The intervention had helped to reduce the use of drugs by an average of 15%, which was less than the 30% they had hoped for immediately following the intervention. However a closer look at the data showed that the results were not uniform across the group. The evaluators found that there was a better understanding of the dangers of drug use and a higher commitment to helping each other stay healthy among the younger females and older male participants. Having the comparison group gave them real confidence in their results. This was good news. Results showed that attitudes had changed and 50% of respondents had reduced their drug use.

Conclusion

The evaluators were able to conclude that the intervention had merit and it was worth doing and replicating. They had to assume that 15% of individuals (range 10%–25%) was a good outcome and that, given that so many of the respondents (50%) had a more positive attitude toward reducing their risk behaviors, the intervention had worked. They planned to replicate the intervention and offer more individuals access to it. They would use the experience of this first trial to tweak it but they did not need to make any major changes.

SUMMARY

■ Descriptive statistics summarize and describe the data. Frequencies, percentages, measures of central tendency (mean, median, mode), and measures of dispersion (standard deviations, variance) are used for descriptive analyses.

■ The method of analysis is determined by the characteristics of the data and the combination levels of measurement across the outcome and the intervention variable. The most commonly used analysis for comparing two groups is the mean.

■ Data must be interpreted based on criteria developed at the start of the process and on the standards that were established by the evaluation team and the stakeholders.

■ The data must be interpreted to reflect their practical significance and importance to the stakeholders in light of their values and standards.

DISCUSSION QUESTIONS AND ACTIVITIES

1. Identify a small data set. Summarize using a data-analysis software package. Write a short report describing the data in terms of each of the variables. What analyses did you use? What conclusions did you draw from your findings? To what extent do your conclusions follow the evidence?

2. Conduct a literature review and find two research articles. Read the articles and write a short summary describing the variables in the data and the analyses that were conducted. How were the results of the analysis displayed? What conclusions did the authors draw from their results? What additional analysis would you recommend?

3. Review the preceding case study and state one to two outcome evaluation questions you would answer. What data would you collect and how would you analyze it?

QUALITATIVE (PART 2)

Qualitative-data analysis is the systematic examination of evidence that is collected as a result of the research based on the collection of nonnumerical data and data that does not lend itself to quantitative data analysis. It is the process of sorting and categorizing the data using the appropriate tools and approaches. Krueger and Casey (2000) define *focus-group analysis* as "systematic, verifiable, and continuous" (p. 128), and the same may be said about qualitative data that is produced in narrative form from individual interviews, digital storytelling, and through other forms of inquiry. However, these are not the only approaches to qualitative research and qualitative data collection. This section of the chapter will describe methods often used in public health in addition to discussing focus groups and individual interviews which are the most commonly used text-based data forms.

ANALYZING QUALITATIVE DATA

Qualitative research using interviewing approaches such as focus groups, individual interviews, appreciative inquiry, case studies, digital storytelling, or components of photovoice provides data that are converted into text through transcription. The next step in the process of handling this qualitative data is to reduce the quantity of information through a series of steps. Since the conversations that occur in focus groups and individual interviews are fairly free flowing to allow respondents to provide as much information as possible, there is also the risk that they wonder off and away from the question and the focus of the interview. When this happens, it is necessary to code the transcripts for only useful data thereby leading to a reduction in the data. It is this reduction in the data that allows for meaningful data analysis.

Text-Based Data

The text-based data reduction process may be significant in some studies and minimal in others. Interview and focus-group instruments may provide the basis for the data reduction based on themes of the analysis, or themes may be identified in a grounded theory approach during the coding process. The purpose of the data collection and the overarching research question may also guide the analysis of the data.

The data may be coded by categories such as time, event, person, place, thing, or other characteristic. For example, if the research question required that the data be viewed through a lens of a sequence of events over time, then each question that asked about a specific date would be identified and the events associated with it would be tagged to that date. The data may be generated any number of ways to understand a phenomenon, a behavior, a service, or an incident; but however it is generated, the evaluator must identify and organize the information from the transcript or the text in a coherent manner. Making sense of the data requires a step that entails coding the data according to themes.

Coding Text-Based Data

Coding data is essentially tagging it. The data is tagged and pegged to a theme or a data or event as described earlier. In the analysis of text-based data, coding or tagging the data is done in multiple ways. One approach is to manually highlight the relevant or emerging themes in the category of interest in the printed document using a different color or pattern for each theme. In the example that follows, three different themes are identified, the first theme is the health condition—high blood pressure; the second one is advice from the doctor—pork causes high blood pressure; and third, action the individual had taken—eliminated pork from her diet.

> One person with high blood pressure was told by her doctor that pork causes high blood pressure, so she eliminated pork from her diet

This same pattern would be followed for the whole transcript: whenever the time appears, the same color would be used. The text that is highlighted in the same color or pattern may then be cut out and stacked to sort and organize the data, keeping the themes in designated piles. Throughout the process, coding may lead to changes in the categories and renewed thinking about the analysis. It may sometimes lead to recoding all or parts of the transcript. This strategy for coding data is helpful when the number of focus groups or interviews is small. Just for reference, a one-and-a-half-hour interview can generate up to 30 pages of transcript. Coding and cutting out themes for large numbers of interviews becomes daunting. Luckily for us, there are now easier ways of coding and sorting, which rely on our ability to handle a computer. An important advantage to using a software package for coding and sorting the codes is it then allows multiple opportunities for conceptualizing the analysis and answering different research questions. In the preceding example, using the highlighter, the categories may not work for answering another question and the transcript would have to be reviewed and coded again.

There are a number of computer-assisted data-coding and data-analysis software packages available on the market, some of which are cost free—software such as NVivo® or N6® from QSR, Ethnograph®, and ATLASti® (Figure 10.4). In addition, a cost-free resource, AnSWR (McLennan, Strotman, McGregor, & Dolan, 2004), is available at the CDC website: http://www.cdc.gov/hiv/library/software/answr/.

The AnSWR software for qualitative data analysis allows for the coordination of team based qualitative data analysis, the management of large datasets, structured codebook development, and text coding and intercoder agreement assessments. In addition it allows for formats that allow for data to be imported into both qualitative and quantitative based programs.

When computer-based software is used, themes are coded and text is linked to the data in much the same way as described earlier.

Four major advantages are associated with using a computer-based program:

1. The text that is coded stays linked to the main document.

2. The same segment of text may be coded for more than one theme.

3. The text can be easily recoded if necessary.

4. Intergroup analysis is facilitated because demographic attributes can be attached to the text.

FIGURE 10.4.   *Screen Shot of Qualitative-Data Coding from*
NVivo® QSR

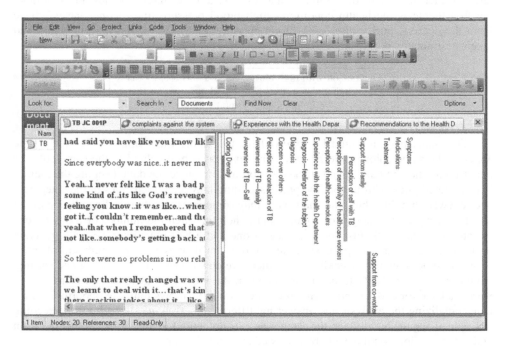

Coding and interpreting qualitative data is an iterative process that requires that the data be reviewed as it is being collected. It is important that the strategy for coding and analyzing the data is defensible and clearly documented.

In order to improve the reliability of the data-coding process, two to three people may be involved in the coding. Early in the process each person codes one to two interviews. The coders then come together to ensure that themes are being coded consistently and similarly based on a previously determined code/definitions protocol. The coders reconcile the codes, include new codes and definitions as needed, and decide on a single coding strategy that they all use for the rest of the transcribed interviews. Coders periodically review their work together until all the documents are coded. Some software packages provide options for determining inter-coder reliability. Alternative ways to sort and organize qualitative data are diagrams, charts, and graphs (Mason, 2002). A cognitive map that charts the data, much like the charting that can be achieved in computer-based coding, may be useful where interpretive themes are related to each other through tree, sister, and daughter codes, as in NVivo®.

Although determining the frequency of specific responses does not constitute an appropriate analysis of qualitative data, it is worth noting the number of people who mentioned the theme or the topic and the specificity with which different themes are discussed (Krueger &

Casey, 2000), when this is feasible. A more appropriate approach for quantifying qualitative data is to use phrases such as "most people," "some participants," "a few participants."

Once the coding process is complete, the themes are used to answer the evaluation research question and provide any additional insights that the data may reveal. Responses to each question or emergent themes are compiled and the results of the study and the answers to the research questions are written up in the results section of the report so readers can clearly see the data and be able to draw their own conclusions should they wish to do so.

This last step of interpreting the data requires explaining the meaning of the data, reporting the main ideas that the data reveal, identifying important concepts, and answering the research question. The interpretations that are made and the conclusions that are drawn must reflect the data accurately to ensure credibility of the evaluation process.

Evaluators write up their reports by drawing on their knowledge of the data, their field notes, and their interpretation of the data through their own lenses. The write-up includes quotations that support the themes and the interpretation the evaluator is trying to convey. It is important to select quotations that illustrate a shared perception or opinion of the respondents. Select quotes from across the range of the data and use two to three to represent a theme (Krueger & Casey, 2000; Ulin et al., 2005). Quotations should represent the voices of participants. These quotes help readers feel close to the members of the community and increase their understanding of the experience. Quotations may also be used to highlight particular or interesting phenomena that may form the basis for further research but may not be typical of the views of most of the participants in the study. Once the report is written, the researcher reconvenes the whole group and requests a review of the report, giving the evaluation team an opportunity to make any edits and ensure appropriate interpretation of the data. After this process is complete, the report may be made public.

EXAMPLE

USE OF QUOTES IN AN EVALUATION REPORT

The risk of diabetes was repeatedly mentioned as a motivator to healthier eating, and sometimes to increase physical activity. For example, one interviewee talked about losing more than 50 pounds by walking and engaging in healthy dietary changes including drinking more water instead of soft drinks and cutting out fast food. Talking about her motivation for these lifestyle changes, she mentions her concern about being "at risk" for diabetes, with a parent dying from diabetes-related complications and a sibling suffering with the disease. Other respondents shared similar stories of the motivation they experience due to existing or potential health problems. Often the health problems inspired dietary changes rather than changes in physical activity. In the words of a few participants:

"I have really been trying to stay away from [fast food restaurants] and trying to not do those just because I know that they're not healthy. If these guys want a snack, I keep and I try to keep [low fat snacks and cereal bars]. I try to keep decent healthy food like fresh fruit. We get the mandarin orange cups. My kids have ADHD. I am a child of ADHD. Food-wise, I know what are triggers and what are not. Yes, the apples and the fruits have sugars but its natural sugars and they burn off differently and they affect the body differently as opposed to the processed sugars." [Female Adult]

"By me being a diabetic, I can't eat out because they put a lot of salt on stuff and I'm not supposed to have it. That stops me from eating a lot of junk food. That's why I do cook." [Female Adult]

"We try to eat as healthy as we can ... to watch what I give the kids because we have diabetes in the family. They have the chance of getting that ... . I have high cholesterol. They have a chance of getting that. So, what I try to do is to ... watch what we eat. Like cholesterol, make sure it doesn't have that much cholesterol, that much trans fats, and all that stuff. I ... look on the back of the package and read it down. If it's got too much, I'll put it back." [Female Adult]

"What I'm basically doing is I have cut back on a lot of fried food ... .Try to do more baked food, more pasta, more seafood. I got one of them table top grills, more grilled stuff where it's taking the grease from it. I just try to cook with less sugar, less butter ... me and her father is both diabetics so she doesn't stand a chance of not being one so we're trying to prevent that also on behalf of her." [Female Adult]

Document and Record Reviews

The range of materials that may be included in document and record reviews allows for considerable flexibility in the selection of data-analysis tools. The analysis of medical records, minutes of meetings, or television commercials may necessitate the development of checklists on which the presence or absence of the phenomenon under study can be recorded.

Although this approach is primarily qualitative, it may also allow for the data to be categorized in diagrams, charts, and tables to allow for quantitative analysis, including determining means, frequencies, and so forth. In addition, the review can use quotes from participants or descriptions of the services provided. These data are handled in much the same way as text-based data, where themes are identified as the data are coded. Later interpretations of the coding allows the research questions to be answered.

For example, the city wanted to develop policies that reduced the number of injuries on the roads. Policies included converting roads with two way traffic to roads with one way traffic as well as instituting speed bumps to calm the traffic. There were mixed responses to this proposal and some community members were very angry since it meant changing their patterns of driving and making things much more inconvenient. The planners had to make the case for changing the roads to the community. A number of community members went to Metro Council to testify about the very fast moving traffic and the risk to children and adults walking, but there were others who did not agree. There are schools in the neighborhood and some residents were really concerned. The evaluators did a study to determine how serious the problem was in a number of the neighborhoods and to help in the framing of the policy. They looked at traffic-accident records at the local police department as well as hospital records to see if they could find anything. In addition, they did some observation studies, because that would provide them with some primary data, rather than relying entirely on secondary data from the police and hospital records. The detailed reports were provided to the communities that were researched as well as to the policy makers who needed the information. Following a considerable amount of work to convince the small group of people who were holding out, the changes occurred and over time, they began to see the value of the conversion from a two-lane road to a one-way road and the use of traffic calming technologies.

Observational Methods

Observational methods may also utilize checklists or note-based formats with appropriate categories for recording events of interest. These data can be analyzed as quantitative data or can be used as descriptive data depending on the purpose of the study. A limitation of an observation is that there is no interaction with the person or service being observed and, therefore, the conclusions that are drawn may not be valid if the actions or the behavior are not understood. In ethnographic studies, where the use of observational methods is much more advanced than in public health, observation studies are divided into two types, participant observation and nonparticipant observation. In participant observation, the researcher is part of the community (for example) and observes the actions and the behaviors from within with a chance to understand their interpretations from those performing the behavior. In nonparticipant observation, however, the researchers observe and make notes of what they see, but may not have the benefit of understanding how it relates to risk (for example) in the context of that community life. It may not have any significance, yet, it gets interpreted as such. Observational studies utilize checklists that may be combined with other qualitative research methods to provide evidence for making decisions.

In an observational approach to assess skill development based on a set of evaluative criteria, the observation tool lists the skill components, which can be rated on a five-point scale from poor performance of the skill to excellent performance of the skill. The data are analyzed as quantitative data, but, in addition, comments or individual interviews may be used to understand the participants' perceptions and intentions to use the skills following the training. Observational studies may also be used to assess environmental factors for purposes of changing policy and understanding patterns of behavior.

For example, students were interested in understanding the patterns associated with drinking behaviors in a nearby pub. They decided to conduct a study observing the traffic into a pub on various days and times of the week. To do this effectively, they had to consider a number of factors: the time of day, the demographics of the traffic, the time of year. Since it was an observation study, they were not able to record the age of the individual, so that was a limitation of the technique. However, they were able to record features of the individual that helped make a determination of age. So they selected criteria such as child, young adult, adult, and elderly adult. The child was clearly under 18 years of age, and the young adult looked more like a high school or college student, whereas the adult was older but not elderly. They had to define these categories very carefully so they would not make a mistake. The checklist they developed helped them record the information for analysis and ultimately reporting back to the community and the policymakers.

Geographic Information Systems Mapping

Multiple data sets may be used to analyze statistical and socioeconomic demographic data. Prevalence, incidence, and services data at county or zip-code level can be used to analyze trends over time or to create a prevalence map. Socioeconomic variables may be used to understand access to resources for different demographic groups that are most affected. Comparisons of health-related data and census data can be used to understand the extent of the problem. A team of student evaluators analyzed the data from eight counties served by a local nonprofit organization. By comparing their breast-cancer rates with state and national rates, the students were able to identify the counties with the greatest need for breast health services.

GIS mapping provides the opportunity to overlay data to understand interacting variables at multiple levels of analysis. It provides a pictorial perspective of data that are not otherwise available and demonstrates the relationships among variables of interest. The overlay of data may show the clustering of individuals with low-socioeconomic status based on low high-school-completion rates, low-paid jobs, female-headed households, and so forth. This information may provide an excellent complement to photographs and interviews reflecting the circumstances of disadvantaged communities and changes that might occur over time due to systems and policy changes. In a recent intervention to improve the environmental that influences obesity rates, the evaluation team developed a series of GIS maps that reflected changes that occurred as a result of a two-year intervention. The maps reflected the changes in the number of (a) corner stores selling fresh produce, (b) farmer's markets, and (c) individuals who had access to fresh produce through population density maps.

INTERPRETING THE DATA AND REACHING CONCLUSIONS

Interpreting the data to reach conclusions allows the evaluation team to consider the following:

- The evidence for answering the evaluation question(s)

- The meaning of the results

- The practical significance of the results

When a combination of methods is used to answer a research question, the evaluator may have interview transcripts, photographs, digital recordings, and maps that represent different aspects of the data collection. All the data are organized to represent the theme or the question to facilitate interpretation.

Different stakeholder perspectives may influence the interpretation of qualitative data. These interpretations may be influenced by culture; age; demographics; life situation; or status as participants, staff, or funders. Funders, administrative staff, volunteers, and participants may look at the same quotations and draw different conclusions.

The aim in interpreting data and reaching conclusions is to present a balanced report of the conclusions that discusses the value of the initiative to the different stakeholder audiences. The value of the initiative may be both tangible and intangible and is assessed against any one or many of multiple criteria that include

- Relevant information about the initiative (description and context)

- Objective, unbiased, and systematic research

- Performance on indicators of merit in process and outcome measures

- Recognized standards and criteria of performance based on comparison groups and/or other programs

- Cost and efficiency criteria

- Policies, regulations, and laws

- Stakeholder and community values and expectations

- Environmental standards

- Standards of social justice and equity

The compiled data are used to answer each research question in turn, using the objective that supports the research question as the standard for the final interpretation. For example, if the evaluation research question is, "What factors influenced the reduced utilization of the emergency room for nonemergency healthcare and by how much was utilization reduced?" the supporting objective might read, "One year after the clinic opening, utilization of the emergency room for nonemergency care will fall by 15%." Text-based data from individual interviews with members of the community, staff of the emergency room, and other key informants are used to understand the factors that influenced the reduced utilization of the emergency room, but complementary quantitative data are used to determine the level to which this reduction took place.

Conclusions about the value or worth of the intervention are based on the previously set standards, in this case the objectives. If the findings demonstrate that the initiative met or exceeded the standard(s), the initiative is said to be of value. In the example, the value may also be identified in cost-benefit terms to the emergency room as well as to the patients. If the objectives are not met, the conclusion might be that the initiative has little value and the investment was not worth the expenditure. The judgment is based entirely on the data that are collected, analyzed, and interpreted. In some cases, the research may suggest that there is no value since the intervention did not appear to be effective; however, value or worth is not always assessed based on research findings. The value or worth may be independently assessed based on criteria related more to stakeholder and community values and expectations or standards of social justice and equity.

To illustrate how decisions about worth are based on the evaluation conclusions, let us continue with the example. The evaluators involved the community in the process so the results would be viewed as credible and useful for making any changes deemed necessary to improve access to health care. They used individual interviews and focus groups to collect the qualitative data and incorporated ideas from Appreciative Inquiry so they had some idea of what specific changes to make if necessary. The evaluators incorporated additional questions into the data collection. They wanted to know to which population the information most applied. They collected information on clinic and emergency-room utilization patterns and reviewed all the clinic documents and data bases that had been used to collect information from the clinic and the hospital before the clinic opened.

Two coders coded the data by identifying the themes and highlighting them. The initial themes for the analysis of the qualitative data were identified from the questions but included new themes that emerged while the data were being coded. The themes in the analysis included:

- Knowledge of clinic services

- Attitudes and behaviors that relate to utilization of the various clinic services

- Perceived improvement in access to health services

- Attitudes toward the use of emergency rooms for nonemergency care

- Knowledge of the policy/policy change that resulted in the opening of the health clinic

- Knowledge of the impact of the new policy (the clinic and other initiatives to address access to health care) on the community

- Knowledge of health-insurance eligibility criteria

- Actions to increase enrollment under the new eligibility

- Problems associated with enrollment

- Impact and perceived impact of the new facilities on user groups with different demographics

Major and minor themes were identified to simplify the interpretation of the data. The coders compared their coding structure after coding the first three transcripts to make sure they were coding items similarly and were clear about the definitions that each had created if a new theme emerged. Because the interviews included men, women, and youth, coders searched for concepts that represented differences in the perceptions of these groups. They organized the data and the analysis to capture any differences. The different responses from clinic users and key informants were identifiable in the sorting and coding because the transcripts were printed on different-colored paper. The coders identified two or three quotes for each of the themes that represented the breadth of the data. The quantitative data were compiled to show utilization patterns before and after the clinic opened using a time-series design. Graphs and tables showed the data pictorially.

The qualitative and quantitative data together allowed the research question to be answered. The expectation of the objective was that utilization of the emergency room for nonemergency health care would drop by 15%, but the evaluation found that it had dropped 20%. This data came from the review of the records. They also realized that the drop was mostly in children who had asthma and used the emergency room because they had no other source of care before the clinic was opened. The emergency room had recently instituted a care share model with the community center clinical team as part of its new patient centered care model. The team called their patients regularly and were able to provide reminders of what to do when a child showed early signs of asthma symptoms rather than wait too long necessitating a visit to the emergency room. The data also showed these results:

- Community members were familiar with the new policy and had registered their children so they would have access to nonemergency healthcare. They had no trouble enrolling their children.

- Community members knew about the clinic and its services from the outreach workers long before the clinic opened.

- Community members trusted the clinic to provide good care and were satisfied with the care they received 12 months after the clinic opened.

- Community members no longer saw the need to use the emergency room for nonurgent care and praised the staff of the clinic for taking care of them in a timely manner. The recently developed care model had helped build patients' confidence in handling early signs of illness.

- Not all groups utilized the services uniformly. Women and children used the clinic much more than men. Men were still seeking care in the emergency room, and their utilization had not changed in spite of the presence of the clinic. Further analysis of the data would be undertaken to understand their specific needs.

The information from both the quantitative and the qualitative data was good news for the board of directors and the executive director of the nonprofit organization that had gone to great lengths to understand the problem before opening the clinic. The data showed that the clinic's diversion of people from the emergency room resulted in considerable savings in tax dollars. Triangulation of the data-collection sources and methods allowed the evaluation team to be confident of their findings. They concluded that opening the clinic was valuable to the community. The value was demonstrated in lower costs for the hospital, in lower levels of anxiety for the community, and in greater access to satisfactory nonemergency health services. A win-win situation!

The outreach staff of the clinic were delighted with the conclusion of the evaluation overall, but were concerned that the focus-group data showed that men did not feel they knew enough about the clinic and did not think the clinic provided services for them. The outreach staff pointed this finding out to the executive director, and they developed a plan for increasing the number of men using the clinic. Because they had asked participants for concrete steps for improving the initiative and for shaping systems and relationships differently with the new clinic, they had a lot of information to start with.

THE ROLE OF STAKEHOLDERS

As with quantitative-data analysis and interpretations, stakeholders are usually less involved in this stage of the process; however, qualitative-data analysis is more intuitive than quantitative analysis, and with some training they should be able to learn how to do it. Qualitative data is more likely to be learned by an adult if the right training is provided, which is unlike quantitative data that generally requires a substantial foundation in math that is more likely obtained in school. Having stakeholders involved allows the team to check their interpretations of the data as well as to check their assumptions in interpreting the data and drawing conclusions. Stakeholder involvement increases the validity of the findings and the likelihood that the results of the evaluation will be used.

SUMMARY

- Conducting qualitative research using interviewing approaches—focus groups, individual interviews, appreciative inquiry, case studies, digital storytelling, or components of photovoice—provides data that are converted into text through transcription. The resulting document can then be coded to produce themes that form the basis for answering the research questions and drawing conclusions.

- In writing reports, it is important to select quotations that are representative of the theme and that illustrate a shared perception or opinion of the respondents. Quotations may also be used to highlight particular or interesting phenomena that may form the basis for further research but may not be typical of the views of most of the participants in the study.

- Qualitative methods can complement each other to reduce the likelihood of bias and provide a comprehensive understanding of the topic under study.

- Conclusions are drawn against the standards including assessing how and whether the process and outcome objectives were met.

FIGURE 10.5. *Valuable Take-Aways*

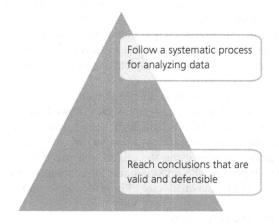

Follow a systematic process for analyzing data

Reach conclusions that are valid and defensible

DISCUSSION QUESTIONS AND ACTIVITIES

1. Identify a 5-to-10-page transcript of a focus-group discussion or an individual interview. Review the transcript and highlight each theme that occurs in a different color. Using scissors, cut out each theme, keeping a part of the text for quotes and context. Write a summary report of your interview data including quotes. What conclusions would you draw from your results? What connections are you making and how might they differ from another person's conclusions? Why might there be a difference?

2. Identify a published qualitative study. Review the results of the data collection, and without looking at the authors' interpretation, write up your own interpretations of the data. Once you have finished your paper, compare your interpretation with that of the author. Did they differ? If so, why do you think they did?

3. Review the published literature for evaluations utilizing GIS mapping. Select one article for this assignment. How was the method used? What kinds of conclusions was the author able to draw? Do you see how the author arrived as the conclusion that he did, if not, what facts, data or evidence would have helped you to figure out what was done?

KEY TERMS

coding
computer coding
data-analysis software
descriptive statistics
frequencies
mean

measures of central tendency
measures of dispersion
mode
standard deviation
transcription
variance

CHAPTER

11

REPORTING EVALUATION FINDINGS

LEARNING OBJECTIVES

- Describe the content of evaluation reports.
- Describe the formats and presentation of evaluation reports.

The final step in the participatory model for evaluation is to report the findings of the evaluation (Figure 11.1). A report provides feedback about the results of the evaluation to multiple stakeholder audiences. It describes the evaluation process and findings and makes recommendations in response to the purpose of the evaluation so that the results will be used.

Patton (2008, p. 37) defines *utilization-focused evaluation* as "evaluation done for and with the specific intended primary users for specific, intended uses." He goes on to say that the entire evaluation process must be conducted carefully if the evaluation is to be useful. He cautions that the report is only one of many mechanisms for facilitating the use of evaluation findings. Reports nonetheless should communicate information for the benefit of the stakeholders for whom the evaluation was intended. Reports provide feedback on the evaluation questions that were asked and information for both accountability and decision-making. They provide necessary and vital accountability not just for the initiative but also for the evaluation team and its stewardship.

Since the evaluation report also includes a complete description of the entity or initiative being evaluated, it provides a justification for the intervention, the resources allocated to the program, the activities undertaken by the program, in addition to the answers to the evaluation questions. Future evaluators have a document that serves as the starting point for the next evaluation providing evidence of what was known at a particular point in time. Having a previous report ensures that evaluations build on each other and do not repeat what was done previously. For example, a process evaluation conducted in year 3 of a 5-year project may have provided sufficient evidence of how the intervention was conceived and implemented in addition to determining the extent to which it was being implemented as

FIGURE 11.1.   *The Participatory Model for Evaluation—Report the Findings*

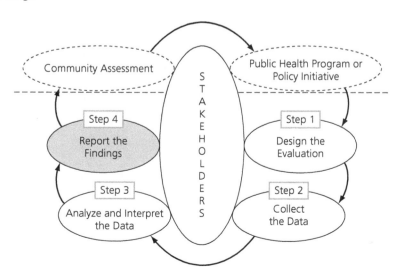

planned. In year 5, it may be much less important to repeat the process evaluation, and more important to determine outcomes of the program using scarce resources to the benefit of the program. If, however, the evaluation team is being called in for the first time in year 5 as often happens, it would be prudent to undertake a process evaluation as well as an outcome evaluation. The questions that are answered will be determined by the needs of the stakeholders and would emerge from the evaluation selection process described earlier in this book. Because there is no one way to conduct an evaluation, so there is no one way to report the findings either. The findings in the report are directly linked to the purpose of the evaluation and to the needs of the stakeholders. For example, if the purpose of the evaluation is to understand the initiative's implementation, then the evaluation approach is a formative or process evaluation depending on the stage of the program. Remember that a formative evaluation is conducted while the initiative is still being developed to ensure that resources are put in place so expected outcomes are more likely to be achieved. Process evaluation on the other hand is conducted primarily after the intervention has a well-developed logic and its ability to get to outcomes has been established. The report would, therefore, provide information that is helpful for determining whether the initiative was being implemented as planned or whether adjustments were required. It may also provide evidence of its sustainability beyond the funded period. If the purpose of the evaluation is to determine the impact of the program, both the evaluation approach and the report would provide information on the effect of the program on the beneficiaries. If the purpose of the evaluation is to determine the cost effectiveness of the initiative compared with others, the report would provide a comparison of multiple programs and a level of detail that may not have been necessary or appropriate in reporting a process evaluation.

In addition to keeping the purpose of the evaluation in mind when writing the report, it is helpful to bear in mind the expectations of stakeholders. Stakeholders may have additional expectations for the final report, which may include, for example, a discussion of issues of social justice. If stakeholders are involved throughout the process, controversial or potentially difficult conclusions can be discussed. Discussing evaluation findings with stakeholders throughout supports the overall intention of improving the likelihood that the report will be used.

Whether the evaluation is conducted for a public health program or a policy initiative, the value of the process is in the ability of the stakeholders to utilize the findings. There are three major reasons why evaluation results are used:

1. The stakeholders have been involved in the process.

2. The report is written in a user-friendly appropriate format.

3. The results are relevant to stakeholders and provide useful information.

If the real value in conducting an evaluation is in using the findings to improve the program, then the report should provide the information in ways that are helpful. The results of evaluations may be used in multiple ways that include revealing new insights into the program and how it works or reordering priorities in program administration or in program direction. The results can lead to a change in the population that is served or to a new direction in policy development. They can result in ending the initiative altogether, or they can persuade stakeholders, policymakers, institutions, professional, or civic groups that the initiative is successful. More and more often evaluation is a requirement for further funding, and the report becomes an indispensable tool in raising money and acquiring resources.

Some of these examples may lead one to believe that an evaluation report must provide information only about an initiative's success. Nothing is further from the truth! An evaluation report must answer the research questions in an objective and unbiased way irrespective of positive or negative findings. In general, reports should be understandable, meaningful, valuable, and accurate, and recommendations should be grounded in and reflect the findings from the data (Patton, 2008). It is imperative that the report's recommendations are within the scope of the agency's work.

This chapter describes the content of the report and suggests formal and alternative ways of providing feedback and the results of the evaluation to a variety of stakeholders. In the participatory model for evaluation, the stakeholder remains central to the process and is a full participant both in the writing of the report and in its delivery.

Evaluation reports must be presented in a manner that facilitates understanding and subsequent use, in a timely way, and by a member of the team, preferably the individual or individuals who have the most credibility with the audience. For example, a youth member of the evaluation team, rather than the team leader, may present the report to the youth who were the subjects of the evaluation because the team leader may have little in common with the group members who should hear and act on the recommendations. In communicating information, we learn that there are three important aspects of transmitting a message: the source, the messenger, and the receiver. When the message and the messenger are both credible, the person receiving and interpreting the message is much more likely to act on it. So using youth to deliver the message is an important strategy for ensuring that the message is received and increases the likelihood of its adoption.

Important considerations in the development of the report are

■ The content

■ The audience

■ The appropriateness of the timing

■ The format of the report

Unlike data collected for research purposes in other settings, evaluations are conducted by the evaluation team for and on behalf of an organization, an agency, a foundation, a board of directors, a federal agency, and so forth. The data from the evaluation research and the reports belong to the organization or agency that commissioned the report. Findings from the study and the evaluation report are released to the person or entity that requested the study and are not released to the public without permission to other stakeholders.

THE CONTENT OF THE REPORT

The content of the evaluation report is derived from the data required to support the message that must be conveyed. The information that is provided in the report answers the evaluation questions and supports the purpose of the evaluation. In addition, the information must be sufficient to clearly describe the program being evaluated, the context, the purposes of the evaluation, the procedures, and the findings (Joint Committee on Standards for Educational Evaluation et al., 1994).

The conclusions of the evaluation describe the value of the initiative to the different stakeholder audiences. The value of the initiative may be both tangible and intangible and is assessed against multiple criteria that include

- The goals and objectives of the initiative as outlined in the evaluation plan

- Expectations for what the initiative should achieve

- Expectations of who should benefit from the initiative

- The reasons for which the evaluation was conducted

- Issues of social justice and equity

In addition to being assessed against expected outcomes, the data are also examined for unexpected outcomes that benefit or hurt the community or participants or nonparticipants in the initiative.

The questions for the evaluation may be identified and categorized as major or minor questions, and the findings may be similarly categorized. Major findings may be significant changes that occurred in individuals, community, and systems as a result of the initiative or may be answers to the questions that were selected as most important for the evaluation process. Major findings may also include unintended consequences that had significant impact on individuals, communities, institutions, or systems. Minor findings may be related to less consequential evaluation questions or unintended consequences of the intervention.

In writing an evaluation report, use simple, direct language and avoid using jargon and unfamiliar acronyms. For example, MCH is a commonly used term in public health, but many people outside the discipline may not know that MCH refers to maternal and child health. MCH would be considered both jargon and an unfamiliar acronym. In writing the report use examples, anecdotes, graphs, charts, diagrams, and quotations to illustrate difficult concepts. They help the reader make sense of some of the narrative.

The evaluation report has eight key components: (1) The cover page, (2) executive summary, (3) an introduction, (4) a description of the evaluation activities, (5) results, (6) analysis, (7) conclusions, and (8) recommendations. In addition, the evaluation report will identify any limitation of the study that will compromise the conclusions and lessons learned. The appendix forms the last part of the report.

The Cover Page

The cover page of the report tells the reader what the title of the report is, who commissioned it, the author(s) and their credentials, and the date on which the report was submitted.

The Executive Summary

The executive summary is usually about one to two pages and captures the main ideas of the evaluation study. For very all-inclusive evaluations, it may be longer, but it should be long enough to provide a good summary of the evaluation and short enough to be read. The goal of the executive summary is to serve as a stand-alone document that captures the main ideas and allows the reader to only go to the full report for details associated with the study. It summarizes the report by providing a synopsis of each section of the report but with a focus on the results and the recommendations. It is often used by board members and executives to highlight the main findings in meetings and when speaking to the media. It does not take the place of the full report.

The Introduction

The introduction to the evaluation report contains a summary of the peer-reviewed scientific literature and published documents that provide information about the distribution, prevalence, incidence, and risk factors associated with the public health problem. It discusses the issue from a national, state, and local perspective. In addition, the introduction includes a summary of findings from the community assessment. Together they provide the rationale for the development of the initiative.

Description of Evaluation Activities

This section contains a report of the major components of the evaluation. It includes a detailed description of the initiative. The logic model summarizes the initiative's theory of change, and the initiative's activities, expected outcomes, outputs, and resources are identified.

EXAMPLE

OUTLINE FOR A DESCRIPTION OF THE INITIATIVE

- Social, political, and cultural context
- Population served
- Goal and objectives
- Theory of change
- Intervention activities
- Intervention logic model

In addition, this section presents the purpose of the evaluation, the evaluation questions, the evaluation plan, and the research design. It discusses stakeholder involvement and roles in the evaluation process.

It provides a detailed description of data-collection strategies, including information about where and how the data were gathered and how the analysis was undertaken. It includes a description of the tools used for data collection. The description of the data analysis specifies the software used and the data-analysis and data-management approaches that were utilized.

The Results and Analysis

From the point of view of the stakeholders, this is probably the most important section. This section discusses the results of the evaluation. It contains a description of the sample from whom the data were drawn for the evaluation, summarizes the findings from the quantitative or qualitative data collection, and presents an appropriate analysis and interpretation of the data. One option for organizing this section is to answer the first evaluation question, then move to the next one until all the questions are answered. This provides some order and allows recommendations to link directly to the findings of the study. In a mixed-methods approach to the evaluation, questions may have been asked in surveys that lend themselves to quantitative or qualitative data-analysis approaches. The appropriate methods for analyzing and interpreting the data must be used.

Quantitative data are generally reported in summary narrative form and are accompanied by charts, tables, graphs, and figures to summarize the data and improve understanding. A summary of the demographic profile of the participants in the sample is the first part of results section followed by an analysis of the survey data. The analysis is presented to the reader recognizing the needs of the stakeholders yet answering the research questions. If the research question required pre/post test surveys, then the analysis would include an appropriate comparison of the before and after intervention data. Alternatively, if the question concerned the level of collaboration among members of a coalition, an appropriate representation of the data would be results from a network analysis and a discussion of findings.

Qualitative data are usually presented in narrative form and accompanied by quotations or photographs that best illustrate the theme that is being described. For example, when the theme being explored was access to healthy foods, participants described what it meant to have access to fruits and vegetables in their communities in a family study conducted as part of the evaluation of an environmental, systems, and policy-change intervention. This quotation provides powerful imagery for the reader: "I think we would eat a lot more fresh vegetables if I could afford it … I like to eat healthy too but a lot of fresh fruits and vegetables tend to cost more so I will cut out on those, just try to get what I can afford, canned or whatever. I feel like if I made more money, I'll be able to buy healthier foods but I don't" [Female Adult].

The Conclusions and Recommendations

The conclusion of the evaluation report discusses the results of the study in the context of the evaluation criteria, which may be the extent to which the objectives of the intervention have been met, or may answer much broader questions related to the value and worth of the initiative. Answering the broader question requires a further level of analysis from just a question like, "did beneficiaries of the intervention benefit, and if so by how much?" It provides the evaluator's judgment of the initiative overall and a critical assessment of the links among the program inputs, activities, outputs, and outcomes. In addition, it provides a fair and balanced examination of the strengths and weaknesses of the initiative.

In a recent evaluation the team adopted a set of criteria (SEPI©) to provide an overall assessment of the initiative. It allowed for a synthesis of the results of the data analysis beyond just answering each research question.

FIGURE 11.2. *Criteria for an Overall Assessment of the Initiative*

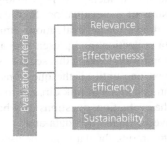

The criteria were (see Figure 11.2):

Relevance: the extent to which the activities designed and implemented were suited to the priorities.

Effectiveness: the extent to which the program has achieved its intended outputs and outcomes.

Efficiency: outputs in relation to inputs.

Sustainability and partnerships: likely sustainability beyond funding and the extent to which the project brings together relevant stakeholders to achieve its goals.

The judgment associated with the conclusions and hence the recommendations that are made incorporate the results of the analysis. In some cases this will be only quantitative, while in others it will be a combination of quantitative and qualitative research. When a combination of methodologies is used the underlying philosophy of triangulation is adopted. Triangulation implies the use of one of more investigators, data sources, or theoretical frameworks in responding to each research question. The results are compared to the standards that have been discussed in previous chapters. They are the standards identified by staff, community members, program participants, and the evaluation team. Factors that strengthen the judgment being made include summarizing believable pathways by which the results could have been reached, suggesting alternative pathways, giving possible reasons why initial—objectives and expectations were not supported by the findings of the evaluation if that was the case, and demonstrating that the results were obtained using systematic and reproducible processes.

The conclusion of an evaluation report

- Presents a list of key findings that highlight important aspects of the evaluation results

- Reflects on the importance of the findings

- Discusses the results of the evaluation in the context of social-justice and other criteria important to stakeholders

■ Identifies unintended consequences, discusses them, and advances solutions for addressing them

■ Suggests new questions that may need to be answered

■ Makes recommendations for decision making and stakeholder and community action

The primary purpose of this section of the report is to communicate actions for consideration by the stakeholders. The actions that are recommended by the evaluation team must be based on the findings from the evaluation process and must be defensible, realistic, and targeted. Recommendations must include not just the recommended actions but reflections on their advantages and disadvantages as well as the cost implications if they are adopted. In addition, Patton (2008, pp. 502–504) identifies political sensitivity, thoughtfulness, and directness as characteristics of recommendations. Recommendations must also support an existing work plan, or be easily incorporated.

For recommendations to be action-oriented they must be specific and considerate of the contextual factors that influence the organization's or agency's operations. For example, a community-based organization's primary activities were to offer HIV/AIDS prevention and treatment services to youth. Based on an assessment of the objectives of the program, the evaluation team determined that the organization had not met its targets. The evaluators made the following recommendations

■ Increase efforts to reach the target population by increasing outreach and services.

■ Increase efforts to improve behavioral risk assessments by the target population by developing mechanisms by which each participant completes the assessment during his or her first visit for prevention case management.

■ Continue to explore strategies to implement the curriculum's use through improving links to youth and appropriate communities.

Recommendations may be influenced by the purpose of the evaluation and hence the intended utilization of the findings. The following examples illustrate how findings are linked to the purpose of the evaluation.

1. *Purpose:* To understand the extent to which the program is being implemented as planned with a view to expanding to serve a larger population.

    Findings: The process evaluation showed that although some parts of the program were well implemented, others lacked sufficient staff support to provide the level of intensity required.

    Recommendations:

    a. Suggest ways that the initiative can realistically increase staffing levels based on the organization's structure and funding

    b. Consider the inclusion of a larger volunteer base to support program activities.

    c. Suggest delaying any expansion of the program until staffing levels are higher.

2. *Purpose:* To determine what effect the initiative had on the program beneficiaries.

Finding: The outcome evaluation results showed that female youth had higher mean scores in almost all the variables that were measured which were significantly different from those of the male youth.

Recommendation: Suggest ways that the initiative can increase the intensity of the offerings for males while ensuring that the females continued to benefit from the program.

3. *Purpose: To determine the initiative's cost effectiveness compared with that of other programs in an assessment of funding priorities.*

Finding: Although the initiative was found to be effective, the cost associated with it was much higher than the cost of similar programs with similar outcomes.

Recommendation: Suggest ways of trimming the cost of the initiative without losing its integrity and its ability to achieve its stated outcomes.

Limitations and Lessons Learned

Limitations of the evaluation and *lessons learned* from conducting the evaluation are identified in this section of the report. It describes any shortcomings of the evaluation and reflections on the research approach, participant recruitment and participation, data collection, and research findings. It includes a discussion of the reliability and validity issues that influenced the research and provides an opportunity to discuss improvements in the evaluation process that may be applicable in similar evaluations.

Appendix

The *appendix* of the evaluation report contains copies of the surveys, consent forms, interview and observation protocols, and similar materials that were used for data collection; it includes any raw data and extensive data analysis that supports the report but may be too much for the body of the report, and contains a list of members of the evaluation team and their roles in the evaluation. The appendix may or may not be read by the person reading the report, so be sure to put any important information in the main body of the report.

THE AUDIENCE FOR THE REPORT

The results of the evaluation are discussed with major stakeholders. The entire evaluation team must participate in this final process. Stakeholders are people who have an interest in knowing the results of the evaluation study, and they constitute the audience for it. These people include:

- Program managers and those who commissioned the evaluation
- Local, state, and federal policymakers and decision makers
- Funding agencies and foundations
- Researchers and program developers

■ Agency board members

■ Members of the staff and volunteers

■ Members of the community who are affected by and /or participate in the offerings of the initiative

The audience determines the format of the report; the level of detail in the report; the type of presentation, whether written or oral; and the timing of the report. In addition to the audience for the report, the specific audience also needs to be considered. Going back to our earlier discussion about communication the report is intended to change a behavior, be it making a decision about the sustainability of the initiative, improving the initiative overall, or aspects of the initiative. The theory behind communication still applies.

Successful reports, which result in action from those hearing them, rely on the right message, given through the right channel, from the right source. In keeping with this philosophy, we must consider the variables that most influence this process. They are age, gender, literacy, knowledge, attitudes, beliefs, and the expected outcomes of the reports. Given all these variables, it is important to consider what each audience would most likely respond to. For example, the program manager and staff of the organization who commissioned the report may want a somewhat different tone and slant of the study and its findings from the politician who wants to take credit for the initiative's success and wants to do a media promotion of the organization and focus entirely on the findings. This expectation guides how the results are presented. The question might be asked, how is the case best made? What results best make the case? What does this audience value the most?

Let's look at another scenario where an important stakeholder group is the youth. They were the focus of the intervention and the evaluation and to get their buy-in for improvements to the intervention and increase the likelihood of success, one of key the audiences for the report is the youth. The youth group is between the ages of 18 and 25 years and is well educated, but they engage in very high-risk behaviors, which need to be addressed by all sectors of the society especially the youth themselves. Given that the group is mixed gender and highly educated, they would be expecting a presentation that has actionable information that is relevant to them. They probably want to see the results of some of the analysis presented in youthful colors and animation. They may also want to have information to take away with them. So, in addition to a formal PowerPoint presentation that is long enough to give them the information they need but short enough to hold their attention, they may want to take some material home that they can put up on one of the social media platforms (e.g., Twitter, Facebook) to share with their peers who were unable to attend the single session.

THE TIMING OF THE REPORT

There are primarily two times for writing an evaluation report: at the end of the contract period or as an interim report during the period of the evaluation. In both cases, the report is presented in time for use. The timing of reports is generally part of the contract that is drawn up at the start of the project. For an outcome evaluation based on a cross-sectional research design, an interim report may be specified in the contract and a final report may be due on completion of the analysis. If the contract period is five years, evaluation reports may be due annually.

In addition, ad hoc reports may be required for decision-making by the board of directors, executive directors, or members of staff at any time during the life of the evaluation contract. This requirement may be negotiated in advance or the team may be asked to provide a report with some notice answering specific questions. Ad hoc reports may be requested for advisory committee or board meetings, especially in the formative stages of a project or in the case of a process evaluation.

The evaluation report should preferably go to the client at least two weeks before the deadline to allow for adequate reflection and appropriate response and for stakeholders to provide input into the recommendations. Allowing sufficient time for review may be especially important when the findings are negative or they provide reason for stakeholders to arrange meetings with the evaluation team prior to a formal presentation. Participation of the stakeholders in this process will increase the likelihood that the report will be read, understood, and used. In an evaluation of a community-based organization, the program manager was given an opportunity to see the final report. As a result, an additional recommendation was included that supported the work of the project manager and provided visibility for the actions that needed to be taken by the organization to meet an important objective. The program manager felt unable to make the recommendation without the support of valid data and the credibility of the evaluation team. Since the outcome of the evaluation meant a review of project finances, the hope was that resources would be made available.

THE FORMAT OF THE REPORT

The final evaluation report can have a variety of forms and formats as determined by the purpose of the evaluation and the person(s) requesting or interested in the report and its findings. A report intended for the board of directors will be different in format, style, and presentation from a report for community members. As stakeholders they both are entitled to a presentation of evaluation findings, but they each have separate expectations for the form it should take.

In addition, the selection of the most appropriate format is guided by the characteristics of the initiative, the appropriateness of the format for a particular audience, and its cost. For example, the board of a nonprofit organization or a foundation may expect a formal printed copy of the report complete with an executive summary, whereas the members of the coalition, who are involved in the day-to-day work of the organization, may prefer a discussion of the main findings with specific recommendations for the actions that are within their control. Consulting with the stakeholders to discuss an appropriate format will improve communication of the results.

Irrespective of the format and whether the evaluation report is in a printed format or delivered orally, start by letting the audience know the focus of the report. The title of the report should make the focus clear.

A formal printed version of the report may be developed for a board of directors, advisory committees, funding agencies, or the executive director and contain a number of components.

The *cover page* contains the title, the name of the organization or agency that commissioned the report, the names of the evaluation team members, and the date of the report.

The *table of contents* lists the topics covered in the order they appear in the report with their associated their page numbers. It is useful to use the features within the References tab of Microsoft Word© to create the Table of Contents. The Word Help within the Microsoft Word© office program provides directions for how to do this.

The *acknowledgments* identify and thank individuals or organizations who contributed to the evaluation, including members of the evaluation team, staff, and participants in the research.

The *list of acronyms* defines short forms and abbreviations of words used in the report that might be unfamiliar to readers. For example, the table of contents from a report which is primarily about maternal and child health services may contain acronyms such as BEmOC or IMNCI. An easy reference for these terms is provided at the beginning of the report (see Table 11.1).

The *executive summary* is a one- to two-page synopsis of the full report. In a very long report, this may be longer, but it is important to keep it short and to the point! The *topics covered* in the executive summary are the background to the evaluation, the methodology, the results, key findings, conclusions, and recommendations. Emphasis is on the results, key findings, conclusions, and recommendations. The main body of the report provides the detail.

The final report may be provided in print form in multiple copies or in electronic form on a flash drive or a combination of the two. It may also be sent by email, if so desired by the stakeholder. The contract often defines the format and the timing of the report if this was discussed. In the absence of any formal negotiation, the evaluation team has the responsibility to determine the format of the report. In addition to presenting the full report accompanied by the executive summary, an oral and PowerPoint® presentation summarizing the report may be presented to stakeholders. This allows for a facilitated discussion of the findings, which may contribute to the use of the report.

An oral presentation contains the full report, yet it generally captures the main ideas more succinctly and in more animated and graphic forms. It is generally divided into three parts. The *introduction* sets the tone for the presentation and allows the presenter to get the audience's full attention. The *middle* explains the evaluation activities (methodology) and presents the results of the study. The *end* provides the recommendations, discusses the next steps, and leaves the audience with a set of specific recommended actions.

If, however, the evaluation report is being developed for members of the community, more appropriate and less formal approaches must be developed. The final report format and content may be discussed and negotiated with stakeholders. Youth may want a different format than other members of the faith community, if the evaluation had been commissioned by the faith community. The content of the report as well as the presentation must take the cultural expectations of the group into consideration and adapt the report and presentation to suit. In a traditional gathering for example, the evaluation the traditional leader will be in charge of the event and the evaluation team gets called on as appropriate, with the evaluation team sitting through all the traditional ceremonies and formalities. A presentation that was expected to take 30 minutes could be embedded within a ceremony that instead

TABLE 11.1. List of Acronyms

BEmOC	Basic Emergency Obstetric Care
CEmOC	Comprehensive Emergency Obstetric Care
CHC	Community Health Center
CHO	Community Health Officer
CHP	Community Health Post
CHW	Any worker within the health system including TBAs (excluding physicians)
CRS	Catholic Relief Services
DHMT	District Health Management Team
DMO	District Medical Officer
HIV/AIDS	Human Immunodeficiency Virus/Acquired Immuno- Deficiency Disease
HMIS	Health Management Information Systems
IMNCI	Integrated Management of Newborn and Childhood Illnesses
IRC	International Red Cross
MCH Aide	Maternal and Child Health Aide
MCHP	Maternal Community Health Post
MOHS	Ministry of Health and Sanitation
NPSE	National Primary School Examination
PBF	Performance Based Financing
PHU	Primary Care Unit
RN	Registered Nurse
SECHN	State Enrolled Community Health Nurse
STI	Sexually Transmitted Infections
TBA	Traditional Birth Attendant
U5	Children 5 years and under
UNICEF	United Nations Children's Fund
VHT	Village Health Team

takes two hours. The evaluation team must make provision for this but be proud that so much attention is given to their report.

The format and the content of the less formal presentations will depend on the community or stakeholder group. Important considerations include reading levels, involvement in the process, and the extent to which recipients understand what the evaluation was about. The more engaged stakeholders are in the evaluation activities, the more likely they are to grasp the details of the methodology.

Appropriate formats for a range of audiences include the following:

- Full report of the evaluation approaches, methodology, findings, recommendations, and conclusions

- One- to two-page executive summary of the full report

- Press release with a focus on the findings and recommendations

- Single-page summary of the major findings and recommendations

- Newspaper-, newsletter-, magazine-, or brochure-style reports highlighting the main findings and recommendations with a focus on what members of the community can do to address the problem

- Community presentations in town hall meetings highlighting the main findings and presenting recommendations that the community can act on immediately and in the long term

- Graphic and/or animated digital-media or radio or television presentations highlighting important findings

- Media presentations that allow the evaluation team to not only present the report but also to discuss its implications with stakeholder groups

- Oral presentations that highlight the main findings and provide audiences the opportunity to ask questions and to clarify conclusions

Additionally, presentations of evaluation findings may occur at conferences and meetings where formal oral, PowerPoint®, and poster presentations may be made summarizing the full report. The focus of the presentation will usually be reflected in the theme of the conference or the meeting. Technical reports and journal articles may also be used to document academic endeavors. An abstract is usually required for academic writings. An abstract consists of

- The background—a brief overview of the purpose of the evaluation

- The numbers, location, and demographic characteristics of participants

- The design of the study and an overview of the type of data collected

- The results of qualitative and/or quantitative research

- The conclusions and recommendations for next steps
- Irrespective of the format that is used, the reporting of evaluation results should
  - Be accurate;
  - Match the reporting to the culture and reading levels of the audience;
  - Provide an appropriate level of detail so the audience understands the approach, the findings, and the recommendations;
  - Include illustrations, photographs, examples, and quotations that provide depth to the data and improve the authenticity and understanding of the report;
  - Communicate respect and fairness to the audience;
  - Provide the audience with clear action-oriented next steps in the recommendations;
  - Use well-designed and effective presentations;
  - Involve stakeholders throughout the process.

Ultimately the evaluation report is a two-way communication between the evaluation team and the stakeholders. The evaluation team ensures that the results are understood; stakeholders get a chance to ask questions, and the evaluation team guides them to implement the recommendations and prepare for the next evaluation cycle.

SUMMARY

Stakeholders must be involved in the development of the report and recommendations as they were throughout the process.

- Evaluation results are used when the stakeholders have been involved in the process; the report is written in a user-friendly, appropriate format; and, most important, the results are relevant to stakeholders and provide useful information.
- The evaluation report contains an explanation of the research study, results, analysis, and recommendations. It includes major and significant findings as well as minor, less consequential findings. It includes a discussion of unintended consequences that had a significant impact on individuals, communities, institutions, or systems, and it discusses issues of social justice.
- The selection of the format for the final presentation and report is guided by the characteristics of the initiative, the information to be provided, the audiences for the report, the delivery channels (print, electronic, in person), and the cost.
- The reporting of evaluation results should be accurate; be appropriate for the culture and reading levels of the audience; include an appropriate level of detail; and use

illustrations, examples, and quotations that provide depth to the findings and improvement to the authenticity of the report.

- The report must communicate respect and fairness to the audience and provide the audience with clear action-oriented next steps.

FIGURE 11.3. *Valuable Take-Aways*

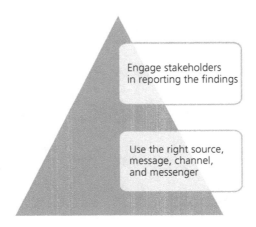

Engage stakeholders in reporting the findings

Use the right source, message, channel, and messenger

DISCUSSION QUESTIONS AND ACTIVITIES

1. You are part of an evaluation team that has just completed a three-year study of a local community organization's initiatives with a lot of different findings. What factors would you take into consideration when preparing the final report?

2. Prepare a report from a study of a youth intervention that you find in the peer reviewed literature in a multimedia format for a selected audience.

3. What ethical dilemmas would you anticipate in presenting evaluation reports to a group of very motivated stakeholders whose jobs depend on your positive findings? How would you handle the reporting process?

KEY TERMS

audience for the report
evaluation findings
evaluation report

executive summary
presentation formats

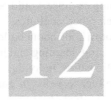

CASE STUDY

THE COMMUNITY ASSESSMENT

The names and data used in this case study are entirely made up and do not refer to any existing persons or situations.

BACKGROUND

The number of persons with diabetes has increased steadily over the past decade. During that time, diabetes has been one of the leading causes of death, and heart disease is often associated with it. Diabetes-associated cardiovascular disease is the largest component of the direct costs of hospitals. Diabetes is a major clinical and public health challenge.

There were high rates of diabetes in a rural community of 250,000 people in Riverside County, and many people had lost limbs because of diabetes-related amputations. Community members wanted to know about the condition, and a team was assembled to conduct a community assessment.

ESTABLISH A TEAM

The team was a demographically diverse group of 15 people who lived or worked or lived and worked in the community. A few people on the team who did not live or work there knew the community well because they had done work with some of the local groups a few years before. But they had stayed in touch with the community and loved to come back for celebrations.

The team agreed on the task. They would conduct a community assessment to understand why this community had such high rates of diabetes, but more than that they wanted to know how to improve community health. The group went around the table and said their names and why they wanted to be there. The project coordinator realized it was a diverse group and decided that a team-building exercise would be a good start. The exercise focused on building an understanding of each other's cultures.

The team adapted an activity from a book about building evaluation capacity. The group discussed how language, food and eating, learning and information processing, the concept of time, communication styles, relationships, individual and community values and norms, work habits, and other practices influence work in general and evaluation in particular. It was a spirited conversation, which helped clarify misconceptions about others' cultures. For example, a few members of the evaluation team had lived and worked in other cultures and had adopted their way of doing things. One was their more casual approach to being at meetings on time. They did not see the importance of being on time and would show up to a meeting that started at 2:00 anytime between 2:30 and 2:45. The team really wanted 2:00 to be 2:00 so they had a discussion about timeliness and how not being on time really was a problem for those who arrived on time. It was not so much respect for others that was considered, as much as what that respect meant. Being late meant they did not respect their time and did not appreciate that they had other responsibilities to attend to. The team resolved to always be on time for meetings!

After the team-building activities, the team took a short break and then reassembled to discuss the task before them. They felt they could contribute to the community assessment. The project director had come across a definition of cultural competence that she liked and wanted to share it: "A set of congruent behaviors, attitudes, and policies that come together in a system, agency, or among professionals and enables that system, agency, or those professionals to work effectively in cross-cultural situations." After the training, the group adopted the definition of competence as a goal for the team. One of the members introduced a game that allowed people to talk about their skills in a nonthreatening way and appreciate the value of each person's contribution to the team. They discovered that they had many skills and talents among them and much in common, and they all felt they had a lot to contribute to the process. Their skills and talents are summarized in Table 12.1; they included

- Experience in writing simple proposals and budgets.

- Experience with conducting interviews and collecting surveys. One person had used photovoice before and found it helpful for engaging more people and understanding the community perspective.

- Experience in collecting and analyzing qualitative and quantitative data.

- Experience in project design and management.

The team members spent some time getting to know one another and working as a team. They did many team building exercises so they would gradually become more comfortable with working with each other. The project coordinator had experience working in teams, and although some of the members had been in meetings together before, they had

TABLE 12.1. **Potential Contributions of Team Members**

Members	Potential Contributions
Project coordinator	Project management, study design, field testing instruments, analyzing and interpreting qualitative data
Community members representing churches, schools, women's groups	Instrument design, data collection, reviewing and interpreting qualitative- and quantitative-analysis results
Staff of state agencies, local government departments, and community-based organizations	Instrument design, data collection, analyzing qualitative and quantitative data
Researcher	Study design, instrument design, analyzing and interpreting quantitative and qualitative data

not worked on the same team. The team-building exercises emphasized respect for each other and valuing each other's cultures and contributions to the project. The team infused community-based participatory research principles into the process. They especially wanted to make sure they built on the strengths and resources of the community, facilitated collaboration among all group members, and developed a learning community that emphasized capacity building.

DETERMINE THE AVAILABILITY OF DATA

The first major task for the team was to ascertain what data were already available nationally. One of the members of the team volunteered to conduct a literature review and came back to the group with a short summary.

There are two major types of diabetes. Type 1, which occurs because of the failure of the body to produce insulin, and Type 2, which results when the body is unable to use the insulin it produces or when the insulin that is present is inefficient. Prediabetes occurs when the levels of glucose in the blood are higher than normal but not high enough to produce a diagnosis of Type 2 diabetes. The risk for Type 2 diabetes increases with age and being a member of a minority population (Jackson et al., 2013). Other risks of diabetes include having diabetes during pregnancy, having high blood pressure, and having high cholesterol levels caused primarily by consuming too much saturated fat and too few vegetables, fruits, and grain products that are high in vitamins and minerals, carbohydrates (starch and dietary fiber), and other substances that are important to good health (Hanity, 2015; Vandam, 2016). In addition, being sedentary and not participating in regular exercise are also considered risk factors. Although obesity occurs among all population groups, obesity is most common among African American women (Jones, 2012).

The team members understood how to focus their community assessment. They wanted to understand

■   Who was most affected by the disease in their community and how they were affected

■   How people's diets affect their health

■   People's perceptions of the connections among diet, obesity, and health

■   People's knowledge, attitudes, and behavior with regard to diabetes, obesity, exercise, general health care, and utilizing health care

■   Environmental factors that influence the availability of fresh fruits and vegetables and opportunities for exercise

■   Cultural factors that influence food intake and exercise

■   Resources available in the community to address the issue

■   Factors influenced by history, and issues of social justice, and equity

DECIDE ON THE DATA-COLLECTION APPROACHES AND METHODS

Team members decided to organize their study around a theory so it would be easier to design an intervention later. They especially liked the ecological model because it allowed them to consider the factors that influenced diabetes at the individual, interpersonal, community, organizational, and policy levels. They wanted to be more specific than the ecological model allowed, so they included constructs from the health-belief model: perceived susceptibility, perceived seriousness of the condition, and barriers to and benefits of addressing the problem. They also used the stages of change from the transtheoretical model. The social cognitive theory was included to provide constructs of reciprocal determinism, outcome expectations, self-efficacy, and self-regulation.

Data-collection Approach

The team members decided that they had a lot to learn. They had skills in both qualitative and quantitative methods, so they focused their attention on the best approaches for getting the information they needed. They understood their population. Most of the women had completed high school, but only a few (1%) had gone to college. They gathered regularly for celebrations and were community oriented. They loved to talk and wanted to be involved in everything that was going on in the community. These characteristics were useful for collecting qualitative data. The team also worked with the local hospital and clinics to get data. They would also get a chance to triangulate their findings, making them more valid.

They decided to use surveys to collect data that were easily categorized and put into numerical format, but they also decided to use individual interviews and digital stories with accompanying photographs. Stories would be dictated by women who had diabetes and who lived with the consequences of poor access to and utilization of health care; their perspectives would add a dimension that the other methods would not have included. GIS maps were drawn of the area with demographic and diabetes information to determine the extent of the overlap between those two.

Data-Collection Instruments

The survey was organized into four major sections and a demographic section. The team identified previous surveys that they thought would be useful and adopted some of the questions. They developed some of their own to create a 50-item survey that included yes/no and scale-type items. Part 1 of the survey asked about women's diets and their perceptions of the connections among diet, obesity, and health. Part 2 asked about their knowledge, attitudes, and behavior with regard to diabetes, obesity, exercise, general health care, and utilizing health care. Part 3 asked questions that tried to get at cultural factors such as body image, family, community, and socialization and how these factors affected food intake and exercise behaviors and patterns. Part 4 focused on environmental factors that possibly affected access to fresh fruits and vegetables and to exercise. The final section included socioeconomic and demographic items, such as age, race, education, marital status, number of children in the household, income, and employment status. African American adult women ages 18–60 were asked to complete the surveys.

Individual key-informant interviews were used primarily to understand the resources available in the community to address the issue and the environmental factors related to access to fresh fruits and vegetables and exercise facilities. In addition, the interviewer solicited information on the history and leadership of the community as well as issues of social justice and equity.

The survey was tested in a pilot study of 30 women who lived in a comparable nearby community and had similar demographics. Two individual interviews were conducted to pilot the key-informant interview guide. The pilot test included testing the use of the consent form.

Interviews were scheduled for a time and place that ensured both confidentiality and safety. Surveys took on average 20 minutes to complete and interviews lasted approximately one hour. Completing the surveys and participating in the in-depth interviews and digital stories were entirely voluntary. Individuals were not compensated for their time.

TRAINING

Members of the research team were trained to serve as interviewers for the individual in-depth interviews through an interactive program that included a discussion of the content and rationale of the study and procedures for documenting participants' responses in the individual interviews. Training gave an overview of the entire research project and an opportunity for participants to provide input into the process and to practice interviewing skills. Training was provided in using the equipment for digital stories. Facilitators who would administer the surveys were also provided an orientation so as to be able to provide accurate information to the community if questions arose about the purpose of the study and the intended use of the data.

RESOURCE PROCUREMENT

Members of the team included members of community-based organizations and state agencies that had some funding for research, so they pooled their resources. They had sufficient money to pay for travel and supplies. The agencies provided in-kind support that covered the production of all the surveys.

ANALYSIS AND INTERPRETATION OF THE DATA

The survey data were analyzed in SPSS® to present traditional descriptive statistics. Data was presented using graphs along with GIS maps. GIS maps showed the distribution of diabetes across the community using data from the hospital and community health-center records and community resources. The prepared maps could then be compared with maps of poverty, unemployment, occupations, educational attainment, household structure, and income to explore the association between diabetes and adverse socioeconomic conditions. The overlay of maps as described suggested potential social, economic, and other risk factors for diabetes and aided in the selection and development of intervention activities.

The data from the digital stories and the individual interviews were analyzed to identify the themes using theoretical and empirical constructs from the literature and embedded in the instruments used for data collection. The qualitative software package NVivo® was used to code the qualitative-data transcripts. There were 30 transcripts.

SUMMARY OF FINDINGS

The community assessment found that the rates of diabetes among Black females who had not completed high school were higher than the rates for White and Hispanic women, with women between the ages of 40 and 64 being the most affected. The number of new cases of diabetes that year was 6.9 per thousand, a jump from 5.9 per thousand in the previous year. Furthermore, the number of obese women had also increased; 30% of women had a BMI greater than 30. A further assessment of risk factors associated with the rates of diabetes in this population included low levels of knowledge about diabetes, its causes, and prevention; poor attitudes about healthy eating and regular exercise; a media market that promoted fast foods. Women described their love of traditional food, which has high levels of saturated fat. The digital stories revealed how much women regretted that they had not paid sufficient attention to eating healthy and exercising more.

This community was what one could call a food desert; only one of the 10 convenience stores within the community sold fruits and vegetables at affordable prices. Most of the respondents were not within walking distance of grocery stores, which were, on average, three miles away. In addition, there were very few affordable exercise facilities. The next step was to design an intervention to provide access to an intervention that would improve their health.

THE INTERVENTION

Background

There were at least three organizations in the community that provided services. One of them, the Community Action Partnerships for Health Organization (CAPHO), was eager to expand its work to include diabetes. CAPHO had been providing services to low-income African American women for 10 years, and they also had noticed the increasing numbers of women who were diagnosed with diabetes in the previous year.

Based on the mission of the organization to "reduce the rates of chronic disease among women who live in the state," they decided they would intervene after they found out the results of the community assessment. The executive director invited her staff to a meeting to assess the organization's capacity to offer an additional service to women. They did a Strengths, Weakness, Opportunities, and Threats (SWOT) analysis to determine the organization's administrative capacity and also to think about the external opportunities and any difficulties that might arise. Once the process was complete, they agreed that although it would stretch their budget, they were already doing some similar interventions as part of other programs. They just needed to add a few new components.

Because they wanted to stay focused on prevention, they decided the goal would be to "reduce the rates of diabetes among low-income African American women in Riverside County." The executive director discussed the proposal with the board of directors, and it was approved. The organization contacted their community advisory committee, which included women in their other programs and staff in other nearby organizations, to discuss their new project. After many meetings, the advisory committee formulated the focus of their prevention program, which would be offered to African American women, the majority of whom were concentrated in three contiguous zip-code areas. They decided they would address two important risk factors for the onset of diabetes: obesity and lack of exercise. They talked with the stakeholders and eventually agreed on the scope of the work and the main overarching question for the intervention they called the Healthy Soon Project: "What effect did the Healthy Soon Project have on women who participated?"

The Healthy Soon Project

There were program pieces of the initiative that CAPHO could do in-house, like provide exercise equipment, but they also wanted women to walk around their neighborhoods to the park, to the stores, and just for pleasure with their friends. They recognized that in the low-income communities, women had limited opportunities to walk. The sidewalks were broken, the park was unsafe, and grocery stores were too far away for a leisurely stroll. The one convenience store that sold fruits and vegetables often kept them in a box under the counter or in the refrigerator too long so they went bad. The team would need to get some other folks into the committee who would work on the policy-development component of the initiative. They had their work cut out for them.

The team did lots of research to help guide them, and the expertise around the table also helped. By incorporating the principles of the ecological model, they were able to address more than one level of influence. To factors at the individual level, they added environmental factors that had been identified in the community assessment. The CAPHO team outlined a set of outcome objectives that provided the direction for the development of the project (and could be used as well later as benchmarks for the evaluation).

Public Health Goal
To reduce the rates of diabetes among low-income African American women in Riverside County.

Program Health Objective
Increase the percentage of African American women who participate in the intervention who are at a healthy weight to 60 percent by 2022.

Program Environmental Objective
Increase to 40 percent the number of stores and other venues that sell affordable produce in low-income neighborhoods by 2019.

The assumption made by the team was that with physical activity and good nutrition women would attain and maintain a healthy weight that would lead to a lower incidence and reduced rates of diabetes within the population. Figure 12.1 illustrates this theory of change.

The team decided to meet once a week until they had the program clearly planned; then they would meet monthly to check in with each other. They set a deadline for launching the program within 6 months. By this time they expected they would have allocated or secured the resources for the program.

The team members wanted to use an evidence-based intervention for their program because they knew that such initiatives were likely to be successful. They first broke down each of the objectives to identify the kinds of outcomes they wanted to see and the types of activities they thought would be appropriate for their population of low-income African American women. The literature suggested that African American women prefer to exercise

FIGURE 12.1.   *Theory of Change*

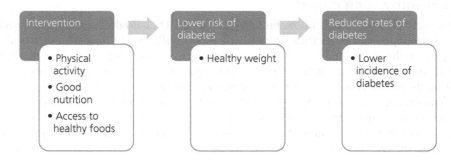

with their friends and families rather than do it by themselves. The team also knew from going into the convenience stores that there was a lot of advertising for alcohol, and women on the committee said that was one reason they discouraged their children from going to the local convenience stores. They thought it was important for the young people to develop better eating habits but there were few options available to them. One way to do that would be to make the stores more child-friendly, which meant making sure they stocked healthy food options as well as fresh fruit and vegetables.

The team conducted a literature search to identify evidence-based programs or evidence-based principles for nutrition and physical-activity programs. They had a list of questions and in addition to getting answers from the literature they talked to members of CAPHO. They wanted to determine

- Whether any interventions had been tested among low-income African American women in a similar community

- Whether any interventions included weight loss or maintaining a healthy weight or a similar outcome

- Whether CAPHO had the human, material, and financial resources needed

The team was able to find recommendations for programs from the American Diabetes Association; the National Institutes of Diabetes, Digestive and Kidney Diseases; and the U.S. Diabetes Prevention Program. The recommendations supported what they wanted to do and gave them additional ideas for activities.

Recommendations included:

- Screening for those who are overweight; are over 45 years of age; have a family history of diabetes and high blood pressure; and belong to a minority racial group.

- Weight loss with a reduced intake of fat; increased intake of dietary fiber; fewer calories.

- Physical activity of moderate intensity for 150 minutes per week.

So, they had what they needed for the first objective but did not have anything for the second objective. They had to find out whether there were evidence-based principles for increasing the number of convenience stores that sold fruits and vegetables and what policy changes would support such an initiative. A search of the literature did not turn up much information, but they knew from conferences they had attended that individuals around the country were developing projects similar to theirs. They contacted some of the organizations to find out what they had done.

The team constructed a table (Table 12.2) that showed the program goals, the expected outcomes, and the intervention approaches.

As they developed the initiative, they wrote subobjectives to reflect proximal benchmarks; and the activity objectives supported the outcome objectives. The team was reminded that activities for the initiative had to meet certain criteria. They had to

- Lead to the change specified in the objective

- Be completed during the specified time frame

TABLE 12.2. **Program Goals, Expected Outcomes, and Intervention Approaches**

Expected Outcome	Intervention Approach
Increase the percentage of African American women who participate in the intervention who are at a healthy weight to 60% by 2022.	
Healthy weight (BMI >19 <27)	Nutrition education; healthy diet; peer-supported and in-gym physical activity and monitoring; increased access to fresh fruits and vegetables
Increase to 40% the number of stores and other venues that sell affordable produce in low-income neighborhoods by 2019.	
Affordable produce	Convenience stores and farmers' markets; laws and policies that support access to affordable healthy foods in underserved neighborhoods; advocates whose primary focus was increasing access to and availability of food

- Have sufficient resources and personnel
- Be appropriate for the culture and expectations of the population for whom they were intended
- Be part of an overall plan to achieve a program's goal

With that set of reminders, the team got to work. See what they did to develop the outcome objectives in Tables 12.3 and 12.4.

With the help of the evaluation experts described in the next section, the team developed a logic model so they could clarify the initiative (Table 12.5).

DESIGN THE EVALUATION

CAPHO's projects had been successful in the past, but this time they wanted to be sure they were reaching their goal, so they discussed bringing an evaluation team in early; by doing so they would be sure to collect the data for the evaluation from the beginning.

A member of the community who had worked with a local community-based organization (CBO) and had been part of their evaluation team suggested Antoinette Pattercake. She was contacted and asked whether she would be available to conduct the study. Just to be sure she would work well with the stakeholders, the team asked her to meet them and provide information about her background, experience, and expertise in conducting evaluations. They were interested in knowing her approach to evaluation and were particularly interested in her ability to work with multiple stakeholders and conduct a participatory evaluation in which they played a major role. They wanted to have a thorough understanding of

TABLE 12.3.   **Outcome Objectives and Initiative Activities for Healthy-Weight Goal**

Outcome Objective	Initiative Activities	Frequency
Increase the proportion of African American women who participate in the intervention who are at a healthy weight to 60% by 2022.		
80 percent of participants in the Healthy Soon Project will report consuming a recommended diet consistently within six weeks of joining the program.	Dietician develops low-fat, high-fiber, low-calorie diets for each participant.	Monthly
	Participants keep a diary of food intake and problem solving that reflects struggles in controlling diet and exercising regularly.	Daily Bimonthly
	Weigh-ins/testimonials and support groups/discussion of how advertising influences food choices.	
80 percent of participants in the Healthy Soon Project will report exercising for a 150 minutes per week within 8 weeks of joining the program.	Recruit friends and family as exercise partners.	Daily
	Strength and toning exercise activities.	
	Participants keep a diary of duration of exercise.	
80 percent of participants in the Healthy Soon Project will maintain prediabetes levels for fasting plasma glucose for 1 year.	Conduct screenings to monitor fasting plasma glucose levels.	Monthly

evaluation when it was all over, so the next time they would feel comfortable taking on their own evaluation studies. Antoinette had her own team of three evaluators who had worked together for five years. She told the group about them and invited members of the community to join the team. Antoinette and her team used the Participatory Model for Evaluation to guide their work.

Before Antoinette's company, Quality Evaluation Inc., took on the task, they developed a scope-of-work document outlining a plan for an evaluation that would be within CAPHO's budget. They wanted to stay within a $50,000 limit. Antoinette knew that would not be a large evaluation, but her evaluators were excited that they would get the chance to do it and to work closely with members of the community. They developed a very modest proposal and planned to keep it small but to make sure that for the first year the questions they would be asking would be, "Was the initiative implemented as planned?" "Was the intended population participating as planned?" They intended to write a grant for funding

TABLE 12.4.   Outcome Objectives and Initiative Activities for Affordable-Produce Goal

Objective	Initiative Activities	Time Frame
Increase to 40% the number of stores that sell affordable produce in low-income neighborhoods by 2019.		
80 percent of local government officials will support the need to increase access to fresh fruits and vegetables in communities by 2017.	Educate policymakers through face-to-face meetings, information brochures, and just-in-time information about the value of having convenience stores sell fresh fruits and vegetables. Build a grassroots coalition to support food security.	Monthly
By 2017 25% more stores will successfully manage fresh produce.	Train store owners in produce management, business management. Provide mentoring for store owners. Provide incentives to offset the cost of the program to store owners. Build programs that encourage purchase of fruits and vegetables— e.g., buy one, get one free; discount coupons.	Ongoing
By 2018 a bill will be passed that provides incentives and other support for carrying fresh foods in convenience stores.	Educate policymakers through face-to-face meetings, information brochures, and just-in-time information.	Monthly
By 2018 a policy will be enacted to reduce the height and number of alcohol-related signs in convenience stores.	Work with store owners to reduce the number and height of advertising for alcohol in local stores.	Weekly

TABLE 12.5. **The Logic-Model Components and Healthy Soon Project Activities**

Logic-Model Component	Healthy Soon Project
Resources (inputs)	▪ $150,000 budget for year 1 ▪ One supervisor and three support staff ▪ Gym facilities ▪ Diabetes screening supplies ▪ Dietician on contract ▪ Farmers
Activities	▪ Nutrition education ▪ Low-calorie/low-fat/high-fiber diet ▪ Glucose monitoring and weigh-ins/food journaling/strength and toning/walking ▪ Farmers' market/fresh fruits and vegetables ▪ Educate policymakers ▪ Enact legislation to reduce advertising for alcohol in convenience stores ▪ Coalition to support access to healthy-foods legislation ▪ Work with store owners to reduce advertising for alcohol ▪ Train store owners in produce and business management ▪ Mentoring for store owners ▪ Incentives to store owners and customers ▪ Community education on risk factors for diabetes
Outputs	▪ African American women participating in nutrition and exercise components ▪ Family members recruited as walking buddies ▪ Farmers participating and providing fruits and vegetables ▪ Farmers' markets ▪ Local store owners trained and fresh-produce sections developed ▪ Satisfaction of store owners, farmers, and project participants ▪ Legal and regulatory frameworks developed ▪ CAPHO/farmers/store owners partnership developed

(Continued)

TABLE 12.5. *(Continued)*

Logic-Model Component	Healthy Soon Project
Expected outcomes (effects)	■ Knowledge of risk factors for diabetes
	■ Increase in the number of stores and other venues that manage and sell fruits and vegetables
	■ Increased consumption of dietician-recommended diets
	■ Exercising for 105 minutes per week
	■ Women maintaining prediabetes levels for fasting glucose
	■ Policy enacted to reduce the level and number of alcohol-related advertisements
	■ Women maintaining healthy weight (BMI > 19 < 27)

the evaluation in subsequent years. They decided to use the first year to develop and test some tools and to collect lots of information to serve as the baseline in addition to conducting the process evaluation. Once the contract was signed, they recruited members of the community to join them. They ended with a team of 10 members. Some of them had participated in the community assessment, so they were clearly motivated to see their project come to fruition.

It was a great team with a lot of enthusiasm. Antoinette and her evaluators attended their first meeting two weeks later, and by asking many questions they found out about the community's concerns. The evaluators tried to understand the fears expressed by the stakeholders and the steps that had been taken to address them.

The purpose of the evaluation was primarily to gain insight into the program's implementation and theory of change, identify any barriers and facilitators to the women's participation, and suggest midterm corrections if necessary. The initiative's theory of change postulated that "if African American women participate in the prescribed nutrition and exercise intervention for a period of 6 weeks and continue the regimen for at least 1 year, they will reduce their risk of getting diabetes." The evaluation would determine whether the program had sufficient intensity to achieve this outcome.

Evaluation Questions

The next step was to use the items from the logic model (Table 12.5) as the framework for stakeholders to think about their questions. As a reminder, Antoinette put the logic model on the wall.

Another member of the group, Kingstee, facilitated the session. The evaluators had two major criteria for identifying questions: they had to clearly state what the stakeholder wanted to know, and they had to link directly to the initiative. The group identified 30 evaluation questions. The program was new, so although they had a combination of process and outcome evaluation questions, they focused on understanding whether the program was

FIGURE 12.2.   *Two-by-Two Table*

Ability to provide understanding of the critical components of program implementation

	High	Low
High	• Were all the components of the plan implemented? • What is the level of implementation of the women's nutrition and exercise initiatives? • What activities have taken place to support the policy to reduce advertisements for alcohol? • What is the knowledge of diabetes risk factors among women who participate in the initiative?	• What human, financial, and material resources were provided and used?
Low	• What educational activities were carried out?	• What activities have taken place to develop the farmers' market?

Ability to contribute to decision-making

being implemented appropriately. Kingstee used the nominal technique to narrow them down to seven and then used a two-by-two table (Figure 12.2) to determine which ones the group considered the most important.

These were the seven questions the group identified:

1. What human, financial, and material resources were provided and used?

2. What educational activities were carried out?

3. Were all the components of the plan implemented?

4. What is the level of implementation of the women's nutrition and exercise initiatives?

5. What activities have taken place to develop the farmers' market?

6. What activities have taken place to support the policy to reduce advertisements for alcohol?

7. What is the knowledge of diabetes risk factors among women who participated in the initiative?

The evaluation team wanted answers to two additional questions:

1. Are the data-collection tools appropriate for assessing program outcomes?

2. Do preliminary findings indicate that the intervention is likely to produce the anticipated outcomes?

As a result of this exercise, the evaluation team focused on the five questions in the top part of the 2x2 table. All five questions had the ability to contribute to decision-making. The questions in the top left quadrant were also considered important for understanding the critical components of the program's implementation. Although the other questions were important, the team had a limited budget, so they had to identify the most important questions, the ones that were critical to the theory of change.

Because the evaluation started early in the program's development, the appropriate type of evaluation would be a formative evaluation, that appears to also be the focus of stakeholders' concerns. Process-evaluation questions are similar to formative-evaluation questions. The difference is that process evaluation is used when the program is more stable than it is when it is being developed, which is when formative evaluation is appropriate. The questions were sorted into formative and outcome questions (Table 12.6) so everybody would be clear about what was being done and to help members of the team learn about evaluation.

Formative and process evaluations assess the context, the reach, the dosage, or the intensity of the initiative and the fidelity with which it is delivered. They assess the initiative at the level of resources/inputs and outputs and determine the effectiveness of the administrative functions of the program. Process and outcome evaluations confirm the theory of change in mature programs. Quality monitoring continues throughout the project.

Indicators and Data Sources

The next task for the team was to develop the indicator table to show what measures would be required (Table 12.7).

TABLE 12.6. Evaluation Question

Were all the components of the plan implemented?

Formative	Outcome
Were all the components of the plan implemented?	What is the knowledge of diabetes risk factors among women who participated in the initiative?
What is the level of implementation of the women's nutrition and exercise initiatives?	
What activities have taken place to support the policy to reduce advertisements for alcohol?	
What human, financial, and material resources were provided and used?	

TABLE 12.7. Indicators and Data Sources

Evaluation Question	Indicator	Source of Data
What human, financial, and material resources were provided and used?	Program in place Personnel hired Space utilized Laboratory invoices ($) Purchase receipt ($)	Record review Audit Attendance records Meeting minutes Database review Interview with accounting staff Observation
What is the knowledge of diabetes risk factors among women who participate in the initiative?	Percentage increase in number of people with knowledge of diabetes	Survey

Ensuring the Quality of the Evaluation

The Quality Evaluation Inc. team discussed the overall research design to assess whether they would be able to determine that the intervention had made a difference. They went back to the project documents and saw that the Healthy Soon intervention would last for six weeks and then the women would be expected to continue exercising on their own and follow the diet plan. They would continue having their weigh-ins and screenings and completing their journals for a year. Therefore, the design they would use to determine the effect of the program was a pre/post quasi-experimental design with a second post-test one year after the women had completed the initial six-week intervention. They were delighted that they had been called into the initiative early enough to collect baseline data and to make sure there was sufficient documentation of the activities. They could then be confident that the intervention had caused the changes they were observing.

CAPHO advertised the program using flyers, announcements in local churches, at day-care centers, and so forth; they had women register to participate in the Healthy Soon Project. After three weeks, they randomly assigned 50 people from the list to be in the intervention group. Another 50 were randomly assigned to be in the control group. The evaluation team was trying to avoid a biased sample. When they compared the two groups later, they found that they were similar, so they had been successful in having comparable groups even though they had started out with women volunteering to participate. Those who volunteer though are not always comparable to those who don't so being able to extrapolate the results beyond this group would be unlikely.

Because the women in the control group had the same risk factors for diabetes, the program wanted to compensate them for their time. In addition, they wanted to help them reduce their risk of diabetes by offering them a reduced intervention. The control group got (a) a single one-hour lecture on diabetes, screening tests, a six-month weigh-in, and they were asked to complete a journal recording any exercise they took and their daily meals; and (b) a free membership to the gym in the second year. Both groups got transportation vouchers whenever they came in for screening.

The evaluators had to also make sure they minimized the threats to internal validity. See Table 12.8 for the steps they took.

COLLECT THE DATA

The evaluation team spent some time discussing how they would use their time profitably to collect all the information they needed. To facilitate the training of team members, each established member of Quality Evaluations Inc. mentored two new members. Mentoring required them working closely with their mentees and teaching them what they were doing. Mentees had to do more than observe; they had books to read and worksheets to complete. By completing the worksheets together, the team knew what information they would need to gather and how they would do it.

The next task was to develop the tools for data collection. For example, the team needed to develop databases so all the information with regard to expenditure and participation were entered. They also wanted to be able to keep a running tally of e-mails that went out to coalition members. Tools had to be developed in this way for each of the indicators.

The team provided training to all the staff so they understood the importance of data collection and how to complete all the tools. Training was provided on how to enter data in the database. The database would be used to track everything: the women's participation, their laboratory results, their weights, and the intensity of their exercise. The database would be useful for answering the second question that the team had: "Do preliminary findings indicate that the intervention is likely to produce the anticipated outcomes?"

Tools developed for ongoing monitoring included:

- A site-visit report
- Journal entries
- An attendance sheet
- A record review sheet

In addition to completing the process evaluation and developing tools for ongoing monitoring, the evaluation team developed some additional materials that they would use as part of the outcome evaluation. One was an interview and the other was a pre/post-test survey.

Site-Visit Report

The site-visit report gathered information about the program components and their level of implementation (Table 12.9). Data was collected throughout the six-week intervention.

TABLE 12.8.   **Addressing Threats to Internal Validity**

Threat to Validity	Actions of the Evaluation Team
Attrition: The loss of participants in the intervention	Participants were told the importance of their participation and encouraged to participate. Incentives were used during and following their successful completion of the 6-week and 1-year evaluations.
History: Events that take place outside the intervention	Participants were asked to include information in their journals about anything they did or heard that was different from the intervention and that would likely change the nature of the intervention for some people and not for others.
Instrumentation: Changes that occur to the reliability and validity of measurement tools	The evaluation team ensured that all the data-collection instruments were reliable and valid.
Maturation: Changes in the study participants caused by natural and physiological changes	The women who participated in this intervention grew older and more experienced during the year they participated in the intervention. These changes occurred in all participants at different levels.
Regression: The study participants are selected on the basis of high or low baseline scores	The team ensured high reliability in testing and that no individual's scores were much higher or much lower than the population mean scores.
Selection: Differences in the study population between the intervention and the control group	The team randomly selected groups for both the intervention and the control groups to ensure their equivalence. In addition, they compared the groups using statistical tests to determine that they were in fact similar.
Statistical-Conclusion Validity: The sample size is too small to show the effect	The sample size was sufficiently large to reduce the threat. Evaluators ensured that their instruments were reliable to reduce errors in measurement. They ensured the standard delivery of the intervention to all participants. The journal entries and staff logs helped track these precautions.
Testing: Changes that occur to participants as a result of the number of times they are tested	Results of the baseline tests were not released to participants. In addition, although the same questions were used in the posttest, the order of the responses were changed.

TABLE 12.9.   Sample Site-Visit Report

Date: _____ Person Conducting the Visit: _____			
Name of Component	Fully Implemented (Y/N)	Participants Registered (Y/N)	Status/Comments

In addition to determining if the component was fully implemented according to previously agreed upon standards, participants registered and any comments were recorded.

Journal Entries

Journal entries were based on a template provided by the evaluation team. The items for the journal entries were

■   Number of minutes on exercise equipment per day

■   Number of minutes walking with peer per day

■   Number of calories consumed per day

■   Food intake per day—quantity and type

■   Use of problem-solving skills to control food intake and to exercise regularly

Attendance Sheet

The attendance sheet (Table 12.10) was used to gather information about participants in all the community-based events both on- and off-site. It was a record of the number of people who attended the events, and it provided a list of people who could be contacted for future evaluations. In addition, the list could be used to provide a database for promoting the initiative's activities and for distributing the community survey. The addresses of the participants provided information about the reach of the program over time.

Record Review Sheet

The record review sheet records recommendations and actions related to the initiative components from board and committee meetings. It includes the date of the review, the title/name of the document, the date of the document, and a summary of the document.

Staff and Participant Interviews

Staff and participant interviews were conducted annually. The first occurred six months after the initiative started. The intent was to understand the programs that were being offered

TABLE 12.10. **Sample Attendance Sheet**

Name of Session: _____

Date: _____

Location: _____

Name	Mailing Address, Zip	Telephone Number	Email Address	Comments
Janet Hairington	334 Wilsden Avenue, 40241	358-648-1285	harrj@yahoo.com	
Koujdo Boateng	204 Cresthill Plains, 40222	301-253-6447	k.boat@gmail.com	

and to elicit recommendations for the annual report. Staff and program participants were interviewed for approximately 60 minutes. The following questions were asked:

- What role do you play in the organization?

- What programs does the Healthy Soon Project offer?

- Who is being served by the program?

- What experiences most represent your feelings about this initiative?

- What do you value most about the program?

- What are the programs processes and successes so far?

- What three things do you especially wish for the program?

- What recommendations do you have for reducing the rate of diabetes among members of this community?

For program participants, an additional question was, "Think back to the past 6 months and being in this program. Tell a story about your experience."

The data from the interviews were analyzed to identify themes using theoretical and empirical constructs embedded in the interview guide used for data collection. The qualitative software package NVivo® was used to code the qualitative-data transcripts.

Survey

In order to determine whether the intervention had made a difference to the women participating, they were compared with the women who were in the control group. A variety of data were collected. To assess the long-term outcome of the initiative—to increase the proportion of African American women who participate in the intervention who are at a healthy weight to 60% by 2022—the evaluators used laboratory tests, surveys, in-depth interviews, and journal reviews to assess knowledge, attitudes, and behavior with regard to diabetes and its prevention at baseline, after the first six weeks, and again one year later.

Among other items, the surveys assessed

- Demographics (age, income, education level, family size, residence, zip code)

- Knowledge of diabetes

- Knowledge of risk factor for diabetes

- Knowledge of the value of physical activity in preventing diabetes

- Knowledge of the value of good nutrition in preventing diabetes

- Attitudes toward getting diabetes

- Perceptions of alcohol advertising in convenience stores

- Levels of physical activity

- Consumption of fruits and vegetables as part of a meal

- Use of convenience stores

- Use of farmers' markets

A 50-item survey was developed from specifically made-up items and previously developed items. The compiled survey was reviewed by all the members of the evaluation team and then sent out to four independent reviewers for their expert opinion. It was reviewed by the Institutional Review Board and pilot-tested with a sample of 30 African American women.

The final survey was distributed as part of the project registration to serve as the baseline and again one year later for the intervention and the control groups. Women in both the intervention and the control groups were asked to complete the survey. All surveys were completed in an average of 20 minutes.

Three statements were included in the survey. The statements "Regular exercise helps to prevent diabetes," and "Good nutrition helps to prevent diabetes" were responded to on a 5-point scale from "strongly disagree" to "strongly agree." The statement "It is okay for people to get diabetes" had a dichotomous yes/no response.

ANALYZE AND INTERPRET THE DATA

Once all the data from the site visits and the survey were collected and collated, the team was ready to answer a couple of the evaluation questions. Quality Evaluation Inc. conducted a site visit to determine the status of the project components two weeks after the start of the initiative. The survey data was collected at baseline from both the intervention and the control groups. It is these two reports that are presented here.

Site Visit

The women in the intervention group had completed a baseline assessment; they were attending the prescribed number of sessions at the fully equipped gym; and they had their initial meeting with the dietician. In addition, participants were expected to recruit a relative or friend to walk with them every evening. Each participant had completed the initial screening tests and was required to complete a journal. The baseline data and the screening tests were also completed for the control group. The records kept by the organization indicated that 50 African American women were enrolled in the study and another 50 were enrolled into the control group. The numbers stayed high for the first six weeks.

Work toward developing the alcohol-advertising legislation had started with a review of existing laws and the development of the legal and regulatory framework. An advocacy coalition had formed that brought together a group of 10 advocates. Farmers had been contacted to develop the farmers' market. The site was being located, and permits were being obtained. A training was being planned and scheduled for the convenience store owners who had agreed to participate in the project, and monthly meetings were held to facilitate the development of the convenience store initiative.

The site visit was conducted by two independent teams from Quality Evaluations Inc., using a protocol with predefined terms and categories for assessment. Each team consisted of an experienced evaluator and a member of the community. The results of each assessment were compared, comments were compiled, and discrepancies were resolved against standards that had been determined previously. For example, the standard for "fully implemented" had been previously defined by the team as being implemented exactly as defined by the protocol. Standards were defined in consultation with the CAPHO executive director because slight changes had been made since the original plans had been written. Table 12.11 is the site-visit report completed by one of the evaluation teams.

Survey

There were 50 participants in the intervention group and 50 in the control group when they completed the survey at baseline. Their ages were comparable, with a mean age of 46.9 years, and the educational level of both groups was a mean of 8.6 years. A few had completed high school (10%), and none had gone to college. They worked in the service industry and many traveled to the nearby beaches to work. The intervention group lived in one of two zip code areas with the highest poverty level in the county, and the control group lived in the other. The average income of the intervention group was $6,900 per year, and the average income for the control group was $ 7,240. The difference was not statistically significant. They were separated by the River Rokel, which is 6 miles wide. Most (75 percent) had children between the ages of 6 and 18 years living at home.

Women in both the intervention and the control groups were given journals to complete at baseline. Two weeks into the project, journals were being completed as prescribed by the intervention group. The initial assessment was that the journals were being completed daily. Individual interviews with staff revealed that the intervention was being implemented as described in the protocols.

Only 15% of the intervention group and 16% of the control group was at a healthy weight, and all met the criteria for prediabetes with marginally high blood glucose levels. Only 15% exercised for approximately 30 minutes per week.

The mean scores for knowledge of the value of physical activity in preventing diabetes was 2.86 for the intervention group and 3.06 for the control group. For the question about knowledge of the value of nutrition in preventing diabetes, the mean score for the intervention group was 2.96, whereas the mean score for the control group was 3.02 (Table 12.12). Neither of the differences in scores was significant.

TABLE 12.11.   **Site-Visit Report at 2 Weeks**

Name of Component	Fully Implemented (Y/N)	Participants Registered (Y/N)	Status/Comments
Physical activity in gym	Y	Y	Gym equipped, open daily for 8 hours, staffed by two certified trainers, 50 participants in each group registered, baseline measures taken; journal entries.
Nutrition	Y	Y	Dietician hired, available 20 hours per week, session length of 1 hour, 50 participants in each group registered, baseline measures taken; journal entries.
Walking with peers	Y	Y	All intervention participants paired; journal entries.
Legal and regulatory framework developed	N		Existing laws reviewed, coalition formed, meetings held quarterly with legislators, monthly newsletter.
Farmers' markets	N		Farmers contacted, establishing schedule, site located.
Convenience store initiative	N		Monthly meetings scheduled, minutes taken, trainer identified, training scheduled.
CAPHO/farmers/store owners partnership developed	N		Monthly meetings scheduled, minutes taken.

TABLE 12.12.   **Intervention Group and Control Group at Baseline on Knowledge About Physical Activity and Nutrition**

Item	Intervention Group (mean)	Control Group (mean)	Significance
Physical activity	2.86	3.06	0.619
Nutrition	2.96	3.02	0.633

TABLE 12.13. **Intervention Group and Control Group at Baseline on Attitude Toward Diabetes**

Response Category	Intervention Group (%)	Control Group (%)
Yes	18 (36)	17 (34)
No	32 (64)	33 (66)
Total	50 (100)	50 (100)

When participants were asked about their attitude toward diabetes, 36% of the intervention group said it was okay for people to get diabetes, whereas in the control group 34% said it was okay (Table 12.13). These data are comparable.

Interpretation

The data showed that the critical components of the initiative were fully implemented and less critical components were not yet implemented in the first month of the initiative. For instance, the six-week exercise/nutrition initiative was fully staffed, participants were recruited for both the intervention group and the control group, and appropriate measurements were being taken. The baseline data revealed no significant difference between the intervention and the control groups. However, approximately a third of individuals in both the intervention group (36%) and the control group (34%) reported not being concerned about getting diabetes, a finding that suggests considerable effort must be devoted to the educational component.

The farmers' market and the convenience store initiatives had not yet been implemented. Meetings had begun among the constituencies, and a coordinator had been named, ensuring that the remaining components were being developed.

The initial study conducted by Quality Evaluation Inc. was to determine whether the preliminary findings indicated that the intervention was likely to produce the anticipated outcomes. Although the study was conducted too early to provide a definitive answer with regard to the outcome, the critical components were in place and the protocols were being followed. The initial samples indicated that the target population group was registered to participate, and baseline laboratory readings suggested, based on evidence from existing research, that the anticipated outcome of a healthy weight could be attained. The team expected they would be able to demonstrate the value of the intervention to the community in lower rates of diabetes risk factors and indicators among those who participated compared to the control group, and to replicate the project to reach many more women in the succeeding years. They expected that in the years to come they would reduce the incidence of diabetes as well.

REPORT THE RESULTS

Quality Evaluation Inc. knew that the executive director and the staff would be interested in knowing how they were doing and wanted to provide feedback to the evaluation team. In consultation with the executive director and the staff, they decided that for this first report they would have 45 minutes of the regular monthly staff meeting to present their findings. The reporting was evenly divided between the original members of the team and the stakeholders who had joined the team. It was an exciting time for them because it was their first evaluation. The team developed a short report and some table and charts; they gave an oral presentation from a set of PowerPoint slides and answered questions. After the presentation, they discussed the evaluation team's findings and next steps. The evaluation team completed the report with the feedback they received and sent the executive director a copy for her records.

During the meeting, three recommendations were added to the list the evaluation team already had. They were all adopted immediately. The most critical was to make sure sufficient educational materials were available for the women. Antoinette had recently found out about a set of materials about prediabetes, so they decided it would be a worthwhile purchase for the organization. Women in the intervention group were provided the additional materials. The other recommendations were ensuring that the farmers'-market and convenience-store components were fully implemented.

An analysis of the evaluation process showed that the team had been able to complete the tasks it had outlined; and they were satisfied they would be able to draw defensible conclusions about the Healthy Soon Project once the intervention was over. They made periodic checks to be sure the data were being collected and to provide any technical assistance that was needed. The team analyzed the data from the intervention and the control groups and provided appropriate reports of the findings. At the end of the first year of the intervention, it was clear that women who had participated in the intervention were able to maintain their healthy eating and physical activity levels. Their relatives and friends seemed also to be benefiting and many had lost weight and felt healthier. The additional components of the intervention seemed to give the women an added advantage over the women in the control group. Once the evaluation was able to demonstrate that the intervention worked with four successive cohorts over a one-year period, the intervention was offered to anybody who came to the program. Successive cohorts of women who participated were also successful. Each year the evaluation team reported any findings from the ongoing data collection and in 2019 reported on the program environmental objective. In 2022 the team reported on the program health objective.

Program Health Objective
Increase the percentage of African American women who participate in the intervention who are at a healthy weight to 60 percent by 2022.

Program Environmental Objective
Increase to 40 percent the number of stores and other venues that sell affordable produce in low-income neighborhoods by 2019.

The evaluation team, Quality Evaluation Inc., reported an increase in the number of stores and other venues that sold affordable produce in low income neighborhoods in 2019 to 48%; and in 2022 that 72% of women who had participated in the initiative were at a healthy weight. The Healthy Soon Project lived up to its name and increased significantly the number of women who were healthy; and contributed to the 10% reduction in the number of individuals who became diabetic across the county compared to previous years.

Through a foundation grant to expand the program, Antoinette's team was able to continue to provide evaluation services to the organization.

DISCUSSION QUESTIONS AND ACTIVITIES

1. Selecting from any of the expected outcomes of the case study, design an evaluation.

2. Consider a program you would like to evaluate. Design a contract that would protect both the evaluator as well as the contractor. What would you include in the contract? What will you need to negotiate?

3. You have been invited to join an evaluation team that is already well established, but you bring a boat load of skills to the team. Don't be modest! In a reflective paper describe your skills and how you will bring them to bear on the evaluation team and the evaluation process itself.

CHAPTER

13

CASE STUDY

PROCESS EVALUATION

The names and data used in this case study do not refer to any existing places, persons, or situations.

Introduction: This case study focuses on process evaluation. It does not represent an example of a specific situation but uses various illustrations to provide the reader with an understanding of some of the thinking that might go into a process evaluation since an evaluation of this kind is unique to each initiative.

Process evaluation, as with all other evaluations, first requires an undertaking of the justification for the intervention and a clear description of the program or policy. The justification is provided by the community assessment and the literature review while the description of the program or policy comes primarily from the stakeholders as described in a previous chapter.

BACKGROUND

This small rural population of 50,000 had experienced very heavy rains and most recently had been through one of the worse hurricanes it had seen in 100 years. Those who were able to leave had left, and 10 years later the community was fractured. Leighster County was devoid of services. As a result, there had been a significant drop in economic fortunes and the young adults had few resources and had developed many negative health behaviors such as smoking and drinking. The mayor who had recently been elected wanted to turn this around and hoped she could bring the community back to its former glory.

She was especially keen to understand how the youth could be helped as she viewed them as the future leaders of the community but recognized they were struggling with many different issues. The mayor set up a community advisory team. It was made up of the mayor, two council members, two faith leaders, four youth, and four members of the business community. She recognized that the team had never worked together and they would need orientation and possibly even training. She also recognized that, over time, the team might change and new members would have to be brought on board. This would be particularly important if the findings required the team to implement projects for which they required expertise on the team.

As the advisory team started they commissioned a community assessment through an evaluation consultancy firm and gave them a contract to assess the extent of the problems. The contract was for nine months and they expected by the end of it to have a full report although they wanted the evaluation firm to report periodically and provide updates to the advisory team. The team consisted of five people with expertise in different areas, but particularly research using mixed methods. They would have to conduct surveys as well as do a few focus group and individual interviews to really understand what was going on in this small but progressive town. The advisory team wanted to be helpful and volunteered their services to support the evaluation. As a result they were given a few roles like participating in conceptualizing the evaluation, coming up with specific questions they wanted to have answered, and helping the evaluation firm validate and interpret their results at the end. Due to the potential for conflict of interest, the advisory team was not asked to participate in any of the data-collection tasks such as recruiting respondents or collecting and analyzing data. The evaluation firm was also careful to protect the confidentiality of the townsfolk.

THEORETICAL FRAMEWORK

Since it was clear that the intervention would have to be comprehensive and address multiple needs, the ecological model was used as the theoretical framework with the social cognitive theory (SCT) and the health-belief model (HBM) overlaid on it to be able to provide some direction at the end of the study (see Figure 13.1).

Taking into consideration the social and environmental factors that influence health allowed the research team to incorporate in its analysis individual, social, and environmental factors. This assessment incorporated constructs from SCT and the HBM. In using the ecological model with the additionally overlaid theories, it allowed the team to make recommendations across a broad spectrum of needs. This study provides data at the individual, interpersonal, community, and policy levels, which will help guide a comprehensive approach to program development. The HBM allowed the team to understand the health threats from consuming drugs and alcohol and the levels of stress that had been reported anecdotally. Stress was being experienced by both the youth and adults. They also needed to think in terms of what barriers were being experienced by the community and the benefits they would perceive as helpful if the negative behaviors were addressed. Another aspect of using the HBM was understanding the extent to which people would feel confident in making the required changes to improve their health. The team wanted to know how to design programs and media interventions in the future that would help stimulate positive behaviors.

FIGURE 13.1. *Model of the Ecological Model interacting With the Health-belief Model and the Social Cognitive Theory*

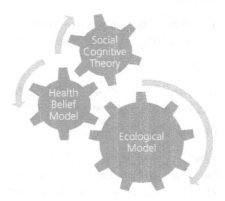

In integrating the constructs of the SCT, the team was interested in assessing some of the community level factors that might be influencing the members of this community in addition to some of the individual level factors. The SCT takes into consideration individual (cognitive, affective, and biological) factors, the behavior itself, and the environment in a dynamic reciprocal model of interaction. It considers the environment and social systems that influence behavior and especially considers how self-reflection, vicarious learning, and self-efficacy could be useful for intervening. Although they did not adopt the full theory, the researcher included social norms as a construct from the theory of planned behavior. They developed a set of instruments combining previously used and validated questions and new questions that met their needs. Since they did not have much time, they did not want to collect more data than was absolutely necessary so they spent some time reviewing questions and selecting those that would be more useful. A pool of experts familiar with the community and conducting community assessments reviewed the final instrument, which was seven pages long and took about 30 minutes to complete. Following that review, the instrument was pilot tested with a small group of adults and young people. Once that was done, the instrument was ready to use. They would validate it for their population later.

COMMUNITY ASSESSMENT FINDINGS

Indeed, and as they had anticipated, the youth (ages 15–18) were the group most affected by the events of the previous years. Since large segments of the population left during the devastating hurricane the educational system had broken down, schools and colleges had closed and the youth found more pleasure in smoking and drinking and other socially deviant behavior than getting an education in a system that was weak and had few resources. Mental health issues were evident among both adults and children and the adults were unable to help their children. The results of the community assessment that were significant and, therefore, would likely form the basis for the first set of interventions were put into a table so the community advisory team had a quick and easy reference. (Table 13.1)

TABLE 13.1.   **Summary of Community Assessment Results**

Variable Measured	Findings
Population of Leighster County	50,000 made up of Caucasians (80%); Hispanics (10%), African Americans (5%) and other groups (5%).
Total sample size	3,000
Sample	15–18; 19–30; 31–40; 41–50; 51–60; 61 and over with each population group sampled
Ages most affected	15–18 years (sample size = 500)
Educational attainment	30% were still in school (grades 9–11); 60% had just completed high school and had high school diplomas; 5% had planned to take GEDs after they dropped out of school in the 11th grade; and 5% had not completed high school or had a GED. 40% of the graduates planned to attend community college and get an Associate's degree and 10% planned to attend the State University.
Role models	Music artists, teachers, and other adults. Most of the role models were seen on a variety of TV reality shows or movies.
Smoking	35% had initiated smoking at 15 years and 5% had smoked illegal substances; 20% were ongoing smokers.
Underage drinking	60% had a least one alcoholic beverage a week; 10% binged.
Unintended injuries	20% reported being involved in a car accident with a friend driving.
Depression	The number of youth and adults who reported feeling stressed or suicidal had increased slightly over the past 10 years. Mental health care had been sought more often (60% reported having seen a psychologist in the past year).
Suicide	Suicide rates were still lower than the national average, but troubling none the less as over time there appeared to be a slight trend upward (7% higher than figures for the previous year). There seemed to be a growing incidence among male youth. 30% of youth reported that their parents sought help from a mental health counselor at least once in the previous year.
Schools and Colleges	There was one community college nearby that most high school graduates attended. Those with degrees from four-year colleges had gone to the State University about three hours north of the town. Most who had left to go to University had not returned.

TABLE 13.1.   (*Continued*)

Variable Measured	Findings
Community support for change	Most of the respondents perceived their situation and health as poor or fair. 60% of the community reported being very supportive of changes to laws and policies that would help make their children safe; 30% were supportive; 10% were neutral.
Policies	Local policies about alcohol sales to minors and driving under the influence of alcohol had not been updated in recent years and did not reflect changes that had been made elsewhere. Law enforcement was also weak.

The community assessment pointed the way. It was clear that any intervention would have to include multiple domains of influence. At the individual level, there needed to be interventions for the youth; their parents needed to provide support but they too needed help; organizations needed to play an important role and the community needed to improve access to services. There were important community, organizational, and policy supports that would be needed.

The community advisory team quickly morphed into the Mayor's Intervention Planning Team (MIPT) but added new members who had expertise in program and policy planning and implementation. Many had a Master's in Public Health or had worked in related fields for many years. Many had taken the CPH exam also. Once the team was assembled and had asked questions about the data and understood all the issues they would have to address, they decided to narrow the scope of the first project, but wanted to make sure they addressed at least three of the domains. They felt they had taken a responsible decision and were more likely to be successful if they addressed individual level and environmental factors that influenced the ability of individuals to adopt healthy behaviors but for the first three years not try to tackle any major policy changes. They knew they were more likely to be successful if they had a comprehensive intervention and encouraged the Bar Association to consider taking that on.

In the process of considering all their options, MIPT invited the evaluation firm to join them. This was a great idea since the evaluators would help ensure that, in addition to the community-assessment data, they used data from work other researchers and practitioners had done to help in their decision-making process. They needed much more information and understanding about the needs than the single community assessment had determined now they were getting down to project planning. They wanted to be sure that the interventions were evidence based. They did an extensive literature review. As the group worked, the evaluators created a working logic model to help them understand how the concept was developing and how all the pieces fitted together. During the planning phase, the evaluator pushed them to think about the assumptions they were making about the intervention and especially about the likelihood of achieving the objectives they identified. They considered the social, cultural, and political factors that could undermine the intervention and identified possible solutions. This additional thinking ensured the likely sustainability of the project.

Planning the Intervention

The team had to make sure they had spent some time considering what the intervention would be and were careful to document everything they did, so the evaluation process would be smooth. The problem they decided to address first was the high rate of alcohol and drug use among the youth (15–18 years). The team knew that with a problem like that, which was influenced by many factors at the individual, interpersonal, community, organizational, and public policy levels, they would also be impacting other important aspects of youth growth and development. They were committed to making a difference and had the support of large sectors of the community including parent organizations, the legal system, schools, and the medical community. This was a problem that impacted many sectors of the society. The group had to consider what it meant for youth to be addicted to drugs and alcohol and the impact that had on society. They had to reconsider the World Health Organization's definition of health as "a complete state of physical, mental and social well-being, and not merely the absence of disease or infirmity" and what that meant for the youth, but also the community as a whole. They had to think about the families but also the impact their behavior had on the larger community. They looked up more and more information as questions came up and as they moved from considering an entirely treatment model to one with a focus on prevention, a public health model albeit with a clinical component to ensure that youth who were addicted to drugs and/or alcohol get appropriate and adequate treatment instead of ending up in the justice system.

As they talked, they realized what it all meant and the team was expanded to reflect the resources they needed to oversee a comprehensive program. The planning team in this small rural community of Leighster brought on board stakeholders who could address many of the issues they identified with a goal of "Improving the quality of life of youth 15–18 years." The team summarized the project in a logic model to help them keep track of their ideas and how the program parts would hang together to create a cohesive intervention. They also had to be sure that they documented all the information that would be helpful for the evaluation. The evaluation team kept pushing them to provide a planning document that was clear and comprehensive and that the level of detail would be sufficient to create an understanding of the various elements and the relationship between them. They needed to be sure the intervention had a complete and sound logic and addressed the contextual factors that might affect implementation. They did an inventory of resources in the community and developed a directory of services and programs.

The MIPT also quickly realized that the initiative was far more complex and much bigger than a few members of a planning team could take on and decided on a process of including organizations that were already set up, but maybe needed some additional resources to expand their services and to be more coordinated so they also limited the waste of resources from duplication. The mayor put out requests for proposals (RFPs) describing the vision, goals, and objectives of the initiative to encourage participation from different sectors. Proposals to undertake projects in all the major areas were received. The committee reviewed proposals for innovative programs for teens addressing drug and alcohol use as well as proposals for improving school performance. It was especially heartening that many had discussed the need for a comprehensive approach and to consider the social determinants of health as the basis for considering their interventions. The committee decided to form a coalition to ensure that the work of the different groups was coordinated, so all the organizations that were accepted and funded under the initiative were required to participate in a coalition with a single set of objectives and the opportunity to share resources with referral systems across projects to ensure access to a continuum of services. This was an innovative way to think about bringing many groups together to achieve a single goal. It made total sense. It also made things easier for the evaluation team.

Think About It!

A coalition was formed with all the funded organizations under one umbrella coalition to ensure coordination of the initiative and a continuum of services for youth in the community. Why do you think this would have made things easier for the evaluation team? What strategies would you adopt to ensure coordination and collaboration for purposes of evaluating this initiative?

The Initiative

Once the groups came together to discuss next steps, the MIPT reviewed the objectives they had sent out in the RFP and made some adjustments. A few were tweaked but overall they wanted to have a reasonable number of objectives that would form the basis of their common work. Taking into consideration the level of resources of the community, their primary concerns and from the results of the Community Assessment, the team framed the following objectives.

1. By the end of the 3-year initiative, the youth would report a 50 percent reduction in alcohol and drug use by youth 15–18.

2. By the end of the 3-year initiative, there would be a 40 percent reduction in the incidence of unintentional injury.

3. Schools will report a 95% graduation rate at the end of each academic year after the first year of the initiative.

4. Five years after the start of the intervention, there would be a 50% reduction in stress levels and suicide among youth 15–18.

In order to achieve these objectives, the partners implemented a series of activities that would address the major problems at multiple levels. The committee decided on a range of interventions that specified changes at different levels of influence (Table 13.2).

In addition, the committee aided by the evaluation team drew a logic model (Figure 13.2) of the overall program recognizing they did it at a high level and it did not contain the detail that would be required for a work plan. It served the purpose for this stage in their planning. Since the evaluation team was a part of the project early on, and all members of the team were well connected in the community, they did not anticipate having any difficulties working with the individual organizations to develop a logic model that provided more detail and their work plan. They would be in contact with the organizations that were funded through the RFP mechanism.

TABLE 13.2. Interventions of the Leighster County Youth Initiative and Equivalent Levels of Influence

Initiative Component	Level(s) of Influence Targeted
Coalition building	Organizational and community
Drug and alcohol prevention programs	Individual and interpersonal
Stress management interventions	Individual and interpersonal
Safe driving for teens intervention	Individual, community, and public policy
School-based interventions to improve academic performance	Individual and organizational

FIGURE 13.2. Leighster County Intervention Logic Model

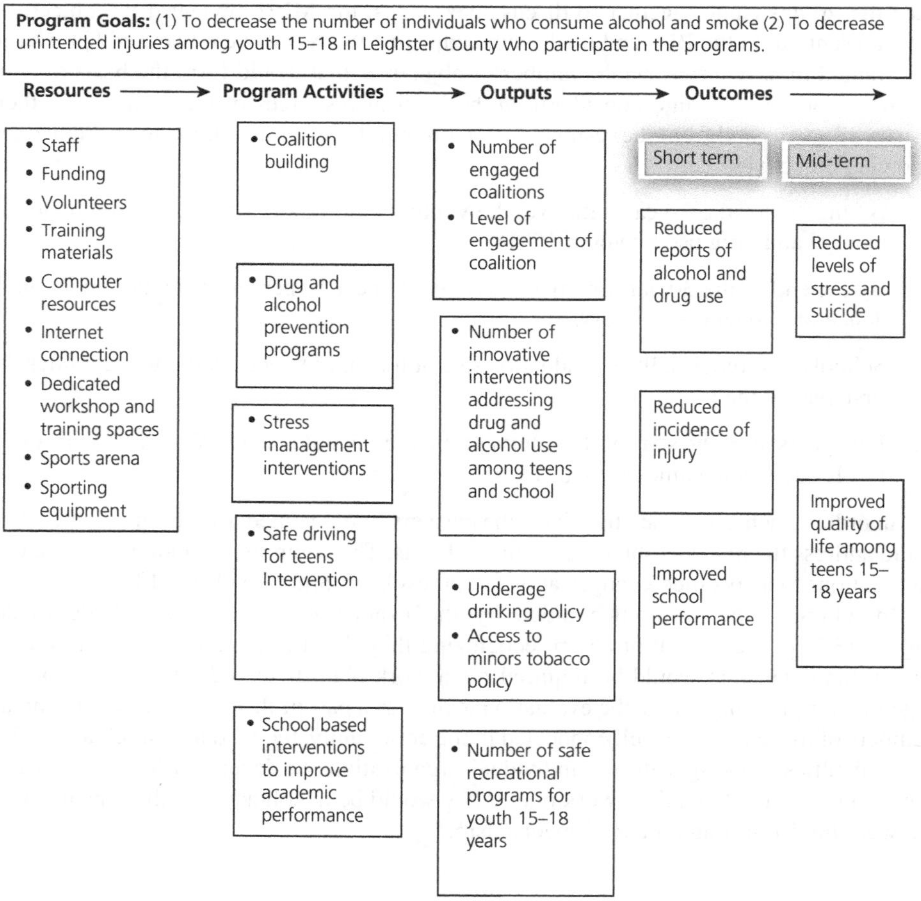

Program Goals: (1) To decrease the number of individuals who consume alcohol and smoke (2) To decrease unintended injuries among youth 15–18 in Leighster County who participate in the programs.

Resources → Program Activities → Outputs → Outcomes →

Resources: Staff, Funding, Volunteers, Training materials, Computer resources, Internet connection, Dedicated workshop and training spaces, Sports arena, Sporting equipment

Program Activities: Coalition building; Drug and alcohol prevention programs; Stress management interventions; Safe driving for teens Intervention; School based interventions to improve academic performance

Outputs: Number of engaged coalitions; Level of engagement of coalition; Number of innovative interventions addressing drug and alcohol use among teens and school; Underage drinking policy; Access to minors tobacco policy; Number of safe recreational programs for youth 15–18 years

Outcomes (Short term): Reduced reports of alcohol and drug use; Reduced incidence of injury; Improved school performance. (Mid-term): Reduced levels of stress and suicide; Improved quality of life among teens 15–18 years

The interventions would require significant resources, among them staff, funding, volunteers, training materials, and dedicated spaces, as well as sports arenas and sporting equipment. The evaluation team would monitor the level of resources, the outputs from the programs, the level of participation of youth and especially those defined as "high risk," those who were in danger of not completing high school.

The Evaluation Team

The initial contract with the evaluation team was to conduct a process evaluation and answering short-term outcome questions when that was appropriate but not getting bogged down with an outcome evaluation until later. They did want to make sure that they had the data for an outcome evaluation later, so the discussion of the need for an outcome evaluation formed part of the contract negotiation and the evaluation team knew to ensure that as they conducted the process evaluation they would also ensure that the data management systems were well established. To be sure that their interventions had an impact on the community, they would collect baseline data if the community assessment data was not sufficient, but they would also identify a similar community they could use as a comparison to increase their confidence in their conclusions about the impact of the mayor's initiative on Leighster County. They knew they had to be careful in selecting the community as well as in monitoring the events in the comparison community since mayors change and communities change based on different stimuli. They had to be sure that any changes were well understood and documented. They had to consider the threats to validity.

Since the focus of the work of the evaluation team would be the process evaluation, the team would provide technical assistance to each of the organizations to ensure they had the data they required to answer the evaluation questions, but more importantly that the organizations continually monitored their projects and made changes that were required quickly so they could be sure that they would achieve their stated outcomes. They had to become learning organizations and ones that responded quickly to changes in participation, personnel, and environmental conditions. Continual monitoring was important to ensure that the intervention was being implemented as intended, resources were provided in a timely manner, and quality control was maintained.

Within the coalition, the relationships between organizations varied from loose relationships, which resulted in only networking opportunities and information sharing, to more established partnerships with written agreements. Those that had mostly networking relationships tended to have different primary missions. Those that formed partnerships were those that had common primary missions and were more likely to have resources that could be shared. For example, the partnerships between the organizations that provided alcohol and drug interventions were stronger with defined areas of work, referring to each other and removing many of the barriers to services that previously existed. Full collaboration included formal work assignments and the utilization of others' resources where necessary (see Figure 13.3). However, irrespective of the strength of the networks between organizations, they went from a group of organizations with very little collaboration to a coalition with a formal agreement and all members involved in decision-making. Over the next few years, they improved their levels of communication and relied on each other to achieve their goals a great deal more.

FIGURE 13.3. *Levels of Collaboration*

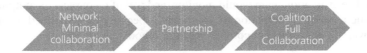

The evaluation team identified the differences in the groups and their relationships with each other and discussed the evaluation plan with each of them. Some groups had not worked with an evaluation team before now, so they had a series of meetings to work out how they would all work together and how they would each contribute to the overall evaluation. The evaluation tools were developed so there would be synergy across the groups and it would be possible to merge the data while preserving the uniqueness of each organization. It was clear that the evaluation team would have to work more closely with some of the groups than with others. They conducted an initial assessment of their evaluation skills, which was followed by training in the basic concepts of evaluation and a detailed explanation of the measurement instruments and how data would be collected. They provided ongoing support to the weaker organizations by attending all their evaluation meetings and helping them think through all their processes asking critical questions along the way. This empowerment evaluation approach was important for ensuring that all the organizations were capable of conducting their own evaluations once the agreed upon contracted evaluation was completed.

THE EVALUATION PLAN

The evaluation team would first conduct a process evaluation and later switch its focus to an outcome/impact evaluation knowing that the intervention was well implemented and that it would have the data for the later evaluation. This case study focuses on the process evaluation of the initiative.

The primary purpose of process evaluation is to understand the implementation aspects of the initiative, how well the program was implemented, the use of resources, level of implementation, reach of the initiative(s), and the satisfaction of stakeholders with implementation. In this case, the following questions were asked by coalition members.

- How well was the coalition run and programs delivered?
- To what extent did the intervention occur at multiple levels of influence (individual, interpersonal, community, organization, and policy)?
- In the case of the coalition, how well was the policy developed and implemented?
- Is the coalition likely to achieve its stated outcomes?
- What are the strengths and weaknesses of the coalition's work?
- Who benefited from the range of interventions that were planned and implemented?
- What changes need to be made to the coalition's work to ensure that it achieves its stated objectives and goals?

The final set of questions is determined by the priorities and preferences of the evaluation team and other stakeholders. In either scenario, the most appropriate questions to ask are based on the level of resources assigned to the evaluation, the stage of the program and the time frame within which the evaluation is being conducted, and the specific needs of the evaluation.

The questions that were selected in consultation with the stakeholders addressed a couple of important overarching questions in process evaluation. The first was about the program's implementation and the second one was about participation and benefits to the youth of Leighster County. Each of the participating organizations had to answer the same questions based on their funded projects and reflected in their logic models. This was a brand-new initiative so it made sense to start by looking at the level of implementation.

Question 1: How well was the coalition run and programs delivered?

Question 2: Who benefited from the range of interventions that were planned and implemented?

Question 3: To what extent did each subgroup benefit from the intervention?

The evaluation team met with each of the 20 grantees soon after they received the first installment of their funding. The first thing each group did was develop individual logic models with stated short-, medium-, and long-term objectives that would be in line with the overall goals and objectives that the MIPT had developed but focused on their organization's mission. These questions have embedded within them many more questions that would need to be answered, and the team must tease out the additional questions that will form a part of the evaluation. The scope of an evaluation was primarily determined by how many additional questions they asked beyond the overarching question. Table 13.3 provides a list of additional questions that the team might consider in support

TABLE 13.3. **Overarching and Subquestions in the Evaluation**

Overarching Evaluation Question	Questions to Be Addressed by the Evaluation
How well was the coalition run and programs delivered?	▪ What interventions were implemented? ▪ Were the interventions implemented as planned? ▪ What were the resources devoted to the interventions? ▪ What changes need to be made to the program or policy to ensure that it achieves its stated objectives and goals?
Who benefited from the range of interventions that were planned and implemented?	▪ Who participated in the intervention ▪ What was the reach of the intervention for each subgroup for who the program was intended?

of answering the overarching question. The evaluation team was expected to provide reports to the mayor's committee that included responses to these questions with data provided by each participating organization in order to come up with an overall assessment of initiative.

In addition to understanding the initiative to address the specific concerns the community had about the youth, the committee decided to have all funded organizations participate in a coalition and there were questions about the levels of participation of its members and its functioning. This added to the work of the evaluation team, but they welcomed it as a challenge. The question that the evaluation team answered was, "how well and to what extent did the groups function as a coalition?"

Process evaluation by its nature relies on the evaluation team developing tools that are specific to the organization and the needs of the evaluation, so the team had to think carefully about the entire evaluation plan that included the specific evaluation questions and the approach to answering them. One of the first steps was to get organized. Developing a table that showed the questions, indicators, data type, data collection approach, and the time line for data collection as outlined in Table 13.4 was a good place to start.

ANSWERING THE EVALUATION QUESTION

One of the questions the evaluation team had to answer was "How well was the coalition run and programs delivered?" The extent to which interventions were implemented gets to the heart of process evaluation. Without appropriate and adequate implementation, the basis for outcome/impact evaluation and drawing valid conclusions about an intervention is lost. So, although it is an important question to ask and answer, it is often not answered in evaluation. Too often we make the mistake of evaluating a program without understanding how well it was implemented and we draw conclusions that may be wrong or inappropriate.

In answering the overarching question, a number of subquestions are answered that would help them frame their report. The additional questions were:

■   What interventions were implemented?

■   Were the interventions implemented as planned?

■   What were the resources devoted to the interventions?

■   What changes need to be made to ensure that it achieves its stated objectives and goals?

The very first step in answering this question is inspecting all the documents associated with the project, discussing it with stakeholders at different levels such as project implementers as well as project participants, and together drawing a logic model that reflects the program as it is being implemented. The work plan, which contains the time line, is also an important document in determining what is being implemented. The information is compared with any previous logic model that may have been developed prior to implementation. Lots of things can happen that can change the program from its original design to its final implementation. In the case of this initiative, the organizations responded to an RFP sent out from the mayor's office. Although their proposals were accepted for funding, there was a period of negotiation that took place that resulted in some changes to their

TABLE 13.4. **Evaluation Questions, Indicators, Data Type, Data Collection Approach, and the Time Line for Data Collection**

Evaluation Question	Indicator	Data Type	Data Collection Approach	Time Line
How well was the coalition run and programs delivered?				
■ Was the intervention implemented as planned?	Approved work plan; implemented work plan of weekly activities; barriers to implementation	Qualitative data; quantitative	Site visits; project application documents; electronic data base of completed activities; coalition reports	Initial review—first 3 months; subsequent monthly reports
■ What were the resources devoted to the program?	Expenditure in dollars; donations of time and effort in hours	Quantitative data	Receipts; auditors reports; survey; databases	Monthly initial review—first 3 months; subsequent monthly reports
Who benefited from the range of interventions that were planned and implemented?				
■ Who participated in the interventions and how often?	Population groups as part of interventions	Qualitative data	Completed sign-in sheets	Initial review—first 3 months; subsequent monthly reports
■ What was the reach of the intervention for each subgroup for whom the program was intended?	Population groups participating in the interventions; project interventions reaching each group	Qualitative data	Weekly work plan reports in electronic database	Initial review—first 3 months; subsequent monthly reports
How well and to what extent did the groups function as a coalition?				
■ Who participated in the coalition?	Initiative-funded organizations	Quantitative data	Meeting notes	Initial data collection
■ How well did the groups function as a coalition?	Items on the survey	Quantitative data	Survey	Initial data collection and six monthly

original plan. In some cases, it was expanded along the same lines as the proposal and the original logic model that was submitted, but for other organizations working within their mission, new programs were proposed and added. The ultimate goal was to ensure that there were adequate services and overall the organizations would achieve the initiative's goals of reach and intensity. The initiative needed to have both depth and substance. The committee needed to be sure that sufficient youth would be reached with appropriately placed services of sufficient intensity to make a difference. They understood they had three years to show that the investment in the community would pay off. The terms of the coalition were also included in each organization's contract so activities around coalition building, coordination, and communication were similarly added.

The organization we will use in this example provided mental health services to youth 15–18 years in a predominantly Hispanic neighborhood that had been devoid of services for a very long time, and long before the hurricane came through the town. The services were open to all members of the community regardless of race or gender.

The Cinapsih Wellness Center (CWC)

The primary findings from the community assessment that the Cinapsih Wellness Center wanted to address in their initiative were

1. The number of youth and adults who reported feeling stressed or suicidal had increased slightly over the past 10 years. Mental health care had been sought more often (60% reported having seen a psychologist in the past year).

2. Suicide rates were lower than the national average, but troubling nonetheless because over time there appeared to be a slight trend upward (7% higher than figures for the previous year). There seemed to be a growing incidence among male youth. Thirty percent of youth reported that their parents sought help from a mental health counselor at least once in the previous year.

This data was alarming in itself and although the original sample only contained 10% of Hispanic youth, they were disproportionately affected and the data for this population reflected a problem that they needed to help tackle. They would be one of five funded interventions across the community that addressed mental health issues and they would form a group of health centers that provided coordinated services to the youth with clearly established referral systems. As a member of the coalition, they would have the opportunity to refer youth to those programs, also. For example, youth who were suicidal were often lonely and needed safe places to meet other youth. Sports activities break down barriers among youth since they don't often make friends easily. Since CWC did not have sufficient space for a full basketball court or an indoor soccer pitch they did what they could to offer stress reduction. They offered activities such as yoga and tai chi and offered the youth referrals to other stress relieving programs that they identified. Other organizations offered basketball and indoor soccer, both games Hispanic youth liked to participate in and they would be able to play on their school teams during the semester. The staff at CWC understood the trauma their families experienced from the natural disasters but also on a daily basis as their families are ripped apart by immigration legislation that criminalized them for wanting to make a new life. In addition to mental health support for the youth, the health center provided group counseling and family support to help families heal and help the youth to reduce their need for mental health services over time. In addition, they hoped that providing mental health services on a consistent basis, using trained staff to teach youth that they could do better in school, graduate, possibly go to college, and be able to have productive lives free from alcohol and drugs. It all fitted together perfectly with the goals of the mayor's initiative.

The CWC services were colocated with other organizations in a school-based health center and they had been instituted on the recommendation of the evaluation team after the review of a recent article (Walker, Kerns, Lyon, Bruns & Cosgrove, 2010) that found that student GPAs improved gradually over the length of the project if mental health services which included drop-in, crisis management, and the management of prescribed medications were provided.

The logic model reflecting the interventions provided by the health center included

1. One-on-one psychological counseling

2. Family counseling

3. Group counseling

4. Referral services to support organizations with complementary programs

5. Buddy support teams to reduce the risk of suicide

6. In-house stress reduction activities such as meditation, yoga, tai chi, and martial arts

7. School-based in-house and outreach mental health services

It was the responsibility of the evaluation team to determine the extent to which the organization did what it said it would do and with fidelity. The evaluation team documented and reflected on the existence of the services, the extent to which the services were implemented, and the level of services provided as well as the participation of the community in the different services. Members of the team collected data from work plans, activity reports, registration logs, and other documents; recorded it all on a series of checklists; and eventually developed a table of their findings. They collected information about the outreach activities and the school-based services through interviews with staff and students at the school as well as through a site visit (see Table 13.5).

Another question the evaluation team asked was, "What were the resources devoted to the program?" What data would we need to answer this question? What are the resources that need to be considered? If we considered the earlier activities, the following resources would most likely have to be in place:

- Staff

- Funding

- Volunteers

- Training materials

- Computer resources

- Internet connection

- Dedicated office, workshop, training, and activity spaces

However, this list might not be complete or it might not have been expanded sufficiently on some of the items to have a clear understanding of what resources were devoted to the program. For example, funding does not explain how much money was received in grants,

TABLE 13.5. **Baseline Level of Services and Participation in the Cinapsih Wellness Center Activities**

Health Center Programs	Number per Week	Number of Participants	Gender of Participants	Race of Participants
One-on-one psychological counseling	3 each	45 (total number registered for services)	Male (70%) Female (30%)	Hispanic (90%)
Family counseling per counselor	2	25	Female (50%) Male (50%)	Hispanic (90%)
Group counseling per counselor	2	12	Female (70%) Male (30%)	Hispanic (70%)
Referrals to support organizations with complementary programs	50	20	Male (70%) Female (30%)	Hispanic (80%)
Buddy support team meetings	5–7	30	Male (70%) Female (30%)	Hispanic (90%)
In-house stress reduction activities	14 (2 daily)	30	Female (50%) Male (50%)	Hispanic (50%)
School based outreach	2	15	Female (90%) Males (10%)	Hispanic (20%)

in-kind services, and donations. Time donated should be estimated carefully to account for hours as well as hourly fees. In addition, an item like sporting equipment does not say enough about what type and how many pieces of equipment were purchased. If the goal is ultimately to conduct a cost-benefit analysis when it is important to have a very clear and accurate description of the costs associated with the program, a fair amount of due diligence must go into collecting and documenting this information. An inventory could be completed at baseline and updated as new items are added. Examples of tables documenting human-resources (staff) costs and staffing levels are shown in Tables 13.6(a) and (b).

Another important question to address during the implementation of a program and especially as the activities are being established is "What changes need to be made to ensure that it achieves its stated objectives and goals?" What additional questions does this conjure up in your mind? The evaluation team wanted to be able to document any barriers that the organization encountered, but more importantly how they were able to resolve them and improve the outcomes of the program. If we go back to Table 13.5, you will note that

TABLE 13.6a.   Personnel Salaries and Annual Cost

Personnel	Description	Number	Hours worked per Week	Monthly Salary	Annual Cost
Staff	Program staff	4	40	$ 40,000	$1,920,000
	Supervisory staff	2	40	$ 50,000	$1,200,000
	Outreach staff	4	40	$30,000	$1,440,000
	Clinical staff—psychologists	3	40	$60,000	$2,160,000
Totals		13		$460,000	$5,720,000

TABLE 13.6b.   Volunteers and Effort

Personnel	Description	Number	Hours worked per Week	Monthly Savings	Annual Savings
Volunteer	Communications Coordinator	1	20	$25,000	$300,000
	Trainer	1	20	$40,000	$480,000
Total savings		2	40	$65,000	$780,000

the participation of Hispanic youth in some of the interventions was lower. For example, although most of them (90%) attended individual, one-on-one counseling, only 70% of those who attended group counseling were Hispanic youth when it was anticipated in the planning period that they would all attend.

In conducting focus groups with the youth to determine what affected their level of participation, it was discovered that many of them did not like to share personal and family problems with their peers and youth they did not know very well in a group setting. It has to do with their culture and what their culture determined were things that could be shared in public spaces and what was private and shared only with family members. Youth from other races had less difficulty doing this. To compensate for this loss and to ensure that Hispanic youth still got the level of counseling needed to heal, the program offered more family counseling sessions increasing the number of family sessions offered from two to three per week allowing families to sign up with any of the clinical staff. In addition, the center had projected that at least 100 youth would receive services a week. The numbers (Table 13.5) that evaluation found were far short of this target, so the outreach team were called in!

The evaluation team would investigate the barriers using a combination of data-collection approaches including satisfaction surveys to determine why youth were not using the center.

When designing the survey, the team had to remember that only information that would be helpful to make decisions about how to improve participation in the program would be collected. If the survey were too general and appeared to ask questions that had little to do with the level of participation in the activities of the center, they would probably not get many of the youth to complete it. The evaluation team clearly defined the objective of the survey, the questions they wanted answered, and the scale they would use to collect the data. They decided on a Likert Scale and framed the questions so the response categories were, 1 = strongly disagree, 2 = disagree, 3 = agree, and 4 = strongly agree. An additional item, 5 = I do not know, was added. Questions were asked about their perceptions regarding recruitment for the program by the outreach staff and the media, orientation, individual family and group counseling sessions, referral systems, and in-house stress reduction activities.

One set of questions on the survey that asked about the perception of the youth to their recruitment into the program focused on how they got the information about the program and their perceptions of the program based on that information and what others around them were saying (Table 13.7).

In addition, they conducted individual interviews with the staff and reviewed the HR files to determine their level of training and experience for the various positions they held as well as any shortcomings they recognized in providing the services. In a couple of cases, the clinical staff were not as fluent in some of the dialects that clients used since the population they served had come from various parts of the Caribbean and Latin America and spoke with slightly different accents. To ensure they get to outcomes, they would provide additional training. Courses were identified on line that staff were encouraged to register for to improve their language skills.

The evaluation team wanted to be sure that, in reviewing the program and determining what changes needed to be made to improve the implementation of the program, they had all the information they needed. They had to keep the goals and objectives of the overall initiative firmly in mind and ensure that each organization's work would ultimately make a difference.

The Coalition

The evaluation team had never before been asked to evaluate coalitions and thought it would be a good opportunity to learn what it entailed. The team had all the skills it needed but called on colleagues who were more familiar with this work to get their advice. The team did some research of its own and looked up how coalitions had been evaluated in the past and adopted one of the models of evaluation. They were up for the task. The team identified a tool that was based on the work of Taylor-Powell, Rossing and Geran (1998) which they liked. The tool was called, "Partnerships and Collaborations: Diagnostic Tool for Evaluating Group Functioning," which they found at http://www.buildinitiative.org/. Although there was no information about its reliability and validity, the team thought it asked the right questions and it seemed straightforward enough, so they decided to use it to conduct an initial assessment of the groups and also at six monthly follow-ups to see if the groups' perceptions changed over time as they got more familiar with the processes and used to working together.

TABLE 13.7. Survey Questions From the Section on Recruitment in Assessing Levels of Participation in the Cinapsih Wellness Center Programs and Activities

Section 1: Recruitment

The following questions ask about your perceptions regarding recruitment into programs and activities at the Cinapsih Wellness Center in the Russell Neighborhood.

Place a check in the box that best represents your response to the item in the first column.
  1 = strongly disagree, 2 = disagree, 3 = agree, 4 = strongly agree and 5 = I do not know

Item	1	2	3	4	5
I heard about the Cinapsih Wellness Center from programs and notices I heard in the media.					
I heard about the Cinapsih Wellness Center from a member of the center staff.					
I know about the programs and activities offered by the center.					
I had all my questions about the programs and activities answered in a timely manner.					
The programs and activities offered by the center are appropriate for me and my family.					
The programs and activities offered by the center are offered at a time that I and my family can participate easily.					
Overall, I believe the programs and activities are good for people in my community.					

In the space below, please tell us how we can encourage youth to participate in the programs and activities at the center.

The diagnostic tool asked questions about respondent's perceptions of a shared vision, goals and objectives, responsibilities and roles, decision-making, membership, conflict management, leadership, relationships, internal and external communication, and evaluation. The questions were asked on a 7-point scale from negative to positive. For example, a critical aspect of coalition building is trust between members and one of the statements on the scale was, "members do not trust each other (1) to members trust each other (7). It was perfect! They decided they would collect data on the networks that were forming and developing across the group and later on conduct a network analysis. They were excited about the potential for new work. They looked forward to bringing on a new member of the team who had expertise in network analysis once they got to that. In the mean time they would collect as much data as they could. They were particularly conscious of assessing the outcomes of the networks as well so were interested in understanding the benefits of the collaboration and the extent to which it led to new or enhanced services or additional funding from leveraging new resources.

Ensuring the Quality of the Evaluation

Ensuring the quality of the evaluation meant that the evaluation team was guided by the principles of systematic inquiry, competence, integrity, respect for person, and responsibility to the general public (see Chapter 6 for a complete listing). This section shows how these principles were applied to the evaluation of the Leighster County Initiative. The evaluation they were primary responsible for in the first phase was process evaluation, but they needed to ensure that as they collected the data for the process evaluation, they also made sure that for the full evaluation they would be able to conduct a systematic data-based inquiry. For the process evaluation, all the information they used to draw their conclusions about the interventions were based on documents that had been prepared ahead of time, or data that they collected systematically as they needed it. The team ensured that the transfer of information for purposes of analysis was accurate. They did this by having more than one person responsible for data and through constant review reached an acceptable level of interrater reliability. Where there was only one person responsible, they tried to establish intrarater reliability and when there was more than one person, they held each other accountable for the accuracy of the data collection. High inter- and intrarater reliability meant that the observers, those entering and coding data, used the same rubric, coding, or rating scale and arrived at the same (or very similar) results. Interrater and intrarater reliability reflect consistency and accuracy.

Collecting accurate data was important and the evaluators had no defendable knowledge of how the youth felt about the recruitment activities of the CWC until they developed a survey tool which they pilot tested to ensure that it was valid before administering it. In addition, they made certain that the data collection process followed the established protocols, so they adhered to the highest technical standards. In order to strengthen the evaluation, the team also kept in mind an additional set of standards, those of utility, feasibility, propriety, and accuracy. The evaluators wanted to be sure that through the process of ongoing consultation the results would be useful. They kept stakeholders involved in the process throughout. By its very nature, process evaluation provides feedback to the client to improve the program's outputs and subsequent outcomes. In providing information about the strengths and weaknesses of the program but particularly about barriers to implementation, the team was able to help CWC improve the quality of the interventions as well as participation of the youth.

The second principle required that the team was competent to perform the evaluation. In the case of the evaluation team for this project, the team leader had 25 years of experience conducting evaluations of a range of different projects and programs but most recently had overseen the evaluation of a community-wide intervention with many different components and organizations. Her expertise was in outcome evaluation, but she had come to value the importance of process evaluation. She assembled a competent team of researchers with a range of skills in qualitative and quantitative research. Since she really wanted to grow the talent in the area as well, she was committed to training youth in evaluation. She hired two interns to be a part of the team. Her team of 10 altogether would provide both technical expertise to the organizations as well as collect primary data to answer the evaluation questions. The members of the team were cross-disciplinary with a range of backgrounds in public health, sociology, psychology, exercise science, and education. She needed the cross-disciplinary thinking, models, and analysis to be applied to the evaluation. This team was coming together for the long haul and she wanted them to learn from each other. The evaluation team leader needed a team that was culturally competent.

This team understood the realities of the community that they were evaluating, the trauma they had experienced, as well as the resources they had. The team was careful to identify and work with the existing leadership structures while making sure members of the team maintained their integrity and they functioned as a competent independent research institution. They recognized the importance of the task and the expectations of many in the community, so they developed skills to work with the tensions produced by the collaboration that was required by the initiative. Among other things, they made sure to use culturally acceptable language, communication, and negotiation. They had to remember that although their group was mixed racially, they would sometimes work with predominantly Hispanic populations on one hand and predominantly White or African American populations on the other who also received services at the center and across the coalition. They had to be flexible, but they had to be culturally astute across all groups. They worked hard to achieve a level of cultural competence that made their work acceptable to all groups through training and diligence.

The evaluation team made sure that in all their dealings with the stakeholders they displayed the utmost concern for the integrity of the process as well as the outcomes. They were honest in their dealings with all the groups even when it was uncomfortable. In one instance there was a conflict of interest when members of the advisory committee wanted very much to be a part of the evaluation. The evaluators had to discuss the importance of ensuring that they maintained the integrity of the research while they involved them in areas that did not present issues of conflict. Other situations arose in which members of the advisory committee had interests in some of the organizations that were members of the coalition and, therefore, being evaluated. Those members were asked to recuse themselves from any discussions of the groups' findings to limit any situations that might have resulted in conflict. The evaluation team was careful in all its dealings to respect the security and dignity of respondents, program participants, clients, and other stakeholders. They were especially careful to ensure that all the data they collected was secured and individual's names were not associated with any findings. In the conduct of the evaluation and data collection, the team maintained the privacy of the respondents. The team abided by ethical standards in the conduct of the evaluation and especially in ensuring that through their work they did not leave the community more traumatized.

Every six months the evaluation team had a retreat to discuss the evaluation process as well as the results they had achieved. This meta-evaluation or, in other words, an evaluation of the evaluation, allowed the team to identify any shortcomings in their work and determine action steps for ensuring the best quality evaluation. They also discussed the next components that had to be tackled in the evaluation plan.

REPORTING THE RESULTS

In reporting the results of the evaluation, there were additional questions the team wanted to include in their report. They had presented multiple reports to stakeholders during the course of the process evaluation. They had worked with the groups to ensure that they understood the results of their organization's work in the context of the larger evaluation. They had helped them improve the implementation of their projects through the results of the process evaluation. All this had happened over the first three years. Now the project was stable and the coalition was functioning well, they looked forward to the next phase, conducting an outcome/impact evaluation. They would have to revise their team to be sure they had the necessary skills in-house or had access to experts in the areas they lacked expertise—for example, in the network analysis they planned. However, now it was time to present the final report to stakeholders. They needed to present the information in such a way as to allow other stakeholders who had not been a part of the process throughout to understand, interpret, and critique their work. Since they had worked closely with members of the community, they were satisfied that this would not be a problem. As a matter of principle, they had also ensured sufficient participation from members of the team such that, as the leader, she would sit back and watch, coming in to only respond to critical politically charged questions or comments from the audience. She had been the eyes and ears of the evaluation team, so she was fully conversant with the hot-button issues that the stakeholders had previously identified. There were not many, but when they came up they got the stakeholders riled up very easily.

The goal of this final report at the end of the initial funded period came as the initiative was well established and the organizations would move to fully implementing their projects focusing on achieving measurable and meaningful outcomes, and the evaluation team would conduct an outcome evaluation based on the outcomes established by the advisory committee. This was still to be negotiated.

The focus for this report was presenting the information so the stakeholders understood whether the initiative for the youth was likely to be successful and produce the changes they hoped to see in them and the community. They understood that three years would not turn around a situation that had built up over 10 years, but they were sure that if they had a good start in the first three years, they would be successful. The specific questions that had to be answered were

1. What are the strengths and weaknesses of the Leighster County Youth Initiative?

2. To what extent did the youth benefit from the resources invested in the initiative?

3. To what extent did the program occur at multiple levels of influence (individual, inter-personal, community, organization, and policy)?

4. What changes need to be made to the program or policy to ensure that it achieves its stated objectives and goals?

The question they had not really answered yet was about the changes that needed to be made to ensure that the initiative achieved its stated goals and objectives. They spent some time in the report discussing the original logic model compared to their findings in the evaluation. It was clear that all the major areas had been covered, or at least the ones the advisory committee had decided to focus on. They had not tackled policy change yet because it seemed to be outside the expertise of most members. They did, however, recommend that the Bar Association get involved with the work of the coalition and possibly take it on. The evaluation team was able to report on the progress they had made so far.

Policy analysis is time consuming and requires a lot of patience and since it was voluntary, they were unable to devote as much time to it. However, they had identified all the sections of the law that addressed issues of alcohol and drug access and use by adolescents. The laws on driving under the influence did not address the issues of age of the driver and they felt this was an important omission and, therefore, an easy one to tackle when the Bar Association met again in the New Year. They wanted to also consider the need for various ordinances to improve access to opportunities for healthy living for adolescents and their families. This included access to open spaces for physical activity as well as relaxation. The community lacked the resources; however, there were some tax incentives that it could consider that would bring in the private sector on much more favorable terms of investment. The community had its work cut out for it and the evaluation team was pleased to include this information in its final report.

At the organizational level, the evaluation team spent a lot of time working with the executive directors and other staff to ensure that they were following the work plans they had developed and that they were monitoring their programs. Most of the changes that needed to be made had been made in the first year. Their work plans were revised annually and updated to reflect any new research or tweaked to take into consideration any new learning. One such change involved when the CWC clinics were run. Early on in the project implementation, clinics had run only during the day with no out-of-hours clinics. Following some formative work, the center started offering clinics in the evenings as well, and staff moved from a 9:00 A.M.–5:00 P.M. schedule to a two-shift schedule allowing the clinic to be open from 8:00 A.M. to 8:00 P.M. daily permitting youth and their families to come in after work and school. The activity center had always offered classes that ran until 9:00 P.M. so no changes were required there.

In addition to answering the specific questions outlined earlier, additional information for decision-making was included in the report to stakeholders based on the following analysis:

Relevance: The extent to which the activities designed and implemented were suited to the priorities.

Effectiveness: The extent to which the program had achieved its intended outputs and outcomes.

Efficiency: Outputs in relation to inputs.

Sustainability and partnerships: Likely sustainability beyond funding and the extent to which the project brought together relevant stakeholders to achieve its goals.

The report provides a list of key findings that highlighted important aspects of the evaluation results and the importance of the findings. Not everything the evaluation found was important and necessary to report. The results discussed the evaluation in the context of social-justice criteria, highlighting where there were gaps in populations being served either in view of their access to the resources provided or their depth of services. The unintended consequences of various findings were highlighted and recommendations for decision-making and stakeholder and community action were presented.

In order to accommodate the different needs for data and their appreciation of the results, the report was presented in a variety of formats. The most used was the more formal report that provided the most information and supporting data. Newsletter articles were published, as were peer-reviewed journal articles, which highlighted the process as well as the challenges of conducting a process evaluation.

The evaluation team signed a new contract with the advisory team, and it was able to plan for conducting a full evaluation. The second phase evaluation was primarily an outcome evaluation but the team integrated some process evaluation for purposes of continual monitoring and to ensure sustainability. The work continued long beyond the mayor's initiative because the team was hired by the larger organizations that were able to secure additional funding to continue to provide evaluation services. New organizations came on board to expand the members of the coalition and, where requested as a matter of good will, the evaluation team worked with them through their start-up phase providing formative evaluation services. Many went on to contract for process evaluation and then outcome/impact evaluation services.

DISCUSSION QUESTIONS AND ACTIVITIES

1. Using the same community assessment data described in this case study, identify a project that you believe would address one of the community's concerns. Design an intervention that you believe addresses the problem. Develop a logic model to show the inputs, activities, and outcomes associated with the intervention.

2. Based on the intervention you have developed above design a process evaluation.

3. As a member of the evaluation team with the responsibility to design the evaluation plan, what steps would you take in designing the process evaluation plan to ensure that it meets the standard of Utility?

APPENDIX

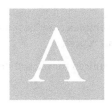

MODEL AGREEMENT BETWEEN EVALUATION CONSULTANT AND TEAM MEMBERS

Agreement between the evaluator and two different categories of consultants (C1 and C2). C1-Supervisor; responsible for data collection and to oversee one additional team in the same region of the country; C2-Data collector; responsible for collecting qualitative data based on semistructured surveys and focus groups.

AGREEMENT

BETWEEN **Evaluation Consultant** and Principal Investigator (hereinafter known as **PI**), AND [name of consultant] (hereinafter known as **[initials]**), of [Address]. The Contracting Organization will hereinafter be known as CO.

WHEREAS **[initials]** has asserted to the PI to the adequacy of his skills and experience, in the field of Data Collection and Analysis, including field research as required by the assignment, with regard to the participation of **[initials]** in the provision of professional services by the [CO]. The Terms of Reference (TOR) forms an integral part of this contract and is show as Attachment A.

Attachment A: Terms of Reference

1. Attend training in field (date).

2. Collect data as prescribed.

3. Complete entry of all data as required for all surveys and forms completed on site as per specifications.

4. Complete and submit draft summary reports within five days of completion of field-work.

5. Complete and submit all deliverables (raw data and final report) within three days of receiving feedback on the draft report.

6. Compete all activities as are required for the satisfactory completion of the Evaluation Study.

IT IS AGREED THAT:

1. **[initials]** will provide such professional services as required by PI consistent with his/her asserted knowledge, training, skills and experience as stated in the Curriculum Vitae made available to PI and the Terms of Reference for the assignment.

2. **[initials]** will be compensated in the sum of [amount]. Payment will be made by [cash/check/direct bank deposit]. This amount includes any additional support that **[initials]** may need to execute his work. Payments shall be subject to the settlement of fee notes by the CO to PI and shall be made in the following instalments totalling 100 percent:

   a. 40 percent is paid upon signing of the contract.

   b. 60 percent will be paid on the submission and confirmation of receipt of all reports and notes CO.

3. PI shall provide the following facilities:

   a. Access to office space at the CO's premises or at the PIs office.

4. **[initials]** will be responsible for all tax liabilities due by him under this contract to responsible authorities of any jurisdiction. **[initials]** hereby unreservedly agrees to indemnify PI in respect of any consequences and/or instances of neglect on his part in this regard.

5. **[initials]** agrees to comply with the ethical, client confidentiality, competence, and personal integrity standards that would normally be expected of a team member of a professional service firm such as FJP. Personal or professional conduct during the duration of this contract that besmirches the reputation of PI shall be deemed to be a breach of contract. In such an event, PI shall issue a formal Letter of Warning to **[initials]**. Failure to satisfactorily address the demands of the letter within one week of its issue shall be deemed a fundamental breach of contract. Any monies remaining under the contract shall be forfeited and the contract terminated without further notice. PI reserves the right to demand the repayment of any monies paid in advance of the delivery of services.

6. **[initials]** agrees to declare, in writing, and in advance of any work for a client, any relationship that may impair or appear to impair his independence from a client. This shall include, but not be limited to

Any financial interest.

Any business relationship.

A close family or dependent relationship with a relevant shareholder or investor or member of a board of directors or trustees or with CO personnel holding positions of management.

Failure by **[initials]** to make a declaration shall be deemed to be neglect of duty and may attract disciplinary action within this contract.

7. **[initials]** agrees to perform the services required of him in a timely manner according to the schedule determined by PI and communicated to **[initials]**.

8. **[initials]** failure to perform the services required by him in a timely manner after the receipt of a statement from **[initials]** to that effect and/or three written requests (by hand or by electronic communication) by PI over a period of two calendar weeks shall be construed as a fundamental breach of contract. Any monies remaining under the contract shall be forfeited and the contract terminated without further notice. PI reserves the right to demand the repayment of any monies paid in advance of the delivery of services.

9. **[initials]**'s failure to perform the services required by him/her as a result of shortcomings on technical skills and/or experience after the receipt of a statement from **[initials]** to that effect and/or after the receipt of three written requests for improvement (by hand or by electronic communication) by PI over a period of two calendar weeks shall be construed as a fundamental breach of contract. Any monies remaining under the contract shall be forfeited and the contract terminated without further notice. PI reserves the right to demand the repayment of any monies paid in advance of the delivery of services.

10. This agreement is subject to the laws of [The Country].

SIGNED PI/DATE_____

SIGNED (**Name of Contractor**) DATE _____

WITNESSED BY/DATE_____

APPENDIX

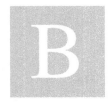

B

MODEL PREAMBLE FOR ADULT INDIVIDUAL INTERVIEWS

You are being asked to participate in a research project. The questions will ask about [purpose of the evaluation]. All those who participate in this study will either be staff in one or more of the programs or have benefited from the programs through receiving services or support. The interview will last approximately 1 hour.

There are no risks to you for participating in this research. We do not expect that any of the questions will be hard for you to answer or cause you any distress. You can refuse to answer any question if it makes you feel uncomfortable.

You will not receive any monetary payment for participating. The information you provide will help to improve programs in your area.

Your participation in this research project is voluntary. You can decide not to answer any of the questions, or you can stop the person interviewing you at any time and say you do not want to continue. If you decide not to participate or you stop answering questions, the services you and/or your child receive will not be affected.

Thank you very much for participating in this study. If you have any questions about this research and you want to know more about what we are doing, please contact: [PI name, address and telephone number]

APPENDIX

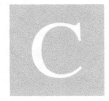

MODEL DEMOGRAPHIC SHEET

This form is to be used for each individual interview to record demographic information ensuring a deeper analysis of the data. The data collected must be relevant to the needs of the project and requirements for analysis. The project represented here was about women of child-bearing age and their school-age children.

Community where interview takes place Name of entity (eg. School, clinic, or other:	Does the respondent live in the same place as the interview? Yes No (circle one) If no, where does the person live?
Age 10–17; 18–24; 25–35; 36–45; >46 years (circle one)	Sex: Male Female Other (circle one) If female, are you pregnant? Yes No (circle one) Do you have a child that is being breastfed? Yes No (circle one)
What is your connection to [organization being evaluated] (Probes: work for the clinic, teach in a sponsored school, volunteer, member of a committee, received training in the past, etc.)	Are you currently employed? If yes, where do you work? If no, how do you earn your living? (Probe: farming, business, etc.)

Do you have any children? Yes/No

If yes, how many_____

What are the ages of your children?

Child 1 _____

Child 2 _____

Child 3 _____

Child 4 _____

Child 5 _____

Other children _____

If the children are school age, do they go to school? (Age 5 upwards) Yes/No

If no, what are the reasons the children do not go to school?

APPENDIX

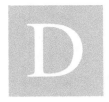

MODEL FIELD NOTES REPORT

Valid and reliable data is a critical component of research. The validity of the conclusions is dependent on the integrity of the research. Record any factors/incidents that affect the collection the data. Turn in the completed form as one of the deliverables of this research. This information will be used to describe any limitations in the data collection phase of the study.

■ Any violations of the interview protocol

■ Problems associated interviewing preidentified respondents

The inclusion criteria is noted on each instrument

Community	Violation (reason for violation and any mitigating circumstances)	Remedy Adopted

Any additional notes

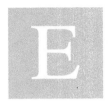

APPENDIX

E

MODEL INTERVIEW REFUSAL REPORT

Note: When potential respondents to an interview refuse to participate, make a note of the reasons for their refusal. Turn in the completed form as one of the deliverables of this research.

Community	Instrument Name	Reason for Refusal	Sex (M/F/other)

APPENDIX

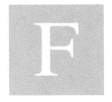

DATA COLLECTION TRAINING MANUAL TEMPLATE

Acronyms

Definitions

Word/Expression	Definition

Background

1. Epidemiological profile of the health problem being investigated.

2. The purpose of this evaluation.

3. Sites of the evaluation.

Evaluation Consultant

    Contact Information

Time Line and Data Collection Schedule

Sample Description

Data Collection Tools

Number of data collection tools and descriptions of each. Purpose for any overlap in questions across questionnaires.

The goal is to collect as much data as possible, paying particular attention to ensuring both validity and reproducibility.

Instrument	Population to Be sampled	Sample Size

CONDUCTING THE INTERVIEW

The next section contains guidelines for conducting the study. The topics discussed in this section are:

- Contacting respondents
- Introducing yourself to a respondent
- Confidentiality
- Building rapport

Contacting Respondents

Mechanism(s) for contacting respondents

Introducing Yourself to a Respondent   Identify yourself and say what your purpose is. A sample of an introduction you might give is provided in the panel to your right. If he/she does not agree to the interview, explain again what the interview is about. Do not force the person to participate. This study is voluntary. Make a note of why any potential participant refused to participate and thank him or her for their time. Complete form found in Appendix E.

> **Sample Introduction Script**
>
> Good morning/Afternoon,
> Dr./Mr./Mrs/Miss/Ma/Pa (as appropriate)
> Thank you for agreeing to participate in our
> study. My name is – – – – – – – – – – – .
> I am from FJP Development and Management
> Consultants in Freetown and we are here to
> conduct an interview as part of research
> study. The study is about the health clinics
> and the elementary schools here and in the
> district. The information we get from you
> and from all the others that we interview
> will be used to improve health and
> education programs and services in your
> community.

Confidentiality The term *confidentiality* refers to our guarantee that information that identifies a person by name, address, or any other identifier is not released to anybody outside the project team and is not used in any reports. Names and other identifiers will not appear on any surveys and materials that allow a link between the individual and a survey/interview data. Separate consent must be obtained for the use of any photographic data involving individuals.

Do not reveal any information that is obtained during the course of an interview to an unauthorized person. Authorized persons are restricted to persons working directly on the project and within the project team. To assure confidentiality, you are asked to protect the interview form, consent form, and any other documentation related to the interview. Only assigned members of the research team will have access to data for the purposes of entering, analyzing, and reporting. The data must be secured under password protected locks.

Building Rapport Having an honest information-filled interview with the respondent begins with the first greeting when you meet the study participant. Developing and maintaining a good rapport with the respondent is critical to collecting valid information.

Provide a friendly atmosphere by showing an interest in the responses that are being given. Take time to reassure him/her of the confidential nature of the information.

> **Assure Confidentiality!**
>
> If a person is nervous or afraid
> to speak, it would result in a
> failure of the interview to
> reflect true behaviors and
> values of the respondent.

If the respondent shows signs of being uncomfortable because he/she cannot answer the question, or is afraid of saying the wrong thing, reassure the person by emphasizing that:

■ There is no right or wrong answer; we are only looking for their opinion.

■ All your answers are confidential.

Use kind and supportive tones in your voice when asking the questions; however, ask questions in a careful and confident manner. It is important that you are not judgmental even if you disagree with the answer. Being judgmental could make the person feel uncomfortable resulting in socially acceptable responses. If a person is nervous or afraid to speak, it would result in a failure of the interview to reflect true behaviors and values of the respondent. Pay particular attention to facial expressions or other body language that indicates your personal feelings about a topic or the response of the individual.

Additional Techniques for Building and Maintaining Rapport The probing procedures listed next are useful in stimulating discussion. Introduce them casually as a natural expression of interest:

Brief assenting comments, such as "Yes, I see," show the respondent that you are giving your attention to the answer. They often stimulate the respondent to talk further.

An expectant pause, accompanied by an inquiring look after the respondent has given only a brief reply often conveys that you are waiting for more information. It often brings forth further response.

Repeating the question, or listing the response categories is useful when the respondent does not understand the question, misinterprets it, seems unable to make up his/her mind, or strays from the subject.

Repeating or paraphrasing the respondent's reply, is useful in helping to clarify the response and prompting the respondent to enlarge upon his/her statement. Be sure you adhere strictly to the respondent's answer.

Neutral questions, in a neutral tone of voice will bring fuller clearer responses. For example:

"I don't understand what you mean."

"Please explain that again for me."

"I am not sure what you mean by that, could you tell me a little more?"

Interviewing Children

Important guidelines for anyone interviewing children during your visit. Be aware that sometimes the settings or circumstances that the children live in or describe may upset or shock you.

Consider Children in Your Approach: Planning and Setting

■ **Plan your interview**. Make sure you know something about the child's community.

■ The **written consent of a parent or guardian** must be given before the interview takes place.

- Unless you are talking about a child's particular experience, it is better to **interview them in a small group**. Individual children may be overawed by a strange adult asking questions. They may feel happier and more relaxed in the presence of their classmates and friends. The shy ones may feel encouraged to come forward and speak. Four to six children in a group is ideal. It is better to interview children of a similar age in one group. If the age range of the group is too wide, the younger children will feel intimidated by the older ones. Try to get a balance of boys and girls but sometimes it may be more appropriate to interview boys and girls separately.

- However, some children will only open up when you interview them one-to-one. Ask children what they prefer. **You should always have a member of the family or community or a teacher that the child trusts present when you interview children, preferably a woman.**

- If you are doing one-on-one interviews, make sure you are visible to others. Do not take a child to a secluded spot. **We have a duty to protect children.**

- The wishes and rights of children need to be balanced against those of parents or guardians. But **children's wishes and best interests should be paramount**—because children have the right to speak out and adults do not have the right to silence them.

- When conducting the interview, think about **choosing the right space**. Put children at ease. They may not feel happy being interviewed in the classroom and might be more comfortable outside for instance. The space should be as private as possible to allow them to talk freely, but it should not be secluded.

- If you are interviewing children in a school situation, you need to get the permission of the head teacher. Children may find it difficult to speak freely in front of their teachers.

Protect Your Interviewees

- **Confidentiality is very important**. Ask the children how they feel about having their names published. If they are uncomfortable, use a fictional name. Respect that some children really want to be named.

- **Do not give children money or presents** as this can have negative consequences for child and family.

Your Behaviors

- Respect cultural norms. **Introductions are important**. Take time over this. Explain who you are and why you want to interview them. Ask children to introduce themselves individually.

- Do not speak down to children or patronize them.

- Think about your **body language**. Maintain eye contact with the children you are talking to unless this is culturally unacceptable.

- **Sit at the same level as the children**. Do not take the biggest and best chair. If the children are sitting on the floor, sit on the floor. If you are working with a group, ask the children to sit in a circle.

■ Being interviewed can be daunting, so spend time letting the children get to know you so they will relax. Play a game with them, do some drawing together if you need to break the ice.

■ **Treat children as equals** and human beings like everyone else. See them as individuals with their own thoughts and concerns.

■ **Listening** is the key to interviewing children. Let them tell their story. Do not interrupt.

■ Do not go in to the interview with preconceived ideas.

■ **Be aware of what you are asking**—be particularly sensitive when asking to see people's homes or asking probing questions. If they are not comfortable to show you or answer, this is their right.

■ Make sure you **finish the interview well**. Don't leave questions hanging. Ask children if they have any questions or if there is anything they have said that they don't want published. Make sure that you send the published article and a few photos to the children.

Empower Children by Ensuring Their Voices Are Heard as They Themselves Intend

■ Explain **how the interview will work** and that they can ask questions if anything is unclear.

■ **Use appropriate language**. Listen to how they speak. Make sure they understand you. Don't use jargon.

■ **Make your questions open** and unambiguous. Give children the freedom to say what they really want.

■ **Respect children** and value their opinions. They want to be taken seriously and understood—reflect this in your reporting of interviews.

■ Do not put words in children's mouths. Let them speak for themselves without adult interference.

■ Do not push children to speak if they do not want to.

■ If the interview is not going well or children are reluctant to talk, they may not understand what is expected of them or they may not want to take part. Take time to talk to them and find out what the problem is.

■ **Allow children to change their minds**. Sometimes they contradict themselves or lie or make up stories. Adults do this too.

> Empower children by ensuring that their voices are heard as they themselves intend!

- Often you will need to work with a **translator.** Take advice from the contracting agency about how to do this if there are concerns. Before you start the interview, spend time talking to the translator to explain your needs. He needs to translate exactly what the children say and not his version of what they are saying. Explain that you want to hear everything, not just the good side of the story.

Taking Photographs of Your Interviewee

- If you are **working with a photographer**, chose a photographer who likes children. Brief them well. Explain the importance of showing respect for children. Ask him/her to get down to their level, that is, sit on the floor, be at eye level. If a child does not want to be photographed, the photographer must respect his/her wishes.

- **Always consider children's safety**. Sometimes they need to be disguised in photos, particularly if they are vulnerable to abuse.

- Be especially aware of what you are asking when taking photographs. Always ask permission both to photograph the individual as well as his/his home or property. Consider how your actions will be perceived by the community.

- Ensure that your photographs portray people, both adults and children, with dignity.

Answering Respondents' Questions

A small percentage of respondents may be reluctant to participate in the survey or other data collection and would need reassurance. It is your responsibility to "sell" the survey or interview and minimize the number of refusals. Selling the survey/interview should be done in an honest manner stressing the importance of the work.

To convert reluctant respondents, try to identify his/her objections to participating in the survey and tailor your answer accordingly. A thorough understanding of the survey/interview and the goal of the research are the key to a good explanation.

If the respondent asks any questions, it is your responsibility to defer answering the question to the end of the interview.

Taking a Gendered View

Consider gender in your interviewing and data collection; they may reflect experiences and perceptions that might be different for males and females. A gendered approach asks the following questions:

- Who participates in projects and programs and why?

- Are the needs of men and women (boys and girls) known and/or responded to?

- Is there a complementary or competing agenda among beneficiaries?

  - Is this different for men and women?

- Have participants had input into project implementation, monitoring and evaluation? (If yes, who has had input, men or women?)

- Do women discuss as a separate group or together with men?

Getting the Best Data!

Although the data collection is voluntary, getting all the selected respondents to participate and complete the questionnaire or interview is an important goal of any research study. If a respondent says that he or she prefers not to participate, explaining the following points may help you to obtain an interview:

- The importance of the survey and the uses of the information that is gathered.

- The confidentiality of the survey information and that only summary data will be reported.

- Ask the interviewee to begin the interview on a "trial basis." Explain that the person does not have to answer any question he or she does not feel comfortable answering. Also, the interview can be ended any time they desire.

Asking Questions

How to ask the questions:

- Ask the questions and probes as they are worded. Ensure that translations (where appropriate) are accurate and ask the question in the way that was intended. Asking the questions as they are worded (after translation) will ensure that the results are comparable across all interviews and similar information is gathered for all respondents. Get as much information as you can.

- Ask every question. It is important to ask every question and to collect information for each question or as many as possible.

- If the respondent misunderstands or misinterprets a question: Repeat the question and give the respondent a chance to answer. Rephrase the question to improve the understanding but make sure to maintain the sense that was intended.

Ending the Interview

End the interview by thanking your interviewee for giving you their time and ask if they have any questions about the project. If you can't answer a specific question about the project, refer it to one of the project staff. If you promise to get the information and get back to the interviewee, make sure to get contact information from the individual specifically for this purpose. This confirms your commitment to maintaining confidentiality.

Note: If there are questions about services offered by [**name of the organization**] provide them with contact information.

Questions and Answers

What is the survey about? The survey will ask questions about [**describe what is being evaluated**]. Specifically, it asks questions about [**complete as appropriate**].

How will this information be used? The information will be used to design more programs [**target population**].

Who will get the information? [**describe**].

How was I selected for this interview? [**describe**].

Who else is being interviewed? Other people in a similar situation to yourself.

Child Assent Form

For activities with children under 18 years

Project Name

Dear .... *(Fill in name of child)*

[**Name and Purpose of the project being evaluated**]. We would like you to participate in a focus group discussion/interview.

During the period of the focus group or individual interview you will be expected to participate in the process **by answering questions asked about the _____ project.**

If you don't want to take part in this activity, you can decide not to, and nothing bad will happen to you. You will continue to have services and the organization will continue to have a good relationship with you. If you are not comfortable with any question please tell us immediately.

Do you have any questions you'd like to ask me? (Record questions)

APPENDIX

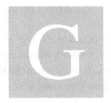

GUIDELINES FOR COMPLETING AN EVALUATION REPORT

The report does not have to be long, but it has to be accurate, complete, and address all the headings listed.

Cover Page (Title of project; person requesting the evaluation; evaluator and credentials; date)

Table of Contents (Generated in Microsoft Word©)

Acronyms

Table of Tables (generated in Microsoft Word©)

Table of Figures (generated in Microsoft Word©)

Executive Summary (summarize your paper in one to two pages)

Background and Introduction

1. Write a background to your project. It should include the following:

   a. A description of the problem you are addressing in the form of a short literature review.

   b. State the health objective—what is it? State the complementary HP 2020 objective.

   c. Draw a logic model describing the inputs, evidence based activities, outputs, and outcomes.

Note: For the literature review, provide a discussion of 6–10 articles in the peer-reviewed literature that provide a context for the topic area/health problem you are addressing. For example: If the health problem you are interested in is diabetes, then do a literature review on diabetes (extent of the problem, cause(s), risk factors associated with it, and attempts to address it (include individual and environmental attempts).

Following the literature review, include a logic model of the hypothetical theory supported program on which your project would be based (if you were implementing this project fully). You may identify a program in the literature that is similar to what you are trying to do (or select an outcome and adapt the program approach to suit you). Make sure to include a reference "adapted/adopted from _____" (name, date).

1. State the purpose of the evaluation and the type of evaluation you are conducting. State if you are conducting a needs assessment, formative, process, or outcome evaluation and provide a justification/rationale for your selection.

2. State the research question(s) your team answered. You are not limited to one question, but all the questions must be directly related to the purpose. If you have questions in more than one category of evaluation you will have to provide the reader with a clear report of how you answered each question. For example, if your research question is an outcome evaluation question and yet you want to include process evaluation measures, you will need to organize your report so that it is reflected clearly.

3. Make a list of the stakeholders associated with your evaluation/needs assessment study and discuss how you involved them in each step of your project (data collection, data analysis and the reporting of the results): This may be hypothetical but must make sense and be complete. Describe an ideal situation if appropriate.

METHODOLOGY

The methodology section describes the approach to answering the research questions. It describes the design of the evaluation, whether you have used an experimental or quasi-experimental design and specifically what the design is. You answer the question how was the data collected? How did you ensure that the data you use for drawing conclusions is valid?

Data Collection

This section describes the data you collected and the analysis that you undertook to answer the evaluation question, explained in more detail next.

Using the materials that you have at your disposal and any that you find helpful, describe your research process and results:

■ Describe the subject of your data collection (people, data base, existing records, etc.). What kind of sample do you have? How did you gather your sample? What approach did you use?

- Describe the data collection approach to your study.
  - Describe how you collected the data for this study (who, what, where, how, and when). Also include:
    - Sample size.
    - Discuss how your project ensured your data was valid and reliable.
  - Provide a complete description of the approach you used to collect the data; describe the methods you used (qualitative/quantitative).
  - Describe the instrument(s) you used, describe the type of data collection tool you used, and the variables that formed the basis for your study. Describe any other databases.
  - Discuss any cultural and ethical considerations data collection.

Data Analysis

- Describe the data analysis process, how you analyzed the data, and what software/ methods/approaches you used.
- Discuss any cultural and ethical considerations data analysis.

Results

Analyze your data and interpret the results of your data analysis. Draw tables, charts, and graphs to clearly show your results. Write a narrative describing each of your tables, charts, and graphs and any other results from your analysis to the reader. The narrative interprets the results for the reader and must be next to graph, chart, or figure that it describes (preferably above it). Each table, graph, or chart must be related to how you arrive at the answer to your evaluation research question. Organize your results by research question, so if you answer more than one question, it is clear which set of data responds to which question. Make sure to start this section describing the demographic data related to your sample.

Recommendations

Based only on the results of your analysis what recommendations would you make for the new policy or program or for improving an existing initiative to address the problem you stated earlier? The literature review might help you with some ideas, if not, do another search and see if you can identify best practices for addressing your problem and use that to help you think about appropriate recommendations. They must be related to your findings and be realistic to the stakeholders.

Reporting Results

Describe how you would provide the results of your study to your stakeholders listed earlier. Select the most relevant stakeholder group for your results—the group that is most likely to act on your findings (the board, the ED, the project participants, etc.) and describe an appropriate approach that you would use for that group; **be specific**:

■ Describe the group.

■ Describe what methods/approach you would use to ensure they understand the study and its major findings.

■ Describe how you will involve stakeholders in this step of the evaluation.

Appendix

The appendix includes samples of the instruments you used to collect the data (e.g., observation and record sheets, etc.) and consent forms.

Additional Comments

1. There must be a logical progression from your problem to drawing conclusions and making recommendations! Your approach to the presentation of your results and dissemination of your report must also be well thought out.

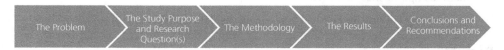

2. Ensure that the concepts and approaches you use are described appropriately and reflect a thorough understanding of evaluation and research principles and approaches.

REFERENCES

Abbatangelo-Gray, J., Cole, G. E., & Kennedy, M. G. (2007). Guidance for evaluating mass communication health initiatives: Summary of an expert panel discussion sponsored by the Centers for Disease Control and Prevention. *Evaluation & the Health Professions, 30,* 229–253.

Ajzen, I., & Fishbein, M. (1980). *Understanding attitudes and predicting social behavior,* Englewood Cliff, NJ: Prentice Hall.

American Evaluation Association. (2008). Guiding principles for evaluators. *American Journal of Evaluation, 29*(3), 233–234.

Andersen, R. M. (1995). Revisiting the behavioral model and access to medical care: Does it matter? *Journal of Health and Social Behavior, 36*(1), 1–10.

Babbie, E. (1990). *Survey research methods.* Belmont, CA: Wadsworth.

Bamberger, M., Rugh, J., & Mabry, L. (2012). Realworld evaluation. Working under budget, time, data, and political constraints. Los Angeles, CA: Sage.

Bandura, A. (1986). *Social foundations of thought and action: A social cognitive theory.* Englewood Cliffs, NJ: Prentice Hall.

Batancourt, J. R., Green, A. R., Carillo, J. E., & Ananeh-Firenpong, O. (2003). Defining cultural competence. A practical framework for addressing racial/ethnic disparities in health and health care. *Public Health Reports, 118,* 293–302.

Baqutayan, S. (2011). *Stress and social support, 33*(1), 29–34.

Belcher, H. J. (1994). *Group participation.* 2nd ed. Thousand Oaks, CA: Sage.

Bender, D. E., & Harbour, C. (2001). Tell me what you mean by "si": Perceptions of quality of prenatal care among immigrant Latina women. *Qualitative Health Research, 1*(6), 780–794.

Carmines, E., & Zeller, R. A. (1979). *Reliability and validity assessment* (vol. *07-017*). Thousand Oaks, CA: Sage.

Centers for Disease Control and Prevention. (1999). *Framework for program evaluation in public health.* Atlanta, GA: Author.

Centers for Disease Control and Prevention. (2007, November 30). *Tiers of evidence: A framework for classifying HIV behavioral interventions.* Retrieved from www.cdc.gov/hiv/topics/research/prs/print/tiers-of-evidence.htm

Cohen, J. (1960). A coefficient of agreement for nominal scales. *Educational and Psychological Measurement, 20,* 37–46.

Commission on Social Determinants of Health. (2008). *Closing the gap in a generation: Health equity through action on the social determinants of health. Final report of the Commission on Social Determinants of Health.* Geneva, Switzerland: World Health Organization.

Cook, T. D., & Campbell, D. T. (1979). *Quasi-experimentation: Design and analysis issues for field settings.* Chicago, IL: Rand McNally.

Cooper, C. P., Jorgensen, C. M., & Meritt, T. L. (2003). Report from the CDC. Telephone focus groups: An emerging method in public health research. *Journal of Women's Health, 12*(10), 945–951.

Creswell, J. W. (2007). *Qualitative inquiry and research design. Choosing among five approaches,* 2nd ed. Thousand Oaks, CA: Sage.

Cutter, S. L., Mitchel, J. T, & Scott, M. S. (2000). Revealing the vulnerability of people and places: A case study of Georgetown county, South Carolina. *Annals of American Geographers, 90,* 713–737.

Delbecq, A. L., Van de Ven, A. H., & Gustafson, D. H. (1975). *Group techniques for program planning.* Glenview. IL: Scott, Foresman.

Dillman, D. A. (2000). *Mail and Internet survey: The tailored design method.* New York, NY: Wiley.

Edbeg, M. (2013). *Essentials of health, culture, and diversity: Understanding people, reducing disparities.* Burlington, MA: Jones & Bartlett.

Fazlay, F. S., Lofton, S. P., Doddato, T. M., & Mangum, C. (2003). Utilizing geographic information systems in community assessment and nursing research. *Journal of Community Health Nursing, 20*(3), 179–191.

Fern, E. (2001). *Advanced focus group research.* Thousand Oaks, CA: Sage.

Fetterman, D. M., Kaftarian, S. J., & Wandersman, A. (1996). *Empowerment evaluation: knowledge and tools for self-assessment and accountability.* Thousand Oaks, CA: Sage.

Feveile, H., Olsen, O., & Hugh, A. (2007). A randomized trial of mailed questionnaires versus telephone interviews. Response patterns in a survey. *BMC Medical Research Methodology 7*(27), 1–7.

Finifter, D. H., Jensen, C. J., Wilson, C. E., & Koenig, B. L. (2005). A comprehensive, multitiered, targeted community needs assessment model. *Family & Community Health 28*, 293–306.

Fishbain, M., & Ajzen, I. (1975). *Belief, attitude, intention and behavior: An introduction to theory and research.* Reading, MA: Addison-Wesley.

Fitzpatrick, J. L., Sanders, J. R., & Worthen, B. R. (2004). *Program evaluation. Alternative approaches and practical guidelines,* 3rd ed. Boston, MA: Pearson.

Frechtling, J. A. (2007). *Logic modeling methods in program evaluation.* San Francisco, CA: Jossey-Bass.

Ghere, G., King, J. A., Stevahn, L., & Minnema, J. (2006). A professional development unit for reflecting on program evaluator competencies. *American Journal of Evaluation, 27,* 108–123.

Giacomini, M. K., & Cook, D. J. (2000). Users' guide to the medical literature: XXIII. Qualitative research in health care. Are the results of the study valid? *Journal of the American Medical Association, 284*(3), 357–362.

Glanz, K., Rimer, B. K., & Viswanath, K. (2008). The scope of health behavior and health education. In K. Glanz, B. K. Rimer, and K. Viswanath (Eds.), *Health behavior and health education: Theory, research and practice* (4th ed., pp. 3–22). San Francisco, CA: Jossey-Bass.

Goodman, R. M., Steckler, A., & Kegler, M. C. (2002). Mobilizing organizations for health enhancement: theories of organizational change, In K. Glanz, B. K. Rimer, & K. Viswanath (Eds.), *Health behavior and health education: Theory, research and practice* (3rd ed., pp. 335–360).San Francisco, CA: Jossey-Bass.

Hancock, T., & Minkler, M. (2007). Community health assessment or healthy community assessment. Whose community? Whose health? Whose assessment? In M. Minkler (Ed.), *Community organizing and community building for health* (3rd ed., pp. 138–157). New Brunswick, NJ: Rutgers University Press.

Harris, M., & López-Defede, A. (2004). *Understanding the social and cultural determinants of tuberculosis: A South Carolina study.* Columbia, SC: Institute for Families in Society.

Herd, D. (2009). Changing Images of Violence in Rap Music Lyrics: 1979–1997. *Journal of Public Health Policy, 30* (4), 395–406.

Hochbaum, G. M. (1958). *Participation in medical screening programs: A psychological study.* Washington, DC: U.S. Department of Health, Education and Medicine.

House, J. S. (1981). *Work, stress and social support.* Reading, MA: Addison-Wesley.

Institute of Medicine. (2001). *The future of public health.* Washington, DC: Institute of Medicine.

Israel, B. A., Eng, E., Schulz, A. J., & Parker, E. A. (Eds.). (2005). *Methods in community-based participatory research for health.* San Francisco, CA: Jossey-Bass.

Jacobson, L. T., & Wetta, R. (2014). Breastfeeding interventions in Kansas: A qualitative process evaluation of program goals and objectives. *Evaluation and Program Planning, 46:* 87–93.

Jekel, J. F., Elmore, J. G., & Katz, D. L. (1996). *Epidemiology, biostatistics and preventive medicine.* Philadelphia, PA: Saunders.

Johnson, E. C., Kirkhart, K. E., Madison, A. M., Noley, G. B., & Solano-Flores, G. (2008). The impact of narrow views of scientific rigor on evaluation practices for underrepresented groups. In N. L. Smith & P. R. Brandon, (Eds.), *Fundamental issues in evaluation.* 261. New York, NY: GuilfordPress.

Joint Committee on Standards for Educational Evaluation, Sanders, J. R., & American Association of School Administrators. (1994). *The program evaluation standards: How to assess evaluations of educational programs*, 2nd ed. Thousand Oaks, CA: Sage.

Keane, C. (2014). A network approach to community health research. In J. G. Burke & S. M. Albert (Eds.), *Methods for community public health research* (pp. 69–104). New York, NY: Springer.

Keiffer, E. C., Salabarria-Pena, Y., Odoms-Young, A. M., Willis, S. K., Baber, K. E., & Gusman, J. R. (2005). The application of focus group methodologies to community- based participatory research. In B. A. Israel, E. Eng, A. J. Schulz, & E. A. Parker (Eds.), *Methods in community-based participatory research for fealth* (pp. 146–166). San Francisco, CA: Jossey-Bass.

King, J. A., Stevahn, L., Ghere, G., & Minnema, J. (2001). Toward a taxonomy of essential evaluator competencies. *American Journal of Evaluation, 22*(2), 229–248.

Kirkhart, K. E. (2005). Through a cultural lens: Reflections on validity and theory in evaluation. In S. Hood, R. Hopson, & H. Frierson (Eds.), *The role of culture and cultural context: A mandate for inclusion, the discovery of truth, and understanding in evaluative theory and practice (pp.* 21–39). Greenwich, CT: IAP- Information Age.

Kretzmann, J. P., & McKnight, J. L. (1993). *Building communities from the inside out: A path towards finding and mobilizing a community's assets.* Evanston, IL: Center for Urban Affairs and Policy Research.

Krueger, R. A., & Casey, M. A. (2000). *Focus groups*, 3rd ed. Thousand Oaks, CA: Sage.

Krueger, R. A., & Casey, M. A. (2009). *Focus groups: A practical guide for applied research.* Thousand Oaks, CA: Sage.

Marmot, M. (2004). *The status syndrome.* New York, NY: Henry Holt.

Mason, J. (2002). *Qualitative researching*, 2nd ed. Thousand Oaks, CA: Sage.

Maxwell, J. A. (2005). *Qualitative research design. An interactive approach*, 2nd ed. Thousand Oaks, CA: Sage.

McLennan, E., Strotman, R., McGregor, J., & Dolan, D. (2004). *AnSWR users guide.* Retrieved from http://www.cdc.gov/hiv/topics/surveillance/resources/software/answr/index.htm

Mercy J., Butchart A., Farrington D., Cerdá, M. (2002). Youth violence. In: E. Krug, L. L. Dahlberg, J. A. Mercy, A. B. Zwi, & R. Lozano (Eds.), World report on violence and health. Page 25–56. Geneva (Switzerland): World Health Organization;

Milstein, B., Wetterhall, S., & Group, C. E. W. (2000). A framework featuring steps and standards for program evaluation. *Health Promotion Practice, 1*(3), 221–228.

Minkler, M., Wallerstein, N., & Wilson, N. (2008). Improving health through community organization and community building. In K. Glanz, B. K. Rimer, & K. Viswanath (Eds.), *Health behavior and health education: Theory, research and practice* (4th ed., pp. 287–312). San Francisco, CA: Jossey-Bass.

Morse, J. M., Barrett, M., Mayan, M., Olson, K., & Spiers, J. (2002). Verification strategies for establishing reliability and validity in qualitative research. *International Journal of Qualitative Methods, 1*(2), 3–22.

National Association of County and City Health Officials (n.d.). *Mobilizing for action through planning and partnerships.* Retrieved September 20, 2009, from http://www.naccho.org/topics/infrastructure/MAPP/index.cfm

Nelson-Barber, S., LeFrance, J., Trumbull, E., & Aburto, S. (2005). Promoting culturally reliable and valid evaluation practice. In S. Hood, R. Hopson, & H. Frierson (Eds.), *The role of culture and cultural context: A mandate for inclusion, the discovery of truth and understanding in evaluative theory and practice* (pp. 61–85). Greenwich, CT: IAP-Information Age.

O'Fallon, L., & Dearry, A. (2002). Community-based participatory research as a tool to advance environmental health sciences. *Environmental Health Perspectives, 110* (Suppl 2), 155–159.

Panet-Raymond, J. (1992). Partnership: Myth or reality? *Community Development Journal, 27*(2), 156–165.

Patton, M. Q. (2008). *Utilization-focused evaluation*, 4th ed. Thousand Oaks, CA: Sage.

Paul, R., & Elder, L. (2012). *The miniature guide to critical thinking concepts and tools.* Tomales, CA: Foundation for Critical Thinking.

Perez, M. A., & Luquis, R. R. (2008). *Cultural competence in health education and health promotion.* San Francisco, CA: Jossey-Bass.

Preskill, H., & Catsambas, T. T. (2006). *Reframing evaluation through appreciative inquiry*. Thousand Oaks, CA: Sage.

Prochaska, J. O., & DiClemente, C. C. (1983). Stages and processes of self-change of smoking: Toward an integrative model of change. *Journal of Consulting and Clinical Psychology, 51,* 390–395.

Public Health Leadership Society. (2002). *Principles of the ethical practice of public health*. New Orleans, LA: Public Health Leadership Society.

Rappaport, J. (1984). Studies in empowerment: Introduction to the issue. *Prevention in Human Services, 3*(2–3), 1–7.

Rissel, C. (1994). Empowerment: The holy grail of health promotion. *Health Promotion International, 9*(1), 39–47.

Rogers, E.M. (2013). Diffusion of Innovation, 5th Edition, Free Press: New York

Rossi, P. H., Lipsey, M. W., & Freeman, H. E. (2004). *Evaluation. A systematic approach*. Thousand Oaks, CA: Sage.

Sallis, J. F., Owen, N., & Fisher, E. B. (2008). Ecological models of health behavior. In K. Glanz, B. K. Rimer, & K. Viswanath (Eds.), *Health behavior and health education: Theory, research and practice* (4th ed., pp. 465–482). San Francisco, CA: Jossey-Bass.

Savage, C. L., Xu, Y., Lee, R., Rose, B. L., Kappesser, M., & Anthony, J. S. (2006). A case study in the use of community based participatory research in public health nursing. *Public Health Nursing, 23*(5), 472–478.

Schulz, A. J., Zenk, S. N., Kannan, S., Israel, B. A., Koch, M. A., & Stokes, C. A. (2005). CBPR approach to survey design and implementation. In B. A. Israel, E. Eng, A. J. Schulz, & E. A. Parker (Eds.), *Methods in community-based participatory research for health* (*pp*. 107–127). San Francisco, CA: Jossey-Bass.

Sector, R. E. (1995). *Cultural diversity in health and illness*, 4th ed. Stamford, CT: Appleton & Lang.

Sharpe, P. A., Greany, M. L., Lee, P. R., & Royce, S. W. (2005). Assets-oriented community assessment. *Public Health Reports, 115,* 205–211.

Shi, L. (2008). *Health Services Research Methods*, 2nd ed. Clifton Park, NY: Thomson/Delmar Learning.

Stufflebeam, D. L., & Shinkfield, A. J. (2007). *Evaluation theory, models, and applications*. San Francisco, CA: Jossey-Bass.

Substance Abuse and Mental Health Administration. (2008). National Registry of Evidence-Based Programs and Practices. Retrieved from http://www.nrepp.samhsa.gov/find.asp

Taylor-Powell, E., Rossing, B., & Geran, J. (1998, July). *Evaluating collaboratives: Reaching the potential* (G3658-8). Madison: University of Wisconsin-Extension.

Tervalon, M., & Murray-Garcia, J. (1998). Cultural humility vs. cultural competence: A critical distinction in defining physician training outcomes in medical education. *Journal of Health Care for the Poor and Underserved, 9*(2), 117–125.

Travers, R., Wilson, M. G., Flicker, S., Guta, A., Bereket, T., McKay, C.,… Rourke, S. B. (2008). The greater involvement of people living with AIDS principle: Theory versus practice in Ontario's HIV/AIDS community-based research sector. *AIDS Care, 20*(6), 615–624.

Trochim, W. (1989). Concept mapping for evaluation and planning. *Evaluation and Program Planning, 12*(1), 1–16.

Ulin, P. R., Robinson, E. T., & Tolley, E. E. (2005). *Qualitative methods in public health: A field guide for applied research*. San Francisco, CA: Jossey-Bass.

United Nations Population Fund. (n.d.). *Guide to working from within; 24 tips for culturally sensitive programming*. Retrieved April 18, 2009, from http://www.unfpa.org/culture/24/cover.htm

U.S. Department of Health and Human Services. (2000). *Healthy People 2010* (2nd ed., 2 vols.). Washington, DC: U.S. Government Printing Office.

U.S. Department of Health and Human Services. (2010). *Healthy People 2020*. Washington, DC: U.S. Government Printing Office.

U.S. Department of Health and Human Services Office of Minority Health (2001). *National standards for culturally and linguistically appropriate services in healthcare*. Washington, DC: U.S. Government Printing Office.

Veach, R. M. (1997). *Medical ethics*, 2nd ed. Sudbury, MA: Jones & Bartlett.

Walker, S. C., Kerns, S. E. U., Lyon, A. R., Bruns, E. J., & Cosgrove, T. J. (2010). Impact of school-based health center on academic outcomes. *Journal of Adolescent Health*, *46*, 251–257.

Wang, C., Burris, M. A., & Ping, X. Y. (1996). Chinese village women as visual anthropologists: A participatory approach to reaching policymakers. *Social Science & Medicine*, *42*(10), 1391–1400.

Windsor, R. A., Baronowski, T., Clark, N., & Cutter, G. (1984) *Evaluation of health promotion and education programs*. Mountain View, CA: Mayfield.

Windsor, R., Clark, N., Boyd, N. R., & Goodman, R. M. (2004). *Evaluation of health promotion, health education and disease prevention programs*, 3rd ed. Boston, MA: McGraw-Hill.

Yonas, M. A. Burke, J. G., Rak, K., Bennett, A., Kelly, V., & Gielen, A.C. (2009). A picture's worth a thousand words: Engaging youth in CBPR using creative arts. *Progress in Community Health Partnerships: Research, Education and Action*, *3*(4), 349–358.

Zenk, S. N., Schulz, A. J., House, J. S., Benjamin, A., & Kannan, S. (2005). Application of CBPR in the design of an observational tool: The neighborhood observational checklist. In B. A. Israel, E. Eng, A. J. Schulz, & E. A. Parker (Eds.), *Methods in community-based participatory research for health* (pp. 167–187). San Francisco, CA: Jossey-Bass.

INDEX

Page references followed by *fig* indicate an illustrated figure; followed by *t* indicate a table.